*HERE'S AMERICA'S FAVORITE
DIET GUIDE*

CALORIES AND
CARBOHYDRATES

*THE BOOK THAT MAKES IT FUN
TO LOSE THOSE EXTRA POUNDS*

Whether you aim to lose five pounds or fifty, the
only safe, healthy way is to eat an adequate, well-
balanced diet, choosing your calories from many
different kinds of foods in order to ensure that
you're getting sufficient vitamins, minerals, and
other nutrients. CALORIES AND CARBOHY-
DRATES contains the most accurate and depend-
able caloric and carbohydrate counts for practi-
cally everything you will eat and drink—thousands and thousands of brand names and basic
foods, including alcoholic beverages and take-out
foods such as your favorites from McDONALD'S
or BURGER KING.

So diet—and enjoy it!

SIGNET Books by Barbara Kraus

Barbara Kraus

CALORIES
and
CARBOHYDRATES

FIFTH REVISED EDITION

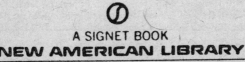

A SIGNET BOOK

NEW AMERICAN LIBRARY

TIMES MIRROR

NAL BOOKS ARE AVAILABLE AT QUANTITY DISCOUNTS
WHEN USED TO PROMOTE PRODUCTS OR SERVICES.
FOR INFORMATION PLEASE WRITE TO PREMIUM MARKETING DIVISION,
THE NEW AMERICAN LIBRARY, INC., 1633 BROADWAY,
NEW YORK, NEW YORK 10019.

SIGNET, SIGNET CLASSICS, MENTOR, PLUME, MERIDIAN AND NAL BOOKS
are published by The New American Library, Inc.,
1633 Broadway, New York, New York 10019

First Signet Printing, August 1973
Second Revised Edition (Seventh Printing), July, 1975
Third Revised Edition (Fourteenth Printing), March, 1979
Fourth Revised Edition (Nineteenth Printing), May, 1981
Fifth Revised Edition (Twenty-fourth Printing), May, 1983

24 25 26 27 28 29 30 31 32

PRINTED IN THE UNITED STATES OF AMERICA

For Carole Anne Pezza

Contents

Introduction

This dictionary of foods lists several thousand brand-name products and basic foods with their caloric and carbohydrate content. The calorie yield of your diet versus the amount of energy you expend is the key to whether you maintain your ideal weight, gain too many pounds or lose weight.

Because of the relationship of weight to health, many individuals are "counting calories" at every meal. Interest has also been directed to the carbohydrate content of the diet in relation to weight control. Comprehensive information on these values in basic foods and brand-name products is not readily available in any one source. Nor is the information regularly reported in portions that are usually eaten or bought at the grocery store. To compound the problem, hundreds of new food items appear in our stores every year.

Arrangement of This Book

Foods are listed alphabetically by brand name or by the name of the food. The singular form is used for the entries, that is, blackberry instead of blackberries. Most items are listed individually though a few are grouped (see p. xii); for example, all candies are listed together so that if you are looking for *Mars* bar, you look first under Candy, then under *M* in alphabetical order. But, if you are looking for a breakfast food such as Oatmeal, you will find it under *O* in the main alphabet. Many cross references are included to assist in finding items called by different names.

Under the main headings, it was often not possible nor even desirable to follow an alphabetical arrangement. For basic foods such as apricots, for example, the first entries are for the fresh product weighed with seeds as it is purchased in the store, then the fruit in small portions as they may be eaten or measured. These entries are followed by the processed products, canned (although it may actually be a bottle or jar), dehydrated, dried and frozen. This basic plan, with adaptations where necessary, was followed for fruits, vegetables and meats.

In almost all entries where data were available the U.S. Department of Agriculture figures are shown first. The Department values represent averages from several manufacturers and are shown for comparison with the values from individual companies or for use where particular brands are not available.

All brand-name products have been italicized and company names appear in parentheses.

Portions Used

The portion column is a most important one to read and note. Common household measures are used insofar as possible. For some items, the amounts given are those commonly purchased in the store, such as 1 pound of meat. These quantities can be divided into the number of servings used in the home and the nutritive values available to each person served can then be readily determined. Of course, any ingredients added to preparing such products must also be taken into account.

The smaller portions given are for foods as served or measured in moderate amounts, such as ½ cup of juice reconstituted, or 4 ounces of meat. Be sure to adjust the calories and carbohydrates to the actual portions you use. For example, if you serve 1 cup of juice instead of ½ cup, multiply the calories and carbohydrates shown for the smaller amount by 2.

Don't fool yourself about the size of portions you use. If you are serious about controlling the calories and carbohydrates in your diet, weigh your foods until you can accurately gauge the weight visually. Remember, the calories and carbohydrates go up with any increase in the weight of foods. Remember, too, that 4 ounces by weight may be very different from 4 fluid ounces or ½ cup. Ounces in the table are always ounces by weight unless specified as fluid ounces, or fractions of a cup or other volumetric measure. Foods that are fluffy in texture, such as flaked coconut and bean sprouts, vary greatly in weight per cup depending on how tightly they are packed into the cup. Such foods as canned green beans also vary when weighed with or without liquid; for example, canned green beans with liquid weigh 4.2 ounces for ½ cup, but drained beans weigh 2.5 ounces for the same ½ cup. Check the weights of your serving portions regularly. Bear in mind that you can cut calories and carbohydrates by cutting the serving size.

It was impossible to convert all the portions to a uniform basis. Some sources were only able to report data in terms of weights with no information on cup or other volumetric measures. I have shown small portions in quantities that might reasonably be expected to be served or measured in the home or institution. Package sizes are useful to show the composition of products as they are purchased and may be divided into the number of serving portions prepared from the entire product, taking into account any added ingredients.

You will find in the portion column the phrases "weighed with bone," or "weighed with skin and seeds" or other inedible parts. These descriptions apply to the products as you purchase them in the markets but the caloric values and the carbohydrate content as shown are for the amount of edible food after you discard the bone, skin, seed or other inedible part. The weight given in the "measure or quantity" column is to the nearest gram or fraction of an ounce.

Data on the composition of foods are constantly changing for many reasons. Better sampling and analytical methods, improvements in marketing procedures and changes in formulas of mixed products, all may alter values for carbohydrates and other nutrients as well as caloric values. Weights of packaged foods are frequently changed. It is essential to read label information to be informed about these matters and to make intelligent use of food tables.

I will be constantly revising and updating this book along with my individual calorie and carbohydrate annual guides (*The Barbara Kraus 1983 Calorie and Carbohydrate Guides to Brand Names and Basic Foods*) to help keep you as up-to-date as possible.

Calories

What is a calorie? It is not a nutrient nor is it a good guide to the nutritive value of food. It is more like a yardstick to measure the energy that a food will yield in the body. You need energy for your body functions as well as for exercise. If your diet contains more calories than your body uses for these purposes, the extra "energy" will be stored as fat.

If your plan is to cut down on calories, the easiest way to do so is to consult the calorie column of this counter and keep an accurate count of your total intake of food and beverages for a period of seven days. If you have not gained or lost weight during that week divide that number by seven and you'll have your maintenance diet expressed in calories. To lose weight, you must reduce your daily or weekly intake of calories below this maintenance level. (To gain, increase the intake.)

One pound of fat is equal to 3,500 calories. Add this number of calories to those you need to balance your energy requirements and you will gain one pound; subtract it, and you will lose a pound.

Carbohydrates

The carbohydrate column shows the amount of this nutrient in grams for the quantities of foods indicated in the portion column. Some dietitians are giving special attention to this nutrient at present in connection with weight control. Carbohydrates include sugars, starches, acids and other nutrients. The values in this book are total carbohydrates, by difference, the basis on which calories from carbohydrates are calculated in the U.S. diet.

Other Nutrients

Do not forget that other nutrients are extremely important in diet planning—protein, fat, minerals and vitamins. Calories yielded by alcohol must also be taken into consideration. From a nutrition viewpoint, perhaps the best advice that can be given to the dieter is to eat a varied diet with all classes of foods represented. Meat, fish, chicken, fats and oils, milk, vegetables, fruits and grain products are all important sources of essential nutrients and some foods from each of these classes of foods should be included in the diet every day. With the great abundance and variety of foods on the grocer's shelves, there is no reason why the dieter should not enjoy a tasty, nutritious and attractive diet. Just eat in moderation and there is no need to eliminate any one food altogether, except in special conditions under a doctor's directions. Choose wisely and eat well.

Sources of Data

Values in this dictionary are based on publications issued by the U.S. Department of Agriculture and on data submitted by manufacturers and processors. The U.S. Department of Agriculture issues basic tables on food composition for use in the United States. The commercial products from U.S.D.A. publications represent average values obtained on products of more than one company. The figures designated "home recipe" are based on recipes on file with the Department of Agriculture. Data on commercial products listed by brand name in this publication are based on values supplied by manufacturers and processors for their own individual products. Very few supermarket brand names, such as Pathmark or private labels were included in this book inasmuch as they are not usually analyzed under these trade names. Every care has been taken to interpret the data and the descriptions supplied by the companies as fully and accurately as possible. Many values have been recalculated to different portions from those submitted in order to bring about greater uniformity among similar items.

Calories in these different sources are not always on a strictly uniform basis. In the Department of Agriculture, calories are calculated using specific factors, which make allowances for losses in digestion and metabolism. The technical explanation of these factors is given in Handbook 74 of the United States Department of Agriculture. Most manufacturers use average factors of 4, 9 and 4 for calories yielded by each gram of protein, fat and carbohydrate respectively; a factor of 7 is used as an average value to calculate the calories from one gram of alcohol. These differences in procedure will give somewhat different results for products of similar composition. Some manufacturers have adopted the values from U.S. Department of Agriculture publications as representative of their own products. In these cases, it will be apparent in the table that the data from the companies match exactly those from U.S.D.A. publications.

Analyses of foods to provide information on nutritive values are extremely expensive to conduct. Many small companies have not been able to afford to have their products analyzed and thus were unable to provide data for this book or were able to provide only the calories or only the carbohydrates. Other companies have simply never gotten around to having the analysis done. New requirements for labeling nutritive values of products may provide information on additional items in the future. Therefore, wherever data for carbohydrates were unavailable, blank spaces were left which may be filled in by the reader at a later time.

Bear in mind that small differences in calorie values on similar products of the same weight are not important in diet planning. They may be due to different methods of calculating the calories or to small differences in the nutritive values of the samples analyzed because no two foods ever have exactly the same composition. Some differences may also be due to the way the food was measured as noted in the case of green beans earlier.

Carbohydrates in this book are usually total carbohydrates by difference. A few manufacturers reported only "available carbohydrates." These values were omitted.

Foods Listed by Groups

Certain foods are reported together rather than as individual items in the main alphabet. For example: Baby Food; Bread; Cake; Cake Icing; Cake Icing Mix; Cake Mix; Candy; Cheese; Cookie; Cookie Mix; Cracker; Gravy; Pie; Pie Filling; Salad Dressing; Sauce; Sausage; Soft Drinks and Syrup.

BARBARA KRAUS

Abbreviations and Symbols

(USDA) = United States Department
    of Agriculture
(HEW/FAO) = Health, Education
    and Welfare/Food
    and Agriculture
    Organization
* = prepared as package directs[1]
< = less than
& = and
" = inch
canned = bottles or jars
    as well as cans
dia. = diameter
fl. = fluid

liq. = liquid
lb. = pound
med. = medium
oz. = ounce
pkg. = package
pt. = pint
qt. = quart
sq. = square
T. = tablespoon
Tr. = trace
tsp. = teaspoon
wt. = weight

italics or name in parentheses = registered trademark, ®
the letters DNA indicate that no data are available.

Equivalents

By Weight
1 pound = 16 ounces
1 ounce = 28.35 grams
3.52 ounces = 100 grams

By Volume
1 quart = 4 cups
1 cup = 8 fluid ounces
1 cup = ½ pint
1 cup = 16 tablespoons
2 tablespoons = 1 fluid ounce
1 tablespoon = 3 teaspoons

[1]If the package directions call for whole or skim milk, the data given here are for whole milk, unless otherwise stated.

Food and Description	Measure or Quantity	Calories	Carbo-hydrates (grams)

A

ABALONE (USDA):
Raw, meat only	4 oz.	111	3.9
Canned	4 oz.	91	2.6

AC'CENT | ¼ tsp. (1 gram) | 3 | 0.

ACEROLA, fresh (USDA) | ½ lb. (weighed with seeds) | 52 | 12.6

ALBACORE, raw, meat only (USDA) | 4 oz. | 201 | 0.

ALCOHOLIC BEVERAGES
(See individual listings)

ALE (See **BEER**)

ALEWIFE (USDA):
Raw, meat only	4 oz.	144	0.
Canned, solids & liq.	4 oz.	160	0.

ALEXANDER COCKTAIL MIX (Holland House) | 6-oz. pkg. | 69 | 16.0

ALLSPICE (French's) | 1 tsp. | 6 | 1.3

ALMOND:
In shell:
(USDA)	10 nuts (25 grams)	60	2.0
(USDA)	1 cup (2.8 oz.)	187	6.1
Shelled:
(USDA):
| Whole | ½ cup (2½ oz.) | 424 | 13.8 |
| Whole | 1 oz. | 170 | 5.5 |

(USDA): United States Department of Agriculture
(HEW/FAO): Health, Education and Welfare/Food and Agriculture Organization
* Prepared as Package Directs

Food and Description	Measure or Quantity	Calories	Carbohydrates (grams)
Whole	13-15 almonds (.6 oz.)	105	3.4
Chopped	1 cup (4½ oz.)	777	25.4
(Blue Diamond)	½ cup	504	19.4
Blanched (Blue Diamond) salted	½ cup	492	15.3
Chocolate-covered (See **CANDY**)			
Flavored (Blue Diamond)	1 oz.	180	9.5
Roasted:			
(USDA) salted	½ cup (2.8 oz.)	492	15.3
(Blue Diamond) diced	1 oz.	176	5.5
(Fisher):			
Dry Roasted	1 oz.	175	5.5
Oil Roasted	1 oz.	178	5.5
(Planters) dry roasted, salted	1 oz.	170	6.0
ALMOND EXTRACT:			
(Durkee) pure	1 tsp.	13	0.
(Virginia Dare) pure, 34% alcohol	1 tsp. (4 grams)	10	0.
ALMOND MEAL, partially defatted (USDA)	1 oz.	116	8.2
ALPHA-BITS, cereal (Post)	1 cup (1 oz.)	173	23.8
AMARANTH, raw (USDA):			
Untrimmed	1 lb. (weighed untrimmed)	103	18.6
Trimmed	4 oz.	41	7.4
AMARETTO DELIGHT COCKTAIL, canned (Mr. Boston) 12½% alcohol	3 fl. oz.	204	27.6
AMARETTO DI SARONNO	1 fl. oz.	82	9.0
AMARETTO SOUR COCKTAIL, canned (Mr. Boston) 12½% alcohol	3 fl. oz.	123	15.6

Food and Description	Measure or Quantity	Calories	Carbohydrates (grams)
A.M. FRUIT DRINK, canned (Mott's)	6 fl. oz.	90	22.0
ANCHOVY, PICKLED, canned (USDA) not heavily salted, drained	2-oz. can	79	.1
ANGEL FOOD CAKE (See **CAKE,** Angel Food)			
ANISE EXTRACT:			
(Durkee) imitation	1 tsp.	16	0.
(Virginia Dare) pure	1 tsp. (4 grams)	22	0.
ANISE SEED, dried (HEW/FAO)	½ oz.	58	6.3
ANISETTE LIQUEUR, (Mr. Boston) 27% alcohol	1 fl. oz.	88	10.8
APPLE, any variety: Fresh (USDA):			
Eaten with skin	1 lb. (weighed with skin & core)	242	60.5
Eaten with skin	1 med., 2½" dia. (about 4 per lb.)	61	15.3
Eaten without skin	1 lb. (weighed with skin & core)	211	55.0
Eaten without skin	1 med., 2½" dia. (about 4 per lb.)	53	13.9
Pared, diced or sliced	1 cup (3.9 oz.)	59	15.5
Pared, quartered	1 cup (4.4 oz.)	68	17.6
Canned (Comstock) sliced	⅙ of 21-oz. can	45	10.0
Dehydrated (USDA):			
Uncooked	1 oz.	100	26.1
Cooked, sweetened	½ cup (4½ oz.)	97	25.0

(USDA): United States Department of Agriculture
(HEW/FAO): Health, Education and Welfare/Food and Agriculture Organization
* Prepared as Package Directs

Food and Description	Measure or Quantity	Calories	Carbohydrates (grams)
Dried:			
(USDA):			
Uncooked	1 cup (3 oz.)	234	61.0
Cooked, unsweetened	½ cup (4½ oz.)	99	25.9
Cooked, sweetened	½ cup (4.9 oz.)	157	40.9
(Del Monte) uncooked	1 cup (2 oz.)	151	37.1
(Sun-Maid) chunks	2-oz. serving	150	40.0
Frozen, sweetened, slices, not thawed (USDA)	10-oz. pkg.	264	68.9
APPLE BROWN BETTY, home recipe (USDA)	1 cup (7.6 oz.)	325	63.9
APPLE BUTTER:			
(USDA)	1 T. (.6 oz.)	33	8.2
(Smucker's) cider	1 T. (.6 oz.)	38	9.0
APPLE-CHERRY JUICE COCKTAIL, canned, *Musselman's*	8 fl. oz.	110	28.0
APPLE CIDER:			
Canned (Mott's) sweet	½ cup	59	14.6
*Mix, *Country Time*	8 fl. oz.	98	24.5
APPLE-CRANBERRY DRINK (Hi-C):			
Canned	6 fl. oz.	90	21.0
*Mix	6 fl. oz.	72	18.0
APPLE-CRANBERRY JUICE, canned (Lincoln)	6 fl. oz.	104	26.0
APPLE DRINK:			
Canned:			
Capri Sun, natural	6 ¾ fl. oz.	90	22.7
(Hi-C)	6 fl. oz.	92	23.0
*Mix (Hi-C)	6 fl. oz.	72	18.0
APPLE DUMPLING, frozen (Pepperidge Farm)	1 dumpling	280	31.0

Food and Description	Measure or Quantity	Calories	Carbo-hydrates (grams)
APPLE, ESCALLOPED, frozen (Stouffer's)	⅓ of 12-oz. pkg.	138	27.8
APPLE-GRAPE JUICE, canned:			
Musselman's	6 fl. oz.	82	21.0
(Red Cheek)	6 fl. oz.	69	22.6
APPLE JACKS, cereal (Kellog's)	1 cup (1 oz.)	110	26.0
APPLE JAM, sweetened (Smucker's)	1 T.	53	13.5
APPLE JELLY:			
Sweetened (Smucker's)	1 T. (.7 oz.)	57	14.0
Dietetic (See **APPLE SPREAD**)			
APPLE JUICE:			
Canned:			
(Lincoln) cocktail	6 fl. oz.	100	24.0
(Mott's) regular or McIntosh	6 fl. oz.	80	19.0
Musselman's	6 fl. oz.	80	21.0
(Red Cheek)	6 fl. oz.	83	21.2
(Seneca Foods) regular or 100% natural	6 fl. oz.	90	22.0
Chilled (Minute Maid)	6 fl. oz.	100	24.0
*Frozen:			
(Minute Maid)	6 fl. oz.	100	24.0
(Seneca Foods):			
Regular or no added sugar	6 fl. oz.	90	22.0
Natural style	6 fl. oz.	84	22.0
APPLE PIE (See **PIE,** Apple)			
APPLE PIE FILLING (See **PIE FILLING,** Apple)			
APPLESAUCE, canned:			
Sweetened:			
(Del Monte)	½ cup (4.6 oz.)	97	23.7

(USDA): United States Department of Agriculture
(HEW/FAO): Health, Education and Welfare/Food and Agriculture Organization
* Prepared as Package Directs

Food and Description	Measure or Quantity	Calories	Carbo-hydrates (grams)
(Mott's):			
Regular	4-oz. serving	115	27.5
With ground cranberries	4-oz. serving	110	27.0
Musselman's	½ cup (4½ oz.)	96	23.5
Unsweetened, dietetic or low calorie:			
(Diet Delight)	½ cup (4.3 oz.)	50	13.0
(Featherweight) water pack	½ cup	50	12.0
(Mott's) natural style	4-oz. serving	50	11.0
Musselman's, natural	½ cup (4½ oz.)	50	12.0
(Seneca Foods) 100% natural	½ cup (4.4 oz.)	50	12.0
(S&W) *Nutradiet,* water pack	½ cup	55	14.0
APPLE SPREAD, low sugar:			
(Diet Delight)	1 T. (.6 oz.)	12	3.0
(Featherweight):			
Regular	1 T.	16	4.0
Artificially sweetened	1 T.	6	1.0
(Slenderella)	1 T. (.6 oz.)	24	6.0
(Smucker's)	1 T. (.6 oz.)	24	6.0
(Tillie Lewis) *Tasti-Diet*	1 T.	12	3.0
APRICOT:			
Fresh (USDA):			
Whole	1 lb. (weighed with pits)	217	54.6
Whole	3 apricots (about 12 per lb.)	55	13.7
Halves	1 cup (5½ oz.)	79	19.8
Canned, regular pack, solids & liq.:			
(USDA):			
Juice pack	4 oz.	61	15.4
Light syrup	4 oz.	75	19.1
Heavy syrup, halves	½ cup (4.6 oz.)	111	28.4
Heavy syrup, halves	3 med. halves with 1¾ T. syrup (3 oz.)	73	18.7
Extra heavy syrup	4 oz.	115	29.5
(Del Monte):			
Halves, unpeeled	½ cup	101	24.4
Whole, peeled	½ cup	104	25.0

Food and Description	Measure or Quantity	Calories	Carbo-hydrates (grams)
(Libby's) heavy syrup, halves	½ cup	110	26.8
(Stokely-Van Camp)	½ cup (4.6 oz.)	110	27.0
Canned, unsweetened or dietetic, solids & liq.:			
(Del Monte) *Lite*, unpeeled, extra light syrup	½ cup (4.3 oz.)	64	15.1
(Diet Delight):			
Juice pack	½ cup (4.4 oz.)	60	15.0
Water pack	½ cup (4.3 oz.)	35	9.0
(Featherweight):			
Juice pack	½ cup	50	12.0
Water pack	½ cup	25	9.0
(S&W) *Nutradiet*:			
Halves:			
Juice pack	½ cup	50	13.0
Water pack	½ cup	35	9.0
Whole, juice pack	½ cup	40	10.0
Dehydrated (USDA):			
Uncooked, sulfured	4 oz.	376	95.9
Cooked, sugar added, solids & liq.	4 oz.	135	34.6
Dried:			
(USDA):			
Uncooked	1 cup (4.6 oz.)	338	86.5
Uncooked	10 large halves (¼ cup or 1.7 oz.)	125	31.9
Cooked, sweetened	½ cup with liq. (4.7 oz.)	164	42.4
Cooked, unsweetened	½ cup with liq. (4.4 oz.)	106	27.0
(Del Monte)	½ cup (2.3 oz.)	145	39.9
(Sun-Maid)	½ cup (3.5 oz.)	250	60.0
(Sunsweet)	½ cup (3½ oz.)	250	60.0
Frozen, unthawed, sweetened (USDA)	10-oz. pkg.	278	71.2

(USDA): United States Department of Agriculture
(HEW/FAO): Health, Education and Welfare/Food and Agriculture Organization
* Prepared as Package Directs

Food and Description	Measure or Quantity	Calories	Carbo-hydrates (grams)
APRICOT, CANDIED (USDA)	1 oz.	96	24.5
APRICOT NECTAR, canned, sweetened:			
(USDA)	½ cup (4.4 oz.)	71	18.3
(Del Monte)	½ cup (4.4 oz.)	75	18.0
APRICOT-PINEAPPLE NECTAR, canned, dietetic or low calorie (S&W) *Nutradiet*	6 fl. oz.	35	12.0
APRICOT & PINEAPPLE PRESERVE, sweetened (Smucker's)	1 T. (.7 oz.)	53	13.5
APRICOT & PINEAPPLE SPREAD, low sugar:			
(Diet Delight)	1 T. (.6 oz.)	6	3.0
(Featherweight) artificially sweetened	1 T.	6	1.0
(S&W) *Nutradiet*	1 T.	12	3.0
(Tillie Lewis) *Tasti-Diet*	1 T.	12	3.0
APRICOT PRESERVE, sweetened (Smucker's)	1 T. (.7 oz.)	53	13.5
APRICOT SOUR COCKTAIL:			
Canned (National Distillers) *Duet,* 12½% alcohol	2 fl. oz.	48	1.6
Mix (Party Time) dry	½-oz. pkg.	50	11.6
APRICOT SPREAD, low sugar (Smucker's)	1 T.	24	6.0
AQUAVIT (Leroux) 90 proof	1 fl. oz.	75	Tr.
ARTICHOKE, Globe or French (See also **JERUSALEM ARTICHOKE**):			
Raw (USDA) whole	1 lb. (weighed untrimmed)	85	19.2

Food and Description	Measure or Quantity	Calories	Carbo-hydrates (grams)
Boiled (USDA) without salt, drained	4 oz.	50	11.2
Canned (Cara Mia) marinated, drained	6-oz. jar	175	12.6
Frozen:			
(Birds Eye) deluxe hearts	⅓ of 9-oz. pkg.	34	5.5
(Cara Mia)	⅓ of 9-oz. pkg.	35	7.5
ASPARAGUS:			
Raw (USDA) whole spears	1 lb. (weighed untrimmed)	66	12.7
Boiled (USDA) without salt, drained:			
Whole spears	4 spears (½" at base, 2.1 oz.)	12	2.2
Cut spears, 1½"-2" pieces	1 cup (5.1 oz.)	29	5.2
Canned, regular pack: (USDA):			
Green spears, solids & liq.	1 cup (8.6 oz.)	44	7.1
Green spears, drained	1 cup (8.3 oz.)	49	8.0
Green spears only	4 med. spears (2.8 oz.)	17	2.7
Green, liquid only	2 T. liquid	3	.7
White spears, solids & liq.	1 cup (8.6 oz.)	44	8.1
White spears only	4 med. spears (2.8 oz.)	18	2.9
White, liquid only	2 T. liquid	3	.8
(Del Monte):			
Green, spears, solids & liq.	1 cup (8.6 oz.)	47	6.4
Green, spears, drained solids	1 cup (8.5 oz.)	65	7.5
White, spears, solids & liq.	1 cup (8.6 oz.)	48	7.3
White, spears, drained solids	1 cup (8.5 oz.)	55	8.0

(USDA): United States Department of Agriculture
(HEW/FAO): Health, Education and Welfare/Food and Agriculture Organization
* Prepared as Package Directs

Food and Description	Measure or Quantity	Calories	Carbo-hydrates (grams)
(Festal):			
Green, spears, solids & liq.	½ cup	24	3.2
Green, spears, drained solids	½ cup	33	3.8
White, spears, solids & liq.	½ cup	24	3.7
White, spears, drained solids	½ cup	28	4.0
(Green Giant) green, cut spears, solids & liq.	½ of 10½-oz. can	22	2.5
(Le Sueur) green, spears, solids & liq.	¼ of 19-oz. can	20	2.3
(Lindy) green, cut spears, solids & liq.	⅓ of 10½-oz. can	14	1.7
(Stokely-Van Camp):			
Green, spears, solids & liq.	1 cup (8.4 oz.)	45	6.0
Green, cut spears, solids & liq.	1 cup (8.4 oz.)	46	6.0
Canned, dietetic or low calorie:			
(USDA):			
Green, spears, solids & liq.	4 oz.	18	3.1
Green, spears, drained solids	4 oz.	23	3.5
Green, liquid only	4 oz. liquid	10	2.3
White, spears, solids & liq.	4 oz.	18	3.4
(Diet Delight) solids & liq.	½ cup (4.2 oz.)	16	2.0
(Featherweight) cut spears, solids & liq.	½ cup	20	3.0
(S&W) *Nutradiet*, green spears, solids & liq.	½ cup	20	4.0
Frozen:			
(USDA):			
Cuts & tips, unthawed	4 oz.	26	4.1
Cuts & tips, boiled, drained	½ cup (3.2 oz.)	20	3.2
Spears, unthawed	4 oz.	27	4.4
Spears, boiled, drained	4 oz.	26	4.3
(Birds Eye):			
Cuts, 5-minute style	⅓ of 10-oz. pkg.	25	3.0
Spears, regular or jumbo	⅓ of 10-oz. pkg.	28	3.4

Food and Description	Measure or Quantity	Calories	Carbo-hydrates (grams)
(Green Giant) cut spears, in butter sauce	⅓ of 9-oz. pkg.	41	2.6
(McKenzie):			
Cuts & tips	3.3-oz. serving	30	3.8
Spears	4-oz. serving	29	8.0
(Seabrook Farms):			
Cuts & tips	3.3-oz. serving	30	3.8
Spears	⅓ of 12-oz. pkg.	29	8.0
(Stouffer's) soufflé	⅓ of 12-oz. pkg.	118	8.0

ASPARAGUS SOUP, cream of, canned:

*(USDA):			
Prepared with equal volume milk	1 cup (8.5 oz.)	144	16.3
Prepared with equal volume water	1 cup (8.5 oz.)	65	10.1
*(Campbell) condensed	10-oz. serving	100	12.0

AUNT JEMIMA SYRUP
(See **SYRUP**)

AVOCADO, peeled, pitted, all commercial varieties (USDA):

Whole	1 fruit (10.7 oz., weighed with seed & skin)	378	14.3
Cubed	1 cup (5.3 oz.)	251	9.5
Puree	1 cup (8.1 oz.)	384	14.5

***AWAKE** (Birds Eye) | 6 fl. oz. | 88 | 21.2

AYDS:

Butterscotch	1 piece (6.6 gms.)	27	5.7
Chocolate, chocolate mint or vanilla	1 piece (6.6 gms.)	26	5.5

(USDA): United States Department of Agriculture
(HEW/FAO):   Health, Education and Welfare/Food and Agriculture
              Organization
* Prepared as Package Directs

Food and Description	Measure or Quantity	Calories	Carbo-hydrates (grams)

B

BABY FOOD:

Food and Description	Measure or Quantity	Calories	Carbo-hydrates (grams)
Advance (Similac)	1 fl. oz.	15	1.5
Apple & apricot (Beech-Nut):			
Junior	7¾-oz. jar	93	24.4
Strained	4¾-oz. jar	57	14.0
Apple-banana juice (Gerber) strained	4.2 fl. oz.	57	13.7
Apple betty (Beech-Nut):			
Junior	7¾-oz. jar	173	41.4
Strained	4¾-oz. jar	106	25.4
Apple-blueberry (Gerber):			
Junior	7½-oz. jar	111	26.2
Strained	4½-oz. jar	74	17.5
Apple-cherry juice:			
Strained:			
(Beech-Nut)	4⅕ fl. oz.	50	14.0
(Gerber)	4.2 fl. oz.	57	13.7
Toddler (Gerber)	4 fl. oz.	52	12.7
Apple cranberry juice (Beech-Nut) strained	4½ fl. oz.	55	13.6
Apple dessert, dutch (Gerber):			
Junior	7¾-oz. jar	160	35.0
Strained	4¾-oz. jar	97	21.2
Apple-grape juice:			
Strained:			
(Beech-Nut)	4⅕ fl. oz.	56	13.9
(Gerber)	4.2 fl. oz.	57	14.0
Toddler (Gerber)	4 fl. oz.	56	13.6
Apple juice:			
Strained:			
(Beech-Nut)	4⅕ fl. oz.	54	13.6
(Gerber)	4.2 fl. oz.	59	14.0
Toddler (Gerber)	4 fl. oz.	54	13.3
Apple-peach juice, strained:			
(Beech-Nut)	4⅕ fl. oz.	59	14.6
(Gerber)	4.2 fl. oz.	55	13.4
Apple-plum juice (Gerber) strained	4.2 fl. oz.	60	14.4
Apple-prune juice (Gerber)			

Food and Description	Measure or Quantity	Calories	Carbo-hydrates (grams)
strained	4.2 fl. oz.	61	14.7
Applesauce:			
Junior:			
(Beech-Nut)	7¾-oz. jar	97	24.1
(Gerber)	7½-oz. jar	95	22.4
Strained:			
(Beech-Nut)	4¾-oz. jar	60	14.8
(Gerber)	4½-oz. jar	59	13.8
Applesauce & apricots (Gerber):			
Junior	7½-oz. jar	98	22.8
Strained	4½-oz. jar	66	15.5
Applesauce & bananas (Beech-Nut) strained	4¾-oz. jar	63	15.4
Applesauce & cherries (Beech-Nut):			
Junior	7¾-oz. jar	115	28.4
Strained	4¾-oz. jar	71	17.4
Applesauce with pineapple (Gerber) strained	4½-oz. jar	63	14.8
Applesauce & raspberries (Beech-Nut):			
Junior	7¾-oz. jar	102	24.6
Strained	4¾-oz. jar	61	15.1
Apple & yogurt (Gerber) strained	4½-oz. jar	95	21.2
Apricot with tapioca:			
Junior:			
(Beech-Nut)	7½-oz. jar	113	27.9
(Gerber)	7¾-oz. jar	162	38.5
Strained (Gerber)	4¾-oz. jar	97	23.2
Apricot with tapioca & apple juice (Beech-Nut) strained	4¾-oz. jar	72	17.6
Banana-apple dessert (Gerber):			
Junior	7¾-oz. jar	166	38.5
Strained	4¾-oz. jar	94	22.7
Banana dessert (Beech-Nut) junior	7½-oz. jar	165	40.1

(USDA): United States Department of Agriculture
(HEW/FAO): Health, Education and Welfare/Food and Agriculture Organization
* Prepared as Package Directs

Food and Description	Measure or Quantity	Calories	Carbohydrates (grams)
Banana with pineapple & tapioca (Gerber):			
Junior	7½-oz. jar	112	26.0
Strained	4½-oz. jar	64	14.7
Banana & pineapple with tapioca & apple juice (Beech-Nut):			
Junior	7¾-oz. jar	109	26.6
Strained	4¾-oz. jar	67	16.3
Banana with tapioca:			
Junior:			
(Beech-Nut)	7¾-oz. jar	72	27.5
(Gerber)	7½-oz. jar	128	30.0
Strained:			
(Beech-Nut)	4¾-oz. jar	72	16.9
(Gerber)	7½-oz. jar	69	15.9
Banana & yogurt (Gerber) strained	4½-oz. jar	80	16.7
Bean, green:			
Junior (Beech-Nut)	7¼-oz. jar	62	13.0
Strained:			
(Beech-Nut)	4½-oz. jar	38	8.1
(Gerber)	4½-oz. jar	31	5.9
Bean, green, creamed (Gerber) junior	7½-oz. jar	87	17.7
Bean, green, potatoes & ham casserole (Gerber) toddler	6¼-oz. jar	132	14.6
Beef (Gerber):			
Junior	3½-oz. jar	98	.4
Strained	3½-oz. jar	93	.3
Beef & beef broth (Beech-Nut):			
Junior	7½-oz. jar	235	.4
Strained	4½-oz. jar	152	.3
Beef with beef heart (Gerber) strained	3½-oz. jar	90	.5
Beef dinner, high meat, with vegetables (Gerber):			
Junior	4½-oz. jar.	125	8.4
Strained	4½-oz. jar	111	7.4
Beef & egg noodle (Beech-Nut):			
Junior	7½-oz. jar	122	17.0
Strained	4½-oz. jar,	72	9.9

Food and Description	Measure or Quantity	Calories	Carbo-hydrates (grams)
Beef & egg noodles with vegetable (Gerber):			
Junior	7½-oz. jar	137	18.9
Strained	4½-oz. jar	85	11.9
Beef lasagna (Gerber) toddler	6¼-oz. jar	109	15.6
Beef liver (Gerber) strained	3½-oz. jar	98	2.9
Beef & rice with tomato sauce (Gerber) toddler	6¼-oz. jar	131	17.0
Beef stew (Gerber) toddler	6-oz. jar	110	12.4
Beef with vegetables & cereal, high meat (Beech-Nut):			
Junior	4½-oz. jar	132	8.0
Strained	4½-oz. jar	132	8.1
Beet (Gerber) strained	4½-oz. jar	47	10.0
Biscuit (Gerber)	11-gram piece	42	8.5
Carrot:			
Junior:			
(Beech-Nut)	7½-oz. jar	67	13.8
(Gerber)	7½-oz. jar	54	10.7
Strained:			
(Beech-Nut)	4½-oz. jar	40	8.3
(Gerber)	4½-oz. jar	31	6.3
Cereal, dry:			
Barley:			
(Beech-Nut)	½-oz. serving	54	9.9
(Gerber)	4 T. (½ oz.)	53	10.4
High protein:			
(Beech-Nut)	½-oz. serving	55	7.1
(Gerber)	4 T. (½ oz.)	53	5.9
High protein with apple & orange (Gerber)	4 T. (½ oz.)	55	7.7
Mixed:			
(Beech-Nut)	½-oz. serving	55	9.9
(Gerber)	4 T. (½ oz.)	54	9.7
Mixed with banana (Gerber)	4 T. (½ oz.)	55	10.6
Oatmeal:			
(Beech-Nut)	½-oz. serving	56	9.7
(Gerber)	4 T. (½ oz.)	56	9.2

(USDA): United States Department of Agriculture
(HEW/FAO): Health, Education and Welfare/Food and Agriculture Organization
* Prepared as Package Directs

Food and Description	Measure or Quantity	Calories	Carbohydrates (grams)
Oatmeal & banana (Gerber)	4 T. (½ oz.)	56	9.8
Rice:			
(Beech-Nut)	½-oz. serving	49	9.9
(Gerber)	4 T. (½ oz.)	55	10.7
Cereal, dry:			
Rice with banana (Gerber)	4 T. (½ oz.)	56	10.7
Cereal or mixed cereal:			
With applesauce & banana:			
Junior (Gerber)	7½-oz. jar	131	26.4
Strained:			
(Beech-Nut)	4½-oz. jar	80	17.3
(Gerber)	4½-oz. jar	83	16.7
& egg yolk (Gerber):			
Junior	7½-oz. jar	109	15.1
Strained	4½-oz. jar	70	9.6
With egg yolks & bacon (Beech-Nut):			
Junior	7½-oz. jar	163	14.9
Strained	4½-oz. jar	113	8.9
Oatmeal with applesauce & banana (Gerber):			
Junior	7½-oz. jar	119	23.0
Strained	4½-oz. jar	73	13.8
Rice with applesauce & banana, strained:			
(Beech-Nut)	4¾-oz. jar	96	21.4
(Gerber)	4¾-oz. jar	96	21.3
Rice with mixed fruit (Gerber) junior	7¾-oz. jar	161	36.1
Cherry vanilla pudding (Gerber):			
Junior	7½-oz. jar	147	32.0
Strained	4½-oz. jar	87	18.9
Chicken (Gerber):			
Junior	3½-oz. jar	137	.2
Strained	3½-oz. jar	139	.3
Chicken & chicken broth (Beech-Nut):			
Junior	7½-oz. jar	228	.4
Strained	4½-oz. jar	128	.3
Chicken & noodles:			
Junior:			
(Beech-Nut)	7½-oz. jar	86	16.6

Food and Description	Measure or Quantity	Calories	Carbohydrates (grams)
(Gerber)	7½-oz. jar	117	16.8
Strained:			
(Beech-Nut)	4½-oz. jar	59	10.5
(Gerber)	4½-oz. jar	77	11.1
Chicken & rice (Beech-Nut) strained	4½-oz. jar	72	12.0
Chicken with vegetables, high meat (Gerber):			
Junior	4½-oz. jar	132	7.5
Strained	4½-oz. jar	126	7.8
Chicken with vegetables & cereal (Beech-Nut):			
Junior	7½-oz. jar	150	14.9
Strained	4½-oz. jar	90	8.9
Chicken soup, cream of (Gerber) strained	4½-oz. jar	77	10.4
Chicken stew (Gerber) toddler	6-oz. jar	145	12.3
Chicken sticks (Gerber) junior	2½-oz. jar	120	1.0
Cookie (Gerber):			
Animal-shaped	6½-gram piece	28	4.3
Arrowroot	5½-gram piece	25	3.7
Corn, creamed:			
Junior:			
(Beech-Nut)	7½-oz. jar	142	30.9
(Gerber)	7½-oz. jar	128	26.2
Strained:			
(Beech-Nut)	4½-oz. jar	85	18.5
(Gerber)	4½-oz. jar	82	16.8
Cottage cheese with pineapple juice (Beech-Nut):			
Junior	7¾-oz. jar	178	32.1
Strained	4¾-oz. jar	111	22.3
Custard:			
Apple (Beech-Nut):			
Junior	7½-oz. jar	132	27.7
Strained	4½-oz. jar	79	16.6
Chocolate (Gerber) strained	4½-oz. jar	106	19.3

(USDA): United States Department of Agriculture
(HEW/FAO):   Health, Education and Welfare/Food and Agriculture
                      Organization
* Prepared as Package Directs

Food and Description	Measure or Quantity	Calories	Carbohydrates (grams)
Vanilla:			
Junior:			
(Beech-Nut)	7½-oz. jar	166	29.0
(Gerber)	7¾-oz. jar	186	33.7
Strained:			
(Beech-Nut)	4½-oz. jar	92	15.7
(Gerber)	4½-oz. jar	106	19.6
Egg yolk (Gerber):			
Junior	3⅓-oz. jar	184	.2
Strained	3⅓-oz. jar	186	.9
Fruit dessert:			
Junior:			
(Beech-Nut):			
Regular	7¾-oz. jar	162	40.3
Tropical	7¾-oz. jar	137	34.1
(Gerber)	7¾-oz. jar	160	38.3
Strained:			
(Beech-Nut)	4½-oz. jar	97	24.0
(Gerber)	4¾-oz. jar	92	22.0
Fruit juice, mixed:			
Strained:			
(Beech-Nut)	4⅕ fl. oz.	59	14.5
(Gerber)	4.2 fl. oz.	58	13.6
Toddler (Gerber)	4 fl. oz.	54	13.2
Fruit, mixed, with yogurt:			
Junior (Beech-Nut)	7½-oz. jar	120	27.3
Strained:			
(Beech-Nut)	4¾-oz. jar	76	17.3
(Gerber)	4½-oz. jar	100	21.6
Guava (Gerber) strained	4½-oz. jar	84	19.9
Guava & papaya (Gerber) strained	4½-oz. jar	85	20.3
Ham (Gerber):			
Junior	3½-oz. jar	114	.4
Strained	3½-oz. jar	105	.5
Ham & ham broth (Beech-Nut) strained	4½-oz. jar	143	.3
Ham with vegetables, high meat (Gerber):			
Junior	4½-oz. jar	105	9.5
Strained	4½-oz. jar	99	8.3

Food and Description	Measure or Quantity	Calories	Carbo-hydrates (grams)
Ham with vegetable & cereal (Beech-Nut):			
Junior	4½-oz. jar	126	7.9
Strained	4½-oz. jar	126	7.9
Hawaiian Delight (Gerber):			
Junior	7¾-oz. jar	187	40.7
Strained	4½-oz. jar	111	24.3
Isomil (Similac) ready-to-feed	1 fl. oz.	20	1.9
Lamb (Gerber):			
Junior	3½-oz. jar	99	.5
Strained	3½-oz. jar	99	.6
Lamb & lamb broth (Beech-Nut):			
Junior	7½-oz. jar	265	.4
Strained	4½-oz. jar	157	.2
Macaroni & cheese (Gerber):			
Junior	7½-oz. jar	135	18.8
Strained	4½-oz. jar	80	10.9
Macaroni & tomato with beef:			
Junior:			
(Beech-Nut)	7½-oz. jar	117	16.4
(Gerber)	7½-oz. jar	119	21.3
Strained:			
(Beech-Nut)	4½-oz. jar	81	10.7
(Gerber)	4½-oz. jar	71	11.5
Mango (Gerber) strained	4¾-oz. jar	97	23.3
MBF (Gerber)			
Concentrate	1 fl. oz. (2 T.)	39	3.7
Concentrate	15-fl.-oz. can	598	56.6
*Diluted, 1 to 1	1 fl. oz. (2 T.)	20	1.9
Meat sticks (Gerber) junior	2½-oz. jar	104	.9
Orange-apple juice, strained:			
(Beech-Nut)	4½ fl. oz.	55	13.5
(Gerber)	4.2 fl. oz.	58	13.5
Orange-apricot juice (Beech-Nut) strained	4.2 fl. oz.	60	13.2
Orange-banana juice (Beech-Nut) strained	4⅕ fl. oz.	58	13.9

(USDA): United States Department of Agriculture
(HEW/FAO): Health, Education and Welfare/Food and Agriculture Organization
* Prepared as Package Directs

Food and Description	Measure or Quantity	Calories	Carbo-hydrates (grams)
Orange juice, strained:			
(Beech-Nut)	4⅕ fl. oz.	56	13.2
(Gerber)	4.2 fl. oz.	57	12.5
Orange-pineapple dessert (Beech-Nut) strained	4¾-oz. jar	107	26.4
Orange-pineapple juice, strained:			
(Beech-Nut)	4⅕ fl. oz.	57	13.6
(Gerber)	4.2 fl. oz.	64	14.8
Orange pudding (Gerber) strained	4¾-oz. jar	101	24.0
Papaya & applesauce (Gerber) strained	4½-oz. jar	82	19.9
Pea:			
Junior:			
(Beech-Nut)	7¼-oz. jar	114	19.1
(Gerber)	7½-oz. jar	127	21.5
Strained:			
(Beech-Nut)	4½-oz. jar	67	11.2
(Gerber)	4½-oz. jar	56	8.6
Pea & carrot (Beech-Nut) strained	4½-oz. jar	61	11.1
Peach:			
Junior:			
(Beech-Nut)	7¾-oz. jar	97	22.9
(Gerber)	7½-oz. jar	94	20.7
Strained:			
(Beech-Nut)	4¾-oz. jar	59	14.0
(Gerber)	4½-oz. jar	64	14.4
Peach & apple with yogurt (Beech-Nut):			
Junior	7½-oz. jar	113	25.1
Strained	4½-oz. jar	68	15.1
Peach cobbler (Gerber):			
Junior	7¾-oz. jar	155	36.8
Strained	4¾-oz. jar	94	22.1
Peach melba (Beech-Nut):			
Junior	7¾-oz. jar	161	39.4
Strained	4¾-oz. jar	99	24.2
Pear:			
Junior:			
(Beech-Nut)	7½-oz. jar	106	26.2
(Gerber)	7½-oz. jar	110	25.4

Food and Description	Measure or Quantity	Calories	Carbo-hydrates (grams)
Strained:			
(Beech-Nut)	4½-oz. jar	64	15.7
(Gerber)	7½-oz. jar	66	15.2
Pear & pineapple:			
Junior:			
(Beech-Nut)	7½-oz. jar	121	29.6
(Gerber)	7½-oz. jar	109	25.4
Strained:			
(Beech-Nut)	4½-oz. serving	73	17.8
(Gerber)	4½-oz. jar	68	15.7
Pineapple dessert (Beech-Nut) strained	4¾-oz. jar	107	26.4
Pineapple with yogurt (Beech-Nut):			
Junior	7½-oz. jar	133	30.0
Strained	4¾-oz. jar	84	19.0
Plum with tapioca (Gerber):			
Junior	7¾-oz. jar	157	37.4
Strained	4¾-oz. jar	91	21.9
Plum with tapioca & apple juice (Beech-Nut):			
Junior	7¾-oz. jar	120	29.3
Strained	4¾-oz. jar	73	17.9
Pork (Gerber) strained	3½-oz. jar	106	.3
Pretzel (Gerber)	6-gram piece	23	4.7
Prune-orange juice (Beech-Nut) strained	4⅕ fl. oz.	66	15.7
Prune with tapioca:			
Junior:			
(Beech-Nut)	7¾-oz. jar	174	40.5
(Gerber)	7¾-oz. jar	172	40.1
Strained:			
(Beech-Nut)	4¾-oz. jar	107	24.8
(Gerber)	4¾-oz. jar	98	22.7
Similac:			
Ready-to-feed or concentrated liquid, with or without added iron	1 fl. oz.	20	2.0

(USDA): United States Department of Agriculture
(HEW/FAO): Health, Education and Welfare/Food and Agriculture Organization
* Prepared as Package Directs

Food and Description	Measure or Quantity	Calories	Carbo-hydrates (grams)
*Powder, regular or with iron	1 fl. oz.	20	2.0
Spaghetti & meatballs (Gerber) toddler	6½-oz. jar	127	18.6
Spaghetti, tomato & beef (Beech-Nut) Junior	7½-oz. jar	131	19.4
Spaghetti with tomato sauce & beef (Gerber) junior	7½-oz. jar	136	22.2
Spinach, creamed (Gerber) strained	4½-oz. jar	56	6.9
Split pea & ham, junior:			
(Beech-Nut)	7½-oz. jar	149	23.4
(Gerber)	7½-oz. jar	151	23.9
Squash:			
Junior:			
(Beech-Nut)	7½-oz. jar	57	11.7
(Gerber)	7½-oz. jar	56	11.1
Strained:			
(Beech-Nut)	4½-oz. jar	34	7.0
(Gerber)	4½-oz. jar	33	6.6
Sweet potato:			
Junior:			
(Beech-Nut)	7¾-oz. jar	118	27.5
(Gerber)	7¾-oz. jar	132	29.5
Strained:			
(Beech-Nut)	4½-oz. jar	68	15.9
(Gerber)	4¾-oz. jar	82	18.2
Turkey (Gerber):			
Junior	3½-oz. jar	130	Tr.
Strained	3½-oz. jar	127	.3
Turkey & rice (Beech-Nut):			
Junior	7½-oz. jar	83	16.6
Strained	4½-oz. jar	59	12.0
Turkey & rice with vegetables (Gerber):			
Junior	7½-oz. jar	131	17.5
Strained	4½-oz. jar	74	9.8
Turkey & vegetables, high meat (Gerber):			
Junior	4½-oz. jar	132	8.1
Strained	4½-oz. jar	127	7.4
Turkey with vegetables & cereal (Beech-Nut) high meat:			
Junior	4½-oz. jar	112	8.9

Food and Description	Measure or Quantity	Calories	Carbo-hydrates (grams)
Strained	4½-oz. jar	112	8.9
Turkey sticks (Gerber) junior	2½-oz. jar	122	1.1
Turkey & turkey broth (Beech-Nut) strained	4½-oz. jar	140	.2
Veal (Gerber):			
Junior	3½-oz. jar	98	.1
Strained	3½-oz. jar	90	.2
Veal & vegetables (Gerber):			
Junior	4½-oz. jar	92	9.2
Strained	4½-oz. jar	85	7.8
Veal with vegetables & cereal, high meat (Beech-Nut) junior or strained	4½-oz. jar	108	8.1
Veal & veal broth (Beech-Nut) strained	4½-oz. jar	143	.2
Vegetable & bacon:			
Junior:			
(Beech-Nut)	7½-oz. jar	141	18.9
(Gerber)	7½-oz. jar	166	19.2
Strained:			
(Beech-Nut)	4½-oz. jar	83	9.9
(Gerber)	4½-oz. jar	96	10.6
Vegetable & beef:			
Junior:			
(Beech-Nut)	7½-oz. jar	123	18.1
(Gerber)	7½-oz. jar	139	20.7
Strained:			
(Beech-Nut)	4½-oz. jar	79	10.9
(Gerber)	4½-oz. jar	85	10.6
Vegetable & chicken:			
Junior:			
(Beech-Nut)	7½-oz. jar	89	15.9
(Gerber)	7½-oz. jar	109	16.8
Strained:			
(Beech-Nut)	4½-oz. jar	58	9.9
(Gerber)	4½-oz. jar	61	8.6
Vegetable & ham, strained:			
(Beech-Nut)	4½-oz. jar	75	10.9

(USDA): United States Department of Agriculture
(HEW/FAO): Health, Education and Welfare/Food and Agriculture Organization
* Prepared as Package Directs

Food and Description	Measure or Quantity	Calories	Carbo-hydrates (grams)
(Gerber)	4½-oz. jar	73	10.7
Vegetable & lamb (Gerber):			
Junior	7½-oz. jar	113	16.4
Strained	4½-oz. jar	73	9.1
Vegetable & lamb with rice & barley (Beech-Nut):			
Junior	7½-oz. jar	120	17.0
Strained	4½-oz. jar	74	10.0
Vegetable & liver (Gerber):			
Junior	7½-oz. jar	90	16.4
Strained	4½-oz. jar	60	9.7
Vegetable & liver with rice & barley (Beech-Nut):			
Junior	7½-oz. jar	91	16.8
Strained	4½-oz. jar	58	9.8
Vegetable & ham (Gerber) junior	7½-oz. jar	126	17.9
Vegetable, mixed:			
Junior:			
(Beech-Nut)	7½-oz. jar	79	17.0
(Gerber)	7½-oz. jar	83	17.0
Strained:			
(Beech-Nut):			
Regular	4½-oz. jar	55	12.0
Garden	4½-oz. jar	66	12.5
(Gerber):			
Regular	4½-oz. jar	52	10.4
Garden	4½-oz. jar	43	6.8
Vegetable & turkey:			
Junior (Gerber)	7½-oz. jar	112	18.3
Strained:			
(Beech-Nut)	4½-oz. jar	77	12.1
(Gerber)	4½-oz. jar	65	9.3
Vegetable & turkey casserole (Gerber) toddler	6¼-oz. jar	147	14.2
BACON, cured:			
Raw (USDA):			
Slab	1 oz. (weighed with rind)	177	.3
Sliced	1 oz.	189	.3

Food and Description	Measure or Quantity	Calories	Carbo- hydrates (grams)
Broiled or fried crisp: (USDA):			
Medium slice	1 slice (7½ grams)	43	.2
Thick slice	1 slice (12 grams)	72	.4
Thin slice	1 slice (5 grams)	30	.2
(Lazy Maple)	3-4 slices (.8 oz.)	140	0.
(Oscar Mayer):			
Regular	.2-oz. slice	35	.1
Thick slice	.4-oz. slice	64	.2
Wafer thin	.14-oz. slice	23	.1
Swift Premium	3-4 slices (.8 oz.)	137	.7
Canned (USDA)	1 oz.	194	.3
BACON BITS:			
(Durkee) imitation	1 tsp. (2 grams)	8	.5
(French's) imitation, crumbles	1 tsp. (2 grams)	6	Tr.
(General Mills) *Bac*Os*	1 T. (.3 oz.)	40	2.0
(Hormel)	1 tsp. (3 grams)	11	.1
(Oscar Mayer) real	1 tsp. (.1 oz.)	6	.1
BACON, CANADIAN:			
Unheated:			
(Hormel) sliced	1-oz. serving	50	.1
(Oscar Mayer) 93% fat free:			
Sliced	.7-oz. slice	30	0.
Sliced	.8-oz. slice	33	0.
Sliced	1-oz. slice	40	0.
Broiled or fried (USDA) drained	1 oz.	79	Tr.
BACON, SIMULATED, cooked:			
(Oscar Mayer) *Lean 'N Tasty:*			
Beef	.3-oz. strip	39	.2
Pork	.4-oz. strip	45	.2
(Swift) *Sizzlean*, pork	.4-oz. strip	50	0.

(USDA): United States Department of Agriculture
(HEW/FAO):   Health, Education and Welfare/Food and Agriculture
Organization
* Prepared as Package Directs

Food and Description	Measure or Quantity	Calories	Carbo-hydrates (grams)
BAGEL (USDA):			
Egg	3″ dia. (1.9 oz.)	162	28.3
Water	3″ dia. (1.9 oz.)	163	30.5
BAKING POWDER:			
(USDA):			
Phosphate	1 tsp. (3.8 grams)	5	1.1
SAS	1 tsp. (3 grams)	4	.9
Tartrate	1 tsp. (2.8 grams)	2	.5
(Calumet)	1 tsp. (3.6 grams)	2	1.0
BALSAMPEAR, fresh (HEW/FAO):			
Whole	1 lb. (weighed with cavity contents)	69	16.3
Flesh only	4 oz.	22	5.1
BAMBOO SHOOT:			
Raw (USDA) trimmed	4 oz.	31	5.9
Canned:			
(Chun King) drained	½ of 8½-oz. can	20	3.0
(La Choy) drained	¼ cup (1½ oz.)	6	1.1
BANANA (USDA):			
Common yellow:			
Fresh:			
Whole	1 lb. (weighed with skin)	262	68.5
Small size	5.9-oz. banana (7¾″ × 1¹¹⁄₃₂″)	81	21.1
Medium size	6.2-oz. banana (8¾″ × 1 ¹³⁄₃₂″)	101	26.4
Large size	7-oz. banana (9¾″ × 1⁷⁄₁₆″)	116	30.2
Mashed	1 cup (about 2 med.)	191	50.0
Sliced	1 cup (about 1¼ med.)	128	33.3
Dehydrated flakes	½ cup (1.8 oz.)	170	44.3
Red, fresh, whole	1 lb. (weighed with skin)	278	72.2

Food and Description	Measure or Quantity	Calories	Carbo-hydrates (grams)
BANANA EXTRACT (Durkee) imitation	1 tsp.	15	0.
BANANA ICE CREAM (Breyer's) red raspberry & strawberry twirl	¼ pt.	150	21.0
BARBECUE SEASONING (French's)	1 tsp. (2½ grams)	6	1.0
BARDOLINO WINE, Italian red (Antinori) 12% alcohol	3 fl. oz.	84	6.3
BARLEY, pearled, dry:			
Light (USDA)	¼ cup (1.8 oz.)	174	39.4
Pot or Scotch:			
(USDA)	2 oz.	197	43.8
(Quaker) Scotch	¼ cup (1.7 oz.)	172	36.3
*BARLEY & MUSHROOM SOUP, frozen (Mother's Own)	8 oz. serving	50	8.0
BASIL:			
Fresh (HEW/FAO) sweet, leaves	½ oz.	6	1.0
Dried (French's) leaves	1 tsp. (1.1 grams)	3	.7
BASS (USDA):			
Black Sea:			
Raw, whole	1 lb. (weighed whole)	165	0.
Baked, stuffed, home recipe	4 oz.	294	12.9
Smallmouth & largemouth, raw:			
Whole	1 lb. (weighed whole)	146	0.
Meat only	4 oz.	118	0.

(USDA): United States Department of Agriculture
(HEW/FAO): Health, Education and Welfare/Food and Agriculture Organization
* Prepared as Package Directs

Food and Description	Measure or Quantity	Calories	Carbohydrates (grams)
Striped:			
Raw, whole	1 lb. (weighed whole)	205	0.
Raw, meat only	4 oz.	119	0.
Oven-fried	4 oz.	222	7.6
White, raw, meat only	4 oz.	111	0.
BAY LEAF (French's) dried	1 tsp. (1.3 grams)	5	1.0
B AND B LIQUEUR (Julius Wile) 86 proof	1 fl. oz.	94	5.7
B.B.Q. SAUCE & BEEF, frozen (Banquet) sliced, *Cookin' Bag*	5-oz. pkg.	126	12.5
BEAN, BAKED, canned:			
(USDA):			
With pork & molasses sauce	1 cup (9 oz.)	383	53.8
With pork & tomato sauce	1 cup (9 oz.)	311	48.5
With tomato sauce	1 cup (9 oz.)	306	58.7
(B & M) *Brick Oven:*			
Pea bean with pork in brown sugar sauce	8-oz. serving	330	49.0
Red kidney in brown sugar sauce	½ of 16-oz. can	330	50.0
Yellow eye bean in brown sugar sauce	½ of 16-oz. can	330	50.0
(Campbell):			
Home style	8-oz. can	270	48.0
With pork & tomato sauce	8-oz. can	260	44.0
(Grandma Brown's) home-baked	8-oz. serving	289	54.1
(Libby's) *Deep Brown:*			
With pork in molasses sauce	½ of 14-oz. can	228	40.6
With pork in tomato sauce	½ of 14-oz. can	220	40.2
Vegetarian, in tomato sauce	½ of 14-oz. can	214	40.8
(Morton House) with tomato sauce	½ of 16-oz. can	270	45.0
(Van Camp) vegetarian style	1 cup	260	48.0
BEAN, BAYO, black or brown (USDA) dry	4 oz.	384	69.4

Food and Description	Measure or Quantity	Calories	Carbo- hydrates (grams)
BEAN, BLACK (USDA) dry	4 oz.	384	69.4
BEAN, BROWN (USDA) dry	4 oz.	384	69.4
BEAN, CALICO (USDA) dry	4 oz.	396	72.2
BEAN, CHILI (See **CHILI**)			
BEAN & FRANKFURTER, canned:			
(USDA)	1 cup (9 oz.)	367	32.1
(Campbell) in tomato & molasses sauce	8-oz. serving	370	43.2
(Hormel) *Short Orders*, 'n Wieners	7½-oz. can	290	29.0
BEAN & FRANKFURTER DINNER, frozen:			
(Banquet)	10¾-oz. dinner	591	63.1
(Morton)	10¾-oz. dinner	528	79.4
(Swanson) *TV Brand*	11¼-oz. dinner	550	75.0
BEAN, GARBANZO, canned, dietetic or low calorie (S&W) *Nutradiet*, solids & liq.	½ cup	105	19.0
BEAN, GREEN or SNAP: Fresh (USDA):			
Whole	1 lb. (weighed untrimmed)	128	28.3
French style	½ cup (1.4 oz.)	13	2.8
Boiled (USDA):			
Whole, drained	½ cup (2.2 oz.)	16	3.3
Pieces, 1½" to 2", drained	½ cup (2.4 oz.)	17	3.7
Canned, regular pack: (USDA):			
Whole, solids & liq.	½ cup (4.2 oz.)	22	5.0
Whole, drained solids	4 oz.	27	5.9

(USDA): United States Department of Agriculture
(HEW/FAO):   Health, Education and Welfare/Food and Agriculture
            Organization
* Prepared as Package Directs

Food and Description	Measure or Quantity	Calories	Carbo-hydrates (grams)
Cut, drained solids	½ cup (2.5 oz.)	17	3.6
Drained liquid only	4 oz.	11	2.7
(Comstock) cut or French style, solids & liq.	½ cup (4 oz.)	23	4.0
(Del Monte):			
Cut, solids & liq.	½ cup (4 oz.)	21	3.8
Cut, drained solids	½ cup (4 oz.)	30	5.3
French style, solids & liq.	½ cup (4 oz.)	18	3.4
French style, drained solids	½ cup (4 oz.)	27	4.9
Seasoned, solids & liq.	½ cup (4 oz.)	22	4.1
Seasoned, drained solids	½ cup (4 oz.)	30	5.5
Whole, solids & liq.	½ cup (4 oz.)	17	2.9
Whole, drained solids	½ cup (4 oz.)	26	4.3
(Festal):			
Cut, solids & liq.	½ cup (4 oz.)	21	3.8
Cut, drained solids	½ cup (4 oz.)	30	5.3
French style, solids & liq.	½ cup (4 oz.)	18	3.4
French style, drained solids	½ cup (4 oz.)	27	4.9
Seasoned, solids & liq.	½ cup (4 oz.)	22	4.1
Seasoned, drained solids	½ cup (4 oz.)	30	5.5
Whole, solids & liq.	½ cup (4 oz.)	17	2.9
Whole, drained solids	½ cup (4 oz.)	26	4.3
(Green Giant) whole, cut or French style, solids & liq.	½ of 8-oz. can	15	2.6
(Kounty Kist) cut, French style or whole, solids & liq.	¼ of 16-oz. can	15	2.7
(Libby's):			
Cut, Blue Lake, solids & liq.	¼ of 16-oz. can	21	4.1
French style, Blue Lake, solids & liq.	¼ of 16-oz. can	21	4.0
(Lindy) cut, French style or whole, solids & liq.	¼ of 16-oz. can	15	2.7
(Stokely-Van Camp) cut, sliced or whole, solids & liq.	½ cup (4.2 oz.)	20	4.0
(Sunshine) solids & liq.	½ cup (4.2 oz.)	20	3.8
Canned, dietetic or low calorie:			
(USDA):			
Solids & liq.	4 oz.	18	4.1
Drained solids	4 oz.	25	5.4
(Diet Delight) solids & liq.	½ cup (4.2 oz.)	20	3.0

Food and Description	Measure or Quantity	Calories	Carbo-hydrates (grams)
(Featherweight) cut or French style, solids & liq.	½ cup	25	5.0
(S&W) *Nutradiet*, cut, solids & liq.	½ cup	20	4.0
Frozen:			
(USDA):			
Cut or French style, unthawed	10-oz. pkg.	74	17.0
Cut or French style, boiled, drained	½ cup (2.8 oz.)	20	4.6
(Birds Eye):			
Cut, 5-minute style	⅓ of 9-oz. pkg.	25	5.0
French, 5-minute style	⅓ of 9-oz. pkg.	30	6.0
French, with sliced mushrooms	⅓ of 9-oz. pkg.	31	6.1
With pearl onions	⅓ of 9-oz. pkg.	32	6.2
Whole, deluxe	⅓ of 9-oz. pkg.	26	5.0
(Green Giant):			
Cut or French, in butter sauce	⅓ of 9-oz. pkg.	31	3.0
With onions & bacon bits	⅓ of 9-oz. pkg.	32	3.6
(McKenzie) French or whole	⅓ of 9-oz. pkg.	29	5.8
(Seabrook Farms) French or whole	⅓ of 9-oz. pkg.	29	5.8
(Southland) cut or French	⅕ of 16-oz. pkg.	25	5.0
BEAN, GREEN, & MUSHROOM CASSEROLE, frozen (Stouffer's)	½ of 9½-oz. pkg.	143	11.9
BEAN, GREEN, WITH POTATOES, canned (Sunshine) solids & liq.	½ cup (4.3 oz.)	34	7.0
BEAN, GREEN, PUREE, canned, dietetic (Featherweight)	1 cup	70	15.0

(USDA): United States Department of Agriculture
(HEW/FAO): Health, Education and Welfare/Food and Agriculture Organization
* Prepared as Package Directs

Food and Description	Measure or Quantity	Calories	Carbo-hydrates (grams)
BEAN, ITALIAN:			
Canned (Del Monte):			
Solids & liq.	1 cup (8 oz.)	57	10.9
Drained solids	½ cup (4 oz.)	43	8.2
Frozen:			
(Birds Eye) 5-minute style	⅓ of 9-oz. pkg.	30	6.0
(McKenzie)	⅓ of 9-oz. pkg.	37	7.1
(Seabook Farms)	⅓ of 9-oz. pkg.	37	7.1
BEAN, KIDNEY OR RED:			
(USDA):			
Dry	1 lb.	1556	280.8
Dry	½ cup (3.3 oz.)	319	57.6
Cooked	½ cup (3.3 oz.)	109	19.8
Canned, regular pack, solids & liq.:			
(Blue Boy)	4 oz.	115	17.8
(Furman) red	½ cup (4½ oz.)	121	21.2
Canned, dietetic or low calorie (S&W) *Nutradiet*, solids & liq.	½ cup	90	16.0
BEAN, LIMA:			
Raw (USDA):			
Young, whole	1 lb. (weighed in pod)	223	40.1
Mature, dry	½ cup (3.4 oz.)	331	61.4
Young, without shell	1 lb. (weighed shelled)	558	100.2
Boiled (USDA) mature, drained	½ cup (3.4 oz.)	131	24.3
Canned, regular pack:			
(Del Monte):			
Solids & liq.	½ cup	76	14.1
Drained solids	½ cup	108	19.7
(Libby's) solids & liq.	½ cup (4.3 oz.)	91	16.0
(Stokely-Van Camp) solids & liq.	½ cup (4.4 oz.)	90	16.5
Canned, dietetic or low calorie:			
(USDA):			
Low sodium, solids & liq.	4 oz.	79	14.6
Low sodium, drained solids	4 oz.	108	20.1
(Featherweight) solids & liq.	½ cup	73	16.0

Food and Description	Measure or Quantity	Calories	Carbo- hydrates (grams)
Frozen:			
(USDA):			
Baby, unthawed	4 oz.	138	26.1
Fordhooks, unthawed	4 oz.	112	21.7
Boiled, drained solids	½ cup (3.1 oz.)	106	20.0
Boiled, Fordhooks, drained	½ cup (3 oz.)	83	16.0
(Birds Eye):			
Baby butter	⅓ of 10-oz. pkg.	140	26.0
Baby, 5-minute style	⅓ of pkg.	120	22.0
Fordhooks, 5-minute style	⅓ of pkg.	100	18.0
Tiny, deluxe	⅓ of 10-oz. pkg.	111	20.0
(Green Giant):			
Baby	¼ of 16-oz. pkg.	124	22.4
Baby, in butter sauce	⅓ of 10-oz. pkg.	107	15.7
Speckled butter bean, Southern recipe	⅓ of 10-oz. pkg.	105	13.2
(Kounty Kist) baby	⅕ of 20-oz. pkg.	154	27.5
(McKenzie):			
Baby	⅓ of 10-oz. pkg.	126	23.6
Baby butter bean	⅓ of 10-oz. pkg.	139	26.1
Fordhook	⅓ of 10-oz. pkg.	98	17.9
Speckled butter bean	⅓ of 10-oz. pkg.	126	23.4
(Seabrook Farms):			
Baby	⅓ of 10-oz. pkg.	126	23.6
Baby butter bean	⅓ of 10-oz. pkg.	139	26.1
Fordhook	⅓ of 10-oz. pkg.	98	17.9
Speckled butter bean	⅓ of 10-oz. pkg.	126	23.4
(Southland) speckled butter bean	⅕ of 16-oz. pkg.	110	20.0
BEAN, MUNG (USDA) dry	½ cup (3.7 oz.)	357	63.3
BEAN, PINTO:			
Dry (USDA)	½ cup (3.4 oz.)	335	61.2

(USDA): United States Department of Agriculture
(HEW/FAO): Health, Education and Welfare/Food and Agriculture Organization
* Prepared as Package Directs

Food and Description	Measure or Quantity	Calories	Carbo-hydrates (grams)
Canned (Del Monte) spicy	½ cup (4.3 oz.)	120	19.0
BEAN, RED MEXICAN, dry (USDA)	4 oz.	396	72.2
BEAN, REFRIED, canned:			
(Del Monte):			
Regular	½ cup (4.3 oz.)	130	20.0
Spicy	½ cup (4.3 oz.)	130	20.0
Old El Paso	½ of 8¼-oz. can	103	17.5
(Ortega) lightly spicy or true bean	½ cup	170	25.0
BEAN SALAD, canned:			
(Green Giant)	¼ of 17-oz. can	92	19.9
(Nalley's)	4½-oz. serving	155	29.4
BEAN, SOUP, canned:			
*(USDA) condensed, with pork, prepared with equal volume water	1 cup (8.8 oz.)	168	21.8
(Campbell):			
Chunky, with ham	11-oz. can	300	35.0
*Condensed, with bacon	11-oz. serving	200	29.0
*Semi-condensed, *Soup For One,* old fashioned with ham	11-oz. serving	220	31.0
*(Grandma Brown's)	8-oz. serving	182	29.1
BEAN SOUP, BLACK, canned:			
*(Campbell) condensed	11-oz. serving	130	21.0
(Crosse & Blackwell) with sherry	½ of 13-oz. can	80	18.0
BEAN SOUP, NAVY (USDA) dehydrated	1 oz.	93	17.8
BEAN SPROUT:			
Fresh (USDA):			
Mung:			
Raw	½ lb.	80	15.0
Raw	½ cup (1.6 oz.)	19	3.5

Food and Description	Measure or Quantity	Calories	Carbo-hydrates (grams)
Boiled, drained	½ cup (212 oz.)	17	3.2
Soy:			
Raw	½ lb.	104	12.0
Raw	½ cup (1.9 oz.)	25	2.9
Boiled, drained	4 oz.	43	4.2
Canned:			
(Chun King) drained	¼ of 16-oz. can	20	2.0
(La Choy) drained	⅔ cup (2 oz.)	7	.8

BEAN, WAX (See BEAN, YELLOW)

BEAN, WHITE (USDA):
Raw:			
Great Northern	½ cup (3.1 oz.)	303	54.6
Navy or pea	½ cup	354	63.8
White	1 oz.	96	17.4
Cooked:			
Great Northern	½ cup (3 oz.)	100	18.0
Navy or pea	½ cup (3.4 oz.)	113	20.4
All other white	4-oz. serving	134	24.0

BEAN, YELLOW or WAX:
Raw, whole (USDA)	1 lb. (weighed untrimmed)	108	24.0
Boiled, drained (USDA) 1″ pieces	½ cup (2.9 oz.)	18	3.7
Canned, regular pack: (USDA):			
Solids & liq.	½ cup (4.2 oz.)	23	5.0
Drained solids	½ cup (2.2 oz.)	15	3.2
Drained, liquid only	4 oz.	12	2.8
(Comstock) solids & liq.	½ cup	22	4.5
(Del Monte):			
Cut, solids & liq.	½ cup (4 oz.)	19	3.4
Cut, drained solids	½ cup	25	4.5
French style, solids & liq.	½ cup (4 oz.)	19	3.6

(USDA): United States Department of Agriculture
(HEW/FAO): Health, Education and Welfare/Food and Agriculture
                        Organization
* Prepared as Package Directs

Food and Description	Measure or Quantity	Calories	Carbo-hydrates (grams)
(Festal):			
Cut, solids & liq.	½ cup	19	3.4
French style, solids & liq.	½ cup (4 oz.)	19	3.6
(Libby's) solids & liq.	½ of 8-oz. can	23	4.4
(Stokely-Van Camp) cut, solids & liq.	½ cup (4.3 oz.)	23	4.0
Canned, dietetic or low calorie:			
(USDA):			
Solids & liq.	4-oz. serving	17	3.9
Drained solids	4-oz. serving	24	5.3
(Blue Boy) solids & liq.	4-oz. serving	28	4.7
(Featherweight) cut, solids & liq.	½ cup	25	5.0
Frozen:			
(USDA):			
Cut, unthawed	4-oz. serving	32	7.4
Boiled, drained	4-oz. serving	31	7.0
(Birds Eye) cut, 5-minute style	⅓ of 9-oz. pkg.	30	4.0
BEAUJOLAIS WINE, French Burgundy (Barton & Guestier) St. Louis, 12% alcohol	3 fl. oz.	60	.1
BEAUNE WINE:			
Clos de Feves, French Burgundy (Chanson) 12% alcohol	3 fl. oz.	83	6.3
St. Vincent, French Burgundy (Chanson) 12% alcohol	3 fl. oz.	84	6.3
BEAVER, roasted (USDA)	4-oz. serving	281	0.
BEECHNUT (USDA):			
Whole	4 oz. (weighed in shell)	393	14.0
Shelled	4 oz. (weighed shelled)	633	23.0

BEEF. Values for beef cuts are given below for "lean and fat" and for "lean only." Beef purchased by the consumer at the

Food and Description	Measure or Quantity	Calories	Carbohydrates (grams)
retail store usually is trimmed to about one-half inch layer of fat. This is the meat discribed as "lean and fat." If all the fat that can be cut off with a knife is removed, the remainder is the "lean only." These cuts still contain flecks of fat known as "marbling" distributed through the meat. Cooked meats are medium done. Choice grade cuts (USDA):			
Brisket:			
Raw	1 lb. (weighed with bone)	1284	0.
Braised:			
Lean & fat	4 oz.	467	0.
Lean only	4 oz.	252	0.
Chuck:			
Raw	1 lb (weighed with bone)	984	0.
Braised or pot-roasted:			
Lean & fat	4 oz.	371	0.
Lean only	4 oz.	243	0.
Dried (see **BEEF, CHIPPED**)			
Fat, separable, cooked	1 oz.	207	0.
Filet mignon. There are no data available on its composition. For dietary estimates, the data for sirloin steak, lean only, afford the closest approximation.			
Flank:			
Raw	1 lb.	653	0.
Braised	4 oz.	222	0.
Foreshank:			
Raw	1 lb. (weighed with bone)	531	0.

(USDA): United States Department of Agriculture
(HEW/FAO): Health, Education and Welfare/Food and Agriculture Organization
* Prepared as Package Directs

Food and Description	Measure or Quantity	Calories	Carbo-hydrates (grams)
Simmered:			
Lean & fat	4 oz.	310	0.
Lean only	4 oz.	209	0.
Ground:			
Lean:			
Raw	1 lb.	812	0.
Raw	1 cup (8 oz.)	405	0.
Broiled	4 oz.	248	0.
Regular:			
Raw	1 lb.	1216	0.
Raw	1 cup (8 oz.)	606	0.
Broiled	4 oz.	324	0.
Heel of round:			
Raw	1 lb.	966	0.
Roasted:			
Lean & fat	4 oz.	296	0.
Lean only	4 oz.	204	0.
Hindshank:			
Raw	1 lb. (weighed with bone)	604	0.
Simmered:			
Lean & fat	4 oz.	409	0.
Lean only	4 oz.	209	0.
Neck:			
Raw	1 lb. (weighed with bone)	820	0.
Pot-roasted:			
Lean & fat	4 oz.	332	0.
Lean only	4 oz.	222	0.
Plate:			
Raw	1 lb. (weighed with bone)	1615	0.
Simmered:			
Lean & fat	4 oz.	538	0.
Lean only	4 oz.	252	0.
Rib roast:			
Raw	1 lb. (weighed with bone)	1673	0.
Roasted:			
Lean & fat	4 oz.	499	0.
Lean only	4 oz.	273	0.

Food and Description	Measure or Quantity	Calories	Carbo-hydrates (grams)
Round:			
Raw	1 lb. (weighed with bone)	863	0.
Broiled:			
Lean & fat	4 oz.	296	0.
Lean only	4 oz.	214	0.
Rump:			
Raw	1 lb. (weighed with bone)	1167	0.
Roasted:			
Lean & fat	4 oz.	393	0.
Lean only	4 oz.	236	0.
Steak, club:			
Raw	1 lb. (weighed without bone)	1724	0.
Broiled:			
Lean & fat	4 oz.	515	0.
Lean only	4 oz.	277	0.
One 8-oz. steak (weighed without bone before cooking) will give you:			
Lean & fat	5.9 oz.	754	0.
Lean only	3.4 oz.	234	0.
Steak, porterhouse:			
Raw	1 lb. (weighed with bone)	1603	0.
Broiled:			
Lean & fat	4 oz.	527	0.
Lean only	4 oz.	254	0.
One 16-oz. steak (weighed with bone before cooking) will give you:			
Lean & fat	10.2 oz.	1339	0.
Lean only	5.9 oz.	372	0.
Steak, ribeye, broiled:			
One 10-oz. steak (weighed before cooking without bone) will give you:			

(USDA): United States Department of Agriculture
(HEW/FAO): Health, Education and Welfare/Food and Agriculture Organization
* Prepared as Package Directs

Food and Description	Measure or Quantity	Calories	Carbo-hydrates (grams)
Lean & fat	7.3 oz.	911	0.
Lean only	3.8 oz.	258	0.
Steak, sirloin, double-bone:			
Raw	1 lb. (weighed with bone)	1240	0.
Broiled:			
Lean & fat	4 oz.	463	0.
Lean only	4 oz.	245	0.
One 16-oz. steak (weighed before cooking with bone) will give you:			
Lean & fat	8.9 oz.	1028	0.
Lean only	5.9 oz.	359	0.
One 12-oz. steak (weighed before cooking with bone) will give you:			
Lean & fat	6.6 oz.	767	0.
Lean only	4.4 oz.	268	0.
Steak, sirloin, hipbone:			
Raw	1 lb. (weighed with bone)	1585	0.
Broiled:			
Lean & fat	4 oz.	552	0.
Lean only	4 oz.	272	0.
Steak, sirloin, wedge & round-bone:			
Raw	1 lb. (weighed with bone)	1316	0.
Broiled:			
Lean & fat	4 oz.	439	0.
Lean only	4 oz.	235	0.
Steak, T-bone:			
Raw	1 lb. (weighed with bone)	1596	0.
Broiled:			
Lean & fat	4 oz.	536	0.
Lean only	4 oz.	253	0.
One 16-oz. steak (weighed before cooking with bone) will give you:			
Broiled:			
Lean & fat	4 oz.	463	0.
Lean only	4 oz.	245	0.

Food and Description	Measure or Quantity	Calories	Carbo-hydrates (grams)
BEEFAMATO COCKTAIL,			
canned (Mott's)	6 fl. oz.	70	15.0
BEEF BOUILLON, cube or powder:			
(Herb-Ox):			
Cube	1 cube (4 grams)	6	.5
Powder	1 packet (4 grams)	8	.8
(Maggi)	1 cube (3½ grams)	6	0.
MBT	1 packet (5½ grams)	14	2.0
BEEF BROTH (See **BEEF SOUP**)			
BEEF, CHIPPED:			
Home recipe (USDA) creamed	½ cup (4.3 oz.)	188	8.7
Frozen, creamed:			
(Banquet) *Cookin' Bag*	5-oz. pkg.	124	10.5
(Stouffer's)	½ of 11-oz. pkg.	231	10.0
(Swanson)	10½-oz. entree	350	15.0
BEEF, CORNED (See **CORNED BEEF**)			
BEEF DINNER OR ENTREE,			
frozen:			
(Banquet):			
Regular, sliced	11-oz. dinner	312	20.9
Regular, chopped	11-oz. dinner	443	32.8
Man-Pleaser:			
Chopped	18-oz. dinner	900	67.2
Sliced	20-oz. dinner	453	63.7
(Morton):			
Country Table, sliced	14-oz. dinner	512	55.7

(USDA): United States Department of Agriculture
(HEW/FAO):   Health, Education and Welfare/Food and Agriculture
                    Organization
* Prepared as Package Directs

Food and Description	Measure or Quantity	Calories	Carbo-hydrates (grams)
Steak House:			
Chopped sirloin	9½-oz. dinner	748	43.2
Rib eye	9-oz. dinner	816	38.4
Sirloin strip	9½-oz. dinner	896	43.2
Tenderloin	9½-oz. dinner	896	43.2
(Swanson):			
Regular, sliced, with gravy & whipped potatoes	8-oz. entree	190	23.0
Hungry Man:			
Chopped	18-oz. dinner	730	70.0
Sliced, dinner	17-oz. dinner	540	51.0
Sliced, entree	12¼-oz. entree	330	23.0
3-course	15-oz. dinner	490	58.0
TV Brand:			
Regular	11½-oz. dinner	370	34.0
Chopped sirloin	10-oz. dinner	460	36.0
(Weight Watchers):			
Beefsteak, 2-compartment	9¾-oz. meal	344	12.0
Sirloin in mushroom sauce, 3-compartment	13-oz. meal	410	16.0
BEEF, DRIED, canned:			
(Hormel) creamed, *Short Orders*	7½-oz. can	160	9.0
(Swift)	1-oz. serving	34	Tr.
BEEF GOULASH, canned:			
(Bounty)	7½-oz. can	203	16.3
(Hormel) *Short Orders*	7½-oz. can	230	16.0
BEEF, GROUND, SEASONING MIX:			
*(Durkee) regular or with onion	1 cup	659	6.5
(French's) with onion	1⅛-oz. pkg.	100	24.0
BEEF HASH, ROAST:			
Canned, *Mary Kitchen* (Hormel):			
Regular	7½-oz. serving	396	17.9
Short Orders	7½-oz. can	370	19.0
Frozen (Stouffer's)	½ of 11½-oz pkg.	262	10.9

Food and Description	Measure or Quantity	Calories	Carbohydrates (grams)
BEEF PEPPER ORIENTAL:			
*Canned (LaChoy):			
Regular	¾ cup	90	12.0
Bi-pack	¾ cup	70	8.0
Frozen (Chun King):			
Dinner	11-oz. dinner	310	43.0
Pouch	12-oz. pouch	160	20.0
BEEF PIE:			
Home recipe (USDA) baked	4¼" pie (8 oz. before baking)	558	42.7
Frozen:			
(Banquet)	8-oz. pie	409	40.9
(Morton)	8-oz. pie	316	31.8
(Stouffer's)	10-oz. pie	552	37.8
(Swanson):			
Regular	8-oz. pie	430	44.0
Hungry Man	16-oz. pie	770	65.0
Hungry Man, steak burger	16-oz. pie	830	69.0
BEEF, POTTED (USDA)	1-oz. serving	70	0.
BEEF PUFFS, frozen (Durkee)	1 piece	47	3.0
BEEF SHORT RIBS, frozen (Stouffer's) boneless, with vegetable gravy	½ of 11½-oz. pkg.	347	2.0
BEEF SOUP:			
Canned, regular pack:			
(Campbell):			
Chunky:			
Regular	9½-oz. can	170	2.0
Regular	10¾-oz. can	190	23.0
With noodles	10¾-oz. can	310	29.0
*Condensed:			
Regular	11-oz. serving	110	15.0
Broth	10-oz. serving	20	2.0

(USDA): United States Department of Agriculture
(HEW/FAO):   Health, Education and Welfare/Food and Agriculture Organization
* Prepared as Package Directs

Food and Description	Measure or Quantity	Calories	Carbo-hydrates (grams)
Broth & barley	11-oz. serving	90	13.0
Broth & noodles	10-oz. serving	80	10.0
Consomme	10-oz. serving	30	2.0
& mushroom	10-oz. serving	90	8.0
& noodles	10-oz. serving	90	9.0
Teriyaki	10-oz. serving	90	11.0
(College Inn) broth	1 cup	18	1.0
(Swanson) broth	7¼-oz. can	18	0.
Canned, dietetic pack			
(Dia-Mel) & noodle	8-oz. serving	70	5.0
*Mix:			
Carmel Kosher	6 fl. oz.	12	1.8
(Lipton) *Cup-A-Soup*, & noodle	6 fl. oz.	50	8.0
BEEF SPREAD, ROAST, canned (Underwood)	½ of 4¾-oz. can	140	Tr.
BEEF STEAK, BREADED, frozen (Hormel)	4-oz. serving	374	12.7
BEEF STEW:			
Home recipe (USDA)	1 cup	218	15.2
Canned, regular pack:			
Dinty Moore (Hormel):			
Regular	7½-oz. serving	184	12.8
Short Orders	7½-oz. can	170	14.0
(Libby's)	8-oz. serving	233	33.8
(Nalley's)	7½-oz. serving	226	17.0
(Swanson)	½ of 15¼-oz. can	150	16.0
Canned, dietetic or low calorie			
(Dia-Mel)	8-oz. can	200	19.0
Frozen:			
(Banquet) *Buffet Supper*	2-lb. pkg.	700	90.9
(Green Giant):			
Bake n' Serve, & biscuits	14-oz. pkg.	368	40.6
Boil in bag	9-oz. pkg.	165	20.2
(Stouffer's)	10-oz. serving	305	15.9
BEEF STEW SEASONING MIX:			
*(Durkee)	1 cup	379	16.7
(French's)	1⅞-oz. pkg.	150	30.0

Food and Description	Measure or Quantity	Calories	Carbo-hydrates (grams)
BEEF STIX, packaged (Vienna)	1-oz. serving	163	1.4
BEEF STOCK BASE (French's)	1 tsp. (4 grams)	8	2.0
BEEF STROGANOFF, frozen (Stouffer's) with parsley noodles	9¾-oz. serving	390	30.7
*BEEF STROGANOFF SEASONING MIX (Durkee)	1 cup	820	71.2
BEER, canned:			
Regular:			
Black Horse Ale, 5% alcohol	12 fl. oz.	162	13.8
Black Label	12 fl. oz.	140	11.3
Buckeye, 4.6% alcohol	12 fl. oz.	144	11.0
Budweiser, 4.9% alcohol	12 fl. oz.	156	12.3
Busch Bavarian	12 fl. oz.	150	11.6
Eastside Lager	12 fl. oz.	145	DNA
Heidelberg, 4.6% alcohol	12 fl. oz.	133	10.7
Knickerbocker, 4.6% alcohol	12 fl. oz.	160	13.7
Meister Brau Premium, regular or draft, 4.6% alcohol	12 fl. oz.	144	11.0
Michelob, 4.9% alcohol	12 fl. oz.	165	16.5
Pabst Blue Ribbon	12 fl. oz.	150	DNA
Pearl Premium, 4.7% alcohol	12 fl. oz.	148	12.5
Primo	12 fl. oz.	142	12.5
Rheingold, 4.6% alcohol	12 fl. oz.	160	13.7
Schmidt, regular or extra special, 4.8% alcohol	12 fl. oz.	165	14.9
Stroh Bohemiam:			
Regular	12 fl. oz.	148	13.6
3.4 low gravity	12 fl. oz.	126	11.6
Tuborg USA, 4.8% alcohol	12 fl. oz.	140	12.1
Light:			
Budweiser	12 fl. oz.	110	6.0
Gablinger's	12 fl. oz.	99	.2
Michelob	12 fl. oz.	134	12.0

(USDA): United States Department of Agriculture
(HEW/FAO): Health, Education and Welfare/Food and Agriculture Organization
* Prepared as Package Directs

Food and Description	Measure or Quantity	Calories	Carbo-hydrates (grams)
Natural Light	12 fl. oz.	110	6.0
Stroh Light	12 fl. oz.	115	7.1
BEER, NEAR:			
Goetz Pale, 0.2% alcohol	12 fl. oz.	78	3.9
Kingsbury, 0.5% alcohol	12 fl. oz.	45	12.7
BEET:			
Raw (USDA):			
Whole	1 lb. (weighed with skins, without tops)	137	31.4
Diced	½ cup (2.4 oz.)	29	6.6
Boiled (USDA) drained:			
Whole	2 beets (2″ dia., 3.5 oz.)	32	7.2
Diced	½ cup (3 oz.)	27	6.1
Sliced	½ cup (3.6 oz.)	33	7.3
Canned, regular pack:			
(Del Monte):			
Pickled, sliced, solids & liq.	½ cup	77	18.1
Pickled, sliced, drained solids	½ cup	81	18.9
Sliced, solids & liq.	½ cup	29	7.0
Sliced, drained solids	½ cup	36	3.6
Whole, tiny, solids & liq.	½ cup	42	9.1
(Greenwood) solids & liq.:			
Harvard	½ cup	70	16.0
Pickled	½ cup	110	27.5
Pickled, with onion	½ cup	115	27.5
(Libby's) solids & liq.:			
Harvard, diced	½ cup (4.2 oz.)	87	20.8
Pickled, sliced	¼ of 16-oz. jar	78	18.5
(Stokely-Van Camp) solids & liq.:			
Cut	½ cup	45	9.5
Diced	½ cup	35	7.5
Harvard	½ cup (4½ oz.)	80	18.0
Pickled	½ cup (4.3 oz.)	95	22.5
Whole	½ cup (4.3 oz.)	45	10.0
Canned, dietetic pack, solids & liq.:			
(Comstock) water pack	½ cup	30	6.5

Food and Description	Measure or Quantity	Calories	Carbo- hydrates (grams)
(Featherweight) sliced	½ cup	45	10.0
(S&W) *Nutradiet*, sliced	½ cup	35	9.0
BEET GREENS (USDA):			
Raw, whole	1 lb. (weighed untrimmed)	61	11.7
Boiled, leaves & stems, drained	½ cup (2.6 oz.)	13	2.4
BEET PUREE, canned, dietetic pack (Featherweight)	1 cup	90	20.0
BENEDICTINE LIQUEUR (Julius Wile) 86 proof	1 fl. oz.	112	10.3
BIG H, burger sauce (Hellman's)	1 T.	71	1.6
BIG MAC (See McDONALD'S)			
BIG WHEEL (Hostess)	1.3-oz. cake	182	21.5
BISCUIT, home recipe (USDA) baking powder	1-oz. biscuit (2″ dia.)	103	12.8
BISCUIT DOUGH, refrigerated (Pillsbury):			
Baking Powder, *1869 Brand*	1 biscuit	100	13.5
Big Country	1 biscuit	95	15.5
Big Country, Good 'N Buttery	1 biscuit	100	14.0
Buttermilk:			
Regular	1 biscuit	50	10.0
Ballard Oven Ready	1 biscuit	50	10.0
1869 Brand	1 biscuit	100	13.5
Extra Lights	1 biscuit	60	10.5
Extra rich, *Hungry Jack*	1 biscuit	65	9.0
Flaky, *Hungry Jack*	1 biscuit	80	13.0
Fluffy, *Hungry Jack*	1 biscuit	100	12.0

(USDA): United States Department of Agriculture
(HEW/FAO):   Health, Education and Welfare/Food and Agriculture
                Organization
* Prepared as Package Directs

Food and Description	Measure or Quantity	Calories	Carbohydrates (grams)
Butter Tastin', 1869 Brand	1 biscuit	100	13.5
Butter Tastin', Hungry Jack	1 biscuit	95	11.0
Country style	1 biscuit	50	10.0
Dinner, baking powder or buttermilk tenderflake	1 biscuit	55	7.5
Flaky, *Hungry Jack*	1 biscuit	90	11.5
Heat 'N Eat, *1869 Brand*	1 biscuit	100	11.5
Oven Ready, *Ballard*	1 biscuit	50	10.0
Prize	1 biscuit	65	9.5
BISCUIT MIX (USDA):			
Dry, with enriched flour	1 oz.	120	19.5
*Baked from mix, with added milk	1-oz. biscuit	91	14.6
BITTERS (Angostura)	1 tsp.	14	DNA
BLACKBERRY:			
Fresh (USDA) includes boysenberry, dewberry, youngsberry:			
With hulls	1 lb. (weighed untrimmed)	250	55.6
Hulled	½ cup (2.6 oz.)	41	9.4
Canned, regular pack (USDA) solids & liq.:			
Juice pack	4-oz. serving	61	13.7
Light syrup	4-oz. serving	82	19.6
Heavy syrup	½ cup (4.6 oz.)	118	28.9
Extra heavy syrup	4-oz. serving	125	30.7
Frozen (USDA):			
Sweetened, unthawed	4-oz. serving	109	27.7
Unsweetened, unthawed	4-oz. serving	55	12.9
BLACKBERRY BRANDY (See **BRANDY, FLAVORED**)			
BLACKBERRY JELLY:			
Sweetened (Smucker's)	1 T. (.7 oz.)	53	13.5
Dietetic (See **BLACKBERRY SPREAD**)			

Food and Description	Measure or Quantity	Calories	Carbo-hydrates (grams)
BLACKBERRY LIQUEUR:			
(Bols) 60 proof	1 fl. oz.	96	8.9
(Hiram Walker) 60 proof	1 fl. oz.	100	12.8
BLACKBERRY PRESERVE or JAM:			
Sweetened (Smucker's)	1 T. (.7 oz.)	53	13.5
Dietetic or low calorie:			
(Dia-Mel)	1 T.	6	0.
(Featherweight)	1 T.	16	4.0
(S&W) *Nutradiet*	1 T.	12	3.0
BLACKBERRY SPREAD, low sugar:			
(Diet Delight)	1 T.	12	3.0
(Featherweight)	1 T.	16	4.0
(Slenderella)	1 T.	24	6.0
(Smucker's)	1 T.	24	6.0
BLACKBERRY WINE (Mogen David) 12% alcohol	3 fl. oz.	135	18.7
BLACK-EYED PEA (See also COWPEA):			
Boiled (USDA) drained	½ cup (3 oz.)	111	20.1
Canned (Sunshine) with pork, solids & liq.	½ cup (4 oz.)	90	16.1
Frozen:			
(Birds Eye)	⅓ of 10-oz. pkg.	130	23.0
(Green Giant) southern recipe	⅓ of 10-oz. pkg.	106	12.7
(McKenzie)	⅓ of 10-oz. pkg.	130	22.7
(Seabrook Farms)	⅓ of 10-oz. pkg.	130	22.7
(Southland)	⅕ of 16-oz. pkg.	120	21.0
BLANCMANGE (See PUDDING or PIE FILLING, Vanilla)			

(USDA): United States Department of Agriculture
(HEW/FAO): Health, Education and Welfare/Food and Agriculture Organization
* Prepared as Package Directs

Food and Description	Measure or Quantity	Calories	Carbo-hydrates (grams)
BLINTZE, CHEESE, frozen (King Kold)	2½-oz. piece	132	21.4
BLOODY MARY MIX:			
Dry (Holland House)	.5-oz. serving	56	14.0
Liquid (Sacramento)	5½-fl. oz. can	39	9.1
BLUEBERRY:			
Fresh (USDA):			
Whole	1 lb. (weighed untrimmed)	259	63.8
Trimmed	½ cup (2.6 oz.)	45	11.2
Canned (USDA) solids & liq.:			
Syrup pack, extra heavy	½ cup (4.4 oz.)	126	32.5
Water pack	½ cup (4.3 oz.)	47	11.9
Frozen (USDA):			
Sweetened, solids & liq.	½ cup (4 oz.)	120	30.2
Unsweetened, solids & liq.	½ cup (2.9 oz.)	45	11.2
BLUEBERRY PIE (See **PIE,** Blueberry)			
BLUEBERRY PRESERVE or JAM:			
Sweetened (Smucker's)	1 T.	53	13.5
Dietetic (Dia-Mel)	1 T.	6	0.
BLUEFISH (USDA):			
Raw:			
Whole	1 lb. (weighed whole)	271	0.
Meat only	4 oz.	133	0.
Baked or broiled	4.4-oz. piece (3½" × 3" × ½")	199	0.
Fried	5.3-oz. piece (3½" × 3" × ½")	308	7.0
BODY BUDDIES, cereal (General Mills):			
Brown sugar & honey	1 cup (1 oz.)	110	25.0
Natural fruit flavor	¾ cup (1 oz.)	100	25.0

Food and Description	Measure or Quantity	Calories	Carbo-hydrates (grams)
BOLOGNA:			
(Best's Kosher):			
Chub	1-oz. serving	90	1.0
Sliced	1-oz. serving	68	1.0
(Eckrich):			
Beef	1-oz. serving	95	1.5
Garlic	1-oz. serving	95	1.5
Ring	1-oz. serving	100	1.5
Ring, pickled	1-oz. serving	95	1.5
Sliced:			
Regular	1-oz. serving	95	1.5
Thick	1.7-oz. slice	160	3.0
Thick	1.8-oz. slice	170	3.0
(Hormel):			
Beef	1-oz. serving	86	.3
Meat	1-oz. serving	85	.2
Ring:			
Coarse ground	1-oz. serving	76	.9
Fine ground	1-oz. serving	82	.6
(Oscar Mayer):			
Beef:			
Regular	.5-oz. slice	45	.4
Regular	.8-oz. slice	72	.7
Garlic	.8-oz. slice	73	.4
Lebanon	.8-oz. slice	51	.4
Thick slice	1.3-oz. slice	118	1.1
German brand	.8-oz. slice	55	.3
Meat:			
Round	.8-oz. slice	73	.7
Square	1-oz. slice	91	.8
Thick, round	1.3-oz. slice	118	1.1
Thin, round	.5-oz. slice	45	.4
Ring, Wisconsin-made:			
Coarse ground	1-oz. serving	81	.4
Fine ground	1-oz. serving	87	.7
(Oscherwitz):			
Chub	1-oz. serving	90	1.0
Sliced	1-oz. serving	68	1.0

(USDA): United States Department of Agriculture
(HEW/FAO): Health, Education and Welfare/Food and Agriculture Organization
* Prepared as Package Directs

Food and Description	Measure or Quantity	Calories	Carbo-hydrates (grams)
(Swift)	1-oz. slice	95	1.5
(Vienna) beef	1-oz. serving	84	.7
BOLOGNA & CHEESE, packaged (Oscar Mayer)	.8-oz. slice	73	.6
BONITO:			
Raw (USDA):			
Whole	1 lb. (weighed whole)	442	0.
Meat only	4 oz.	191	0.
Canned (Star-Kist) in oil:			
Chunk	6½-oz. can	604	0.
Solid	7-oz. can	650	0.
BOO*BERRY, cereal (General Mills)	1 cup (1 oz.)	110	24.0
BORDEAUX WINE (See also individual regional, vineyard, or brand names or **CLARET WINE**) Rouge (Cruse) 10½% alcohol	3 fl. oz.	63	DNA
BORSCHT, canned:			
Regular pack:			
(Gold's)	8-oz. serving	72	17.5
(Mother's) old fashioned	8-oz. serving	90	21.3
Dietetic or low calorie:			
(Gold's)	8-oz. serving	24	17.5
(Mother's):			
Artificially sweetened	8-oz. serving	29	6.1
Unsalted	8-oz. serving	107	25.1
(Rokeach)	8-oz. serving	27	6.7
BOURBON WHISKEY, unflavored (See **DISTILLED LIQUOR**)			
BOYSENBERRY:			
Fresh (See **BLACKBERRY**)			
Frozen (USDA) sweetened	10-oz. pkg.	273	69.3

Food and Description	Measure or Quantity	Calories	Carbo-hydrates (grams)
BOYSENBERRY JELLY, sweetened (Smucker's)	1 T.	53	13.5
BOYSENBERRY PRESERVE or JAM:			
Sweetened (Smucker's)	1 T. (.7 oz.)	53	13.5
Dietetic or low calorie:			
(Slenderella)	1 T. (.6 oz.)	24	6.0
(S&W) *Nutradiet*	1 T.	12	3.0
BOYSENBERRY SPREAD, low sugar (Smucker's)	1 T.	24	6.0
BRAINS, all animals, raw (USDA)	1 oz.	60	17.5
BRAN:			
Crude (USDA)	1 oz.	60	17.5
Miller's (Elam's)	1 oz.	87	13.7
BRAN BREAKFAST CEREAL:			
(Kellogg's)			
All-Bran	⅓ cup (1 oz.)	70	21.0
Bran-Buds	⅓ cup (1 oz.)	70	22.0
Cracklin' Bran	½ cup (1 oz.)	110	20.0
40% bran flakes	¾ cup (1 oz.)	90	23.0
Raisin Bran	¾ cup (1.3 oz.)	110	28.0
(Nabisco) 100% bran	½ cup (1 oz.)	70	21.0
(Post):			
40% bran flakes	⅔ cup (1 oz.)	107	22.6
With raisins	½ cup (1 oz.)	102	21.4
(Quaker) *Corn Bran*	⅔ cup (1 oz.)	109	23.3
(Ralston Purina):			
Bran Chex	⅔ cup (1 oz.)	110	20.0
40% bran flakes	¾ cup (1 oz.)	100	23.0
Honey bran	⅞ cup (1 oz.)	100	24.0
Shoprite:			
40% bran flakes	⅝ cup	104	21.9

(USDA): United States Department of Agriculture
(HEW/FAO): Health, Education and Welfare/Food and Agriculture Organization
* Prepared as Package Directs

Food and Description	Measure or Quantity	Calories	Carbo-hydrates (grams)
Raisin	⅝ cup	101	22.0
(Van Brode):			
40% bran flakes	⅝ cup	104	21.9
Raisin	⅝ cup	101	22.0
BRANDY, unflavored (See **DISTILLED LIQUOR**)			
BRANDY, FLAVORED			
(Mr. Boston):			
Apricot	1 fl. oz.	94	8.9
Blackberry	1 fl. oz.	92	8.6
Cherry	1 fl. oz.	87	8.4
Coffee	1 fl. oz.	100	10.6
Ginger	1 fl. oz.	72	3.5
Peach	1 fl. oz.	94	8.9
BRAUNSCHWEIGER:			
(Oscar Mayer):			
Chub	1-oz. serving	98	1.0
Tube, German brand	1-oz. serving	95	.6
(Swift) 8-oz. chub	1-oz. serving	109	1.4
BRAZIL NUT:			
Whole, in shell (USDA)	1 cup (4.3 oz.)	383	6.4
Shelled (USDA)	½ cup (2½ oz.)	458	7.6
Shelled (USDA)	4 nuts (.6 oz.)	114	1.9
Roasted (Fisher) salted	¼ cup (1 oz.)	193	3.1
BREAD (listed by type or brand name):			
American Granary (Arnold)	.9-oz. slice	70	12.5
Boston Brown (USDA)	1.7-oz. slice (3″ × ¾″)	101	21.9
Bran'nola (Arnold)	1.2-oz. slice	90	15.5
Cracked-wheat:			
(USDA) 20 slices to 1 lb.	.8-oz. slice	60	12.0
(Pepperidge Farm)	1 slice	70	13.0
(Wonder)	1-oz. slice	75	13.6
Crisp Bread, *Wasa:*			
Mora	3¼-oz. slice	333	70.5
Rye:			
Golden	.4-oz. slice	37	7.8

Food and Description	Measure or Quantity	Calories	Carbo-hydrates (grams)
Lite	.3-oz. slice	30	6.2
Sesame	.5-oz. slice	50	10.6
Sport	.4-oz. slice	42	9.1
Date nut roll (Dromedary)	½″ slice	80	13.0
Flatbread, *Ideal*:			
Bran	.2-oz. slice	19	4.1
Extra thin	.1-oz. slice	12	2.5
Whole grain	.2-oz. slice	19	4.0
French:			
(USDA) 20 slices to 1 lb.	.8-oz. slice	67	12.7
(Arnold):			
Francisco	⅟₁₆ of loaf (1 oz.)	80	14.5
Francisco, Vienna	.8-oz. slice	80	14.5
(Pepperidge Farm)	2-oz. slice	150	27.0
(Wonder)	1-oz. slice	75	13.6
Hillbilly (Wonder)	1-oz. slice	70	12.5
Hollywood (Wonder):			
Dark	1-oz. slice	73	12.5
Light	1-oz. slice	75	13.5
Honey bran (Pepperidge Farm)	1 slice	90	13.0
Honey Wheatberry (Arnold)	1.2-oz. slice	90	16.0
Italian:			
(USDA) 20 slices to 1 lb.	.8-oz. slice	63	13.0
(Pepperidge Farm)	2-oz. serving	150	28.0
Low sodium (Wonder)	1-oz. slice	73	13.6
Naturel (Arnold)	.9-oz. slice	65	12.0
Oatmeal (Pepperidge Farm)	1 slice	70	12.5
Profile:			
Dark	1-oz. slice	75	12.5
Light	1-oz. slice	73	13.1
Protogen protein (Thomas')	1 slice	45	8.5
Pumpernickel:			
(Arnold)	1.1-oz. slice	75	14.0
(Levy's)	1-oz. slice	70	14.0
(Pepperidge Farm):			
Regular	1 slice	80	15.0
Party	1 slice	15	3.0

(USDA): United States Department of Agriculture
(HEW/FAO): Health, Education and Welfare/Food and Agriculture
               Organization
* Prepared as Package Directs

Food and Description	Measure or Quantity	Calories	Carbo- hydrates (grams)
Raisin:			
(Arnold) tea	.9-oz. slice	70	13.0
(Pepperidge Farm) cinnamon	1 slice	75	13.5
(Thomas') cinnamon	.8-oz. slice	60	11.7
(Sun-Maid)	1-oz. slice	80	14.5
Roman Meal	1-oz. slice	77	13.6
Rye:			
(Arnold):			
Jewish, with or without caraway seeds	1.1-oz. slice	75	14.0
Melba thin	.7-oz. slice	50	9.5
(Levy's) real, with or without caraway seeds	1-oz. slice	70	13.0
(Pepperidge Farm):			
Regular	1 slice	85	15.5
Party	1 slice	15	3.0
(Wonder)	1-oz. slice	71	13.4
Sahara (Thomas'):			
Wheat	1-oz. piece	70	14.0
White	1-oz. piece	80	16.0
Salt rising (USDA)	.9-oz. slice	67	13.0
Sourdough, *DiCarlo*	1-oz. slice	70	13.6
Toaster cake (See **TOASTER CAKE** or **PASTRY**)			
Wheat (See also Cracked-wheat, *Honey Wheatberry* and Whole Wheat):			
Fresh Horizons	1-oz. slice	54	9.6
Fresh & Natural	1-oz. slice	77	13.6
Home Pride, butter top	1-oz. slice	75	13.1
(Pepperidge Farm)	1-oz. slice	95	17.5
(Wonder)	1-oz. slice	75	15.6
Wheatberry, *Home Pride*	1-oz. slice	70	12.5
Wheat germ (Pepperidge Farm)	1 slice	65	12.0
White:			
(USDA):			
Prepared with 1-4% non- fat dry milk	.8-oz. slice	62	11.6
Prepared with 5-6% non-fat dry milk	.8-oz. slice	63	11.5
(Arnold):			
Brick Oven	.8-oz. slice	65	11.0
Brick Oven	1.1-oz. slice	85	14.5

Food and Description	Measure or Quantity	Calories	Carbo-hydrates (grams)
Country	1.2-oz. slice	95	17.0
Hearthstone, 2-lb. loaf	1.1-oz. slice	85	15.0
Melba thin	.5-oz. slice	40	7.0
Fresh Horizons	1-oz. slice	54	10.0
Home Pride, butter top	1-oz. slice	75	13.1
(Levy's) no salt added	.9-oz. slice	80	14.0
(Pepperidge Farm):			
Large loaf	1 slice	75	13.0
Sandwich	1 slice	65	11.5
Sliced	.8-oz. slice	55	10.5
Sliced	.9-oz. slice	75	12.5
Toasting	1 slice	85	15.5
Very thin slice	1 slice	40	7.5
(Wonder) regular and with buttermilk	1-oz. slice	75	13.6
Whole wheat:			
(USDA):			
Prepared with 2% non-fat dry milk	.8-oz. slice	56	11.0
Prepared with 2% non-fat dry milk	.9-oz. slice	61	11.9
Prepared with water	.9-oz. slice	60	12.3
(Arnold):			
Brick Oven	.8-oz. slice	60	9.5
Brick Oven	1.1-oz. slice	80	13.0
Melba thin	.5-oz. slice	40	6.5
Stone ground, 100%	.8-oz. slice	55	9.5
(Pepperidge Farm):			
Thin sliced	1 slice	70	12.0
Very thin sliced	1 slice	45	7.5‡
(Thomas')	.8-oz. slice	56	10.1
(Wonder) 100%	1-oz. slice	70	11.9
BREAD, CANNED (B&M)			
brown, plain or with raisins	½" slice (1.6 oz.)	80	11.4
BREAD CRUMBS:			
(Contadina) seasoned	½ cup (2.1 oz.)	228	44.3

(USDA): United States Department of Agriculture
(HEW/FAO): Health, Education and Welfare/Food and Agriculture Organization
* Prepared as Package Directs

Food and Description	Measure or Quantity	Calories	Carbo-hydrates (grams)
(4C):			
Plain	2-oz. serving	203	42.6
Seasoned	2-oz. serving	192	38.6
*BREAD DOUGH, frozen (Rich's):			
French	½₀ of loaf	59	11.0
Italian	½₀ of loaf	60	11.0
Raisin	½₀ of loaf	66	12.3
Wheat	.5-oz. slice	60	10.5
White	.8-oz. slice	56	9.4
*BREAD MIX (Pillsbury):			
Applesauce spice	1/12 of loaf	150	28.0
Apricot nut	1/12 of loaf	160	27.0
Banana	1/12 of loaf	150	27.0
Blueberry nut	1/12 of loaf	150	26.0
Cherry nut	1/12 of loaf	170	30.0
Cranberry	1/12 of loaf	160	28.0
Date	1/12 of loaf	160	32.0
Nut	1/12 of loaf	170	28.0
BREAD PUDDING, with raisins, home recipe (USDA)	1 cup (9.3 oz.)	496	75.3
BREADFRUIT, fresh (USDA):			
Whole	1 lb. (weighed untrimmed)	360	91.5
Peeled & trimmed	4 oz.	117	29.7
BREAKFAST BAR (Carnation):			
Almond crunch	1 piece	210	20.0
Chocolate chip	1 piece	200	20.0
Chocolate crunch	1 piece	200	22.0
Peanut butter crunch	1 piece	200	22.0
BREAKFAST DRINK, instant (Pillsbury):			
Chocolate or chocolate malt	1 pouch	130	26.0
Strawberry or vanilla	1 pouch	130	27.0
BREAKFAST SQUARES (General Mills) all flavors	1 bar (1.5 oz.)	190	22.5

Food and Description	Measure or Quantity	Calories	Carbo-hydrates (grams)
BRIGHT & EARLY	6 fl. oz. (6.6 oz.)	90	21.6
BROCCOLI:	—		
Raw (USDA):			
Whole	1 lb. (weighed untrimmed)	89	16.3
Large leaves removed	1 lb. (weighed partially trimmed)	113	20.9
Boiled (USDA):			
½" pieces, drained	½ cup (2.8 oz.)	20	3.5
Whole, drained	1 med. stalk (6.3 oz.)	47	8.1
Frozen:			
(Birds Eye):			
In cheese sauce	⅓ of 10-oz. pkg.	110	8.0
Chopped, spears or baby deluxe spears	⅓ of 10-oz. pkg.	25	4.0
In Hollandaise sauce	⅓ of 10-oz. pkg.	100	2.9
(Green Giant):			
Cuts in cheese sauce, Bake 'N Serve	⅓ of 10-oz. pkg.	91	5.6
Spears in butter sauce	⅓ of 10-oz. pkg.	43	3.7
(Kounty Kist) cut	¼ of 18-oz. pkg.	34	3.8
(Mrs. Paul's) & cheese, batter fried	⅓ of 7¾-oz. pkg.	162	18.6
(McKenzie or Seabrook Farms):			
Chopped	⅓ of 10-oz. pkg.	30	4.1
Spears	⅓ of 10-oz. pkg.	31	4.5
(Stouffer's) au gratin	⅓ of 10-oz. pkg.	113	4.6
BROWNIE (See **COOKIE**)			
BRUSSELS SPROUTS:			
Raw (USDA)	1 lb.	188	34.6
Boiled (USDA) drained, 1¼"-1½" dia.	1 cup (7-8 sprouts, 5.5 oz.)	56	9.9

(USDA): United States Department of Agriculture
(HEW/FAO): Health, Education and Welfare/Food and Agriculture Organization
* Prepared as Package Directs

Food and Description	Measure or Quantity	Calories	Carbohydrates (grams)
Frozen:			
(Birds Eye):			
Regular	⅓ of 10-oz. pkg.	30	5.0
Baby sprouts, deluxe	⅓ of 10-oz. pkg.	42	5.8
(Green Giant):			
Regular	¼ of 16-oz. pkg.	47	7.3
In butter sauce	⅓ of 10-oz. pkg.	53	5.0
Halves in cheese sauce	⅓ of 10-oz. pkg.	61	6.6
(Kounty Kist)	⅕ of 20-oz. pkg.	47	7.3
(Stouffer's) au gratin	⅓ of 10⅞-oz. pkg.	124	10.6
BUCKWHEAT:			
Flour (See **FLOUR**)			
Groats (Pocono):			
Brown, whole	1 oz.	104	19.4
White, whole	1 oz.	102	20.1
BUC*WHEATS, cereal			
(General Mills)	¾ cup (1 oz.)	110	23.0
BULGAR (from hard red winter wheat) (USDA):			
Dry	1 lb.	1605	343.4
Canned:			
Unseasoned	4-oz. serving	191	39.7
Seasoned	4-oz. serving	206	37.2
BULLOCK'S HEART (See **CUSTARD APPLE**)			
BUN (See **ROLL or BUN**)			
BURGER KING:			
Apple pie	3-oz. pie	240	32.0
Cheeseburger	1 burger	350	30.0
Cheeseburger, double meat	1 burger	530	32.0
French fries	1 regular order	210	25.0
Hamburger	1 burger	290	29.0
Onion rings	1 regular order	270	29.0
Shake:			
Chocolate	1 shake	340	57.0
Vanilla	1 shake	340	52.0

Food and Description	Measure or Quantity	Calories	Carbo-hydrates (grams)
Whopper:			
Regular	1 burger	630	50.0
With cheese	1 burger	740	52.0
Double meat	1 burger	850	52.0
Double meat with cheese	1 burger	950	54.0
Junior	1 burger	370	31.0
Junior with cheese	1 burger	420	22.0
BURGUNDY WINE:			
(Great Western) 12% alcohol	3 fl. oz.	70	2.3
(Italian Swiss Colony) 13% alcohol	3 fl. oz.	61	.9
(Louis M. Martini) 12% alcohol	3 fl. oz.	90	.2
(Paul Masson) 12% alcohol	3 fl. oz.	70	2.2
(Taylor) 12½% alcohol	3 fl. oz.	75	3.3
BURGUNDY WINE, SPARKLING:			
(Great Western) 12% alcohol	3 fl. oz.	82	5.1
(Taylor) 12½% alcohol	3 fl. oz.	78	4.2
BURRITO:			
*Canned (Del Monte)	1 burrito	310	39.0
Frozen:			
(Hormel):			
Beef	1 burrito	220	28.4
Cheese	1 burrito	250	32.7
Chicken & rice	1 burrito	199	29.4
Hot chili	1 burrito	210	32.0
(Van de Kamp's) crispy fried with guacamole sauce	6-oz. serving	354	40.0
***BURRITO FILLING MIX,** canned (Del Monte)	1 cup (8.5 oz.)	220	39.0
BUTTER, salted or unsalted:			
(USDA)	¼ lb. (1 stick, ½ cup)	812	.5

(USDA): United States Department of Agriculture
(HEW/FAO): Health, Education and Welfare/Food and Agriculture Organization
* Prepared as Package Directs

Food and Description	Measure or Quantity	Calories	Carbohydrates (grams)
(USDA)	1 T. (⅛ stock, .5 oz.)	100	.1
(Breakstone):			
Regular	1 T. (.5 oz.)	100	<.1
Whipped	1 T. (9 grams)	67	.1
(Meadow Gold)	1 tsp.	35	0.
BUTTER BEAN (See **BEAN, LIMA**)			
BUTTER BRICKLE ICE CREAM BAR (Heath) chocolate covered	2½-fl.-oz. bar	154	18.0
BUTTERFISH, raw (USDA):			
Gulf:			
Whole	1 lb. (weighed whole)	220	0.
Meat only	4 oz.	108	0.
Northern:			
Whole	1 lb. (weighed whole)	391	0.
Meat only	4 oz.	192	0.
BUTTER FLAVORING (Durkee) imitation	1 tsp.	3	
BUTTERMILK (See **MILK**)			
BUTTERNUT (USDA):			
Whole	1 lb. (weighed in shell)	399	5.3
Shelled	4 oz.	713	9.5
BUTTER PECAN ICE CREAM:			
(Breyer's)	¼ pt.	180	15.0
(Good Humor)	4-fl. oz.	150	14.0
BUTTERSCOTCH MORSELS (Nestlé)	1 oz.	150	19.0

Food and Description	Measure or Quantity	Calories	Carbohydrates (grams)

C

CABBAGE:
White (USDA):
  Raw:

Food and Description	Measure or Quantity	Calories	Carbohydrates (grams)
Whole	1 lb. (weighed untrimmed)	86	19.3
Finely shredded or chopped	1 cup (3.2 oz.)	22	4.9
Coarsely shredded or sliced	1 cup (2.5 oz.)	17	3.8
Wedge	3½″ × 4½″	24	5.4
Boiled:			
Shredded, in small amount of water, short time, drained	½ cup (2.6 oz.)	15	3.1
Wedges, in large amount of water, long time, drained	½ cup (3.2 oz.)	17	3.7
Dehydrated	1 oz.	87	20.9
Red:			
Raw (USDA) whole	1 lb. (weighed untrimmed)	111	24.7
Canned, solids & liq.:			
(Comstock) sweet & sour	½ cup	60	13.0
(Greenwood)	½ cup	60	13.0
Savory (USDA) raw, whole	1 lb. (weighed untrimmed)	86	16.5
CABBAGE, CHINESE or CELERY, raw (USDA):			
Whole	1 lb. (weighed untrimmed)	62	13.2
1″ pieces, leaves with stalk	½ cup (1.3 oz.)	5	1.1
CABBAGE, STUFFED, frozen (Green Giant) with beef in tomato sauce	½ of 14-oz. pkg.	209	16.5

(USDA): United States Department of Agriculture
(HEW/FAO): Health, Education and Welfare/Food and Agriculture Organization
* Prepared as Package Directs

Food and Description	Measure or Quantity	Calories	Carbo-hydrates (grams)
CABERNET SAUVIGNON WINE:			
(Louis M. Martini) 12½% alcohol	3 fl. oz.	90	.2
(Paul Masson) 11.9% alcohol	3 fl. oz.	70	.2
CAFE COMFORT, 55 proof	1 fl. oz.	79	8.8
CAKE:			
Not frozen:			
Plain:			
Home recipe, with butter & boiled white icing	⅑ of 9″ square	401	70.5
Home recipe, with butter & chocolate icing	⅑ of 9″ square	453	73.1
Angel food, home recipe	1/12 of 8″ cake	108	24.1
Caramel, home recipe:			
Without icing	⅑ of 9″ square	331	46.2
With caramel icing	⅑ of 9″ square	322	50.2
Chocolate, home recipe, with chocolate icing, 2-layer	1/12 of 9″ cake	365	55.2
Coffee (Tastykake) *Koffee Kakes*, creme filled	1-oz. cake	124	DNA
Crumb (See also **ROLL or BUN**) (Hostess)	1¼-oz. piece	131	21.7
Devil's food, home recipe:			
Without icing	3″ × 2″ × 1½″ piece	201	28.6
Without chocolate icing, 2-layer	1/16 of 9″ cake	277	41.8
Fruit, home recipe:			
Dark	1/30 of 8″ loaf	57	9.0
Light, made with butter	1/30 of 8″ loaf	58	8.6
Honey (Holland Honey Cake) low sodium:			
Fruit and raisin	½″ slice (.9 oz.)	80	19.0
Orange and premium unsalted	½″ slice (.9 oz.)	70	17.0
Pound, home recipe:			
Equal weights flour, sugar, butter and eggs	3½″ × 3½″ slice (1.1 oz.)	142	14.1
Traditional, made with butter	3½″ × 3½″ slice (1.1 oz.)	123	16.4

Food and Description	Measure or Quantity	Calories	Carbohydrates (grams)
Sponge, home recipe	1/12 of 10″ cake	196	35.7
White, home recipe:			
Made with butter, without icing, 2-layer	1/9 of 9″ wide, 3″ high cake	353	50.8
Made with butter, with coconut icing, 2-layer	1/12 of 9″ wide, 3″ high cake	386	63.1
Yellow, home recipe, made with butter, without icing, 2-layer	1/9 of cake	351	56.3
Frozen:			
Apple walnut (Sara Lee)	1/8 of 12.8-oz. cake	165	21.6
Banana (Sara Lee)	1/8 of 13¾-oz. cake	175	26.9
Banana nut layer (Sara Lee)	1/8 of 20-oz. cake	232	26.5
Black forest (Sara Lee)	1/8 of 21-oz. cake	203	27.9
Carrot (Sara Lee)	1/8 of 12¼-oz. cake	152	18.9
Cheesecake:			
(Morton) *Great Little Desserts*:			
Cherry	6½-oz. cake	476	53.6
Cream cheese	6½-oz. cake	489	46.2
Pineapple	6½-oz. cake	484	55.4
Strawberry	6½-oz. cake	491	57.2
(Rich's) Viennese	1/16 of 42-oz. cake	230	24.5
(Sara Lee):			
Blueberry, cream cheese:			
Regular	1/6 of 19-oz. cake	233	35.3
For 2	½ of 11.3-oz. cake	425	66.6
Cherry, cream cheese:			
Regular	1/6 of 19-oz. cake	225	35.2
For 2	½ of 11.3-oz. cake	423	69.3

(USDA): United States Department of Agriculture
(HEW/FAO): Health, Education and Welfare/Food and Agriculture Organization
* Prepared as Package Directs

Food and Description	Measure or Quantity	Calories	Carbo-hydrates (grams)
Cream cheese:			
Large	⅙ of 17-oz. cake	231	25.9
Small	⅓ of 10-oz. cake	281	29.9
French, cream cheese	⅛ of 23½-oz. cake	274	24.9
Strawberry, cream cheese:			
Regular	⅙ of 19-oz. cake	223	33.6
For 2	½ of 11.3-oz. cake	420	67.9
Strawberry, French, cream cheese	⅛ of 26-oz. cake	258	27.5
Chocolate (Sara Lee):			
Regular	⅛ of 13¼-oz. cake	199	28.1
Bavarian	⅛ of 22½-oz. cake	285	22.6
German	⅛ of 12¼-oz. cake	173	19.3
Layer, 'n cream	⅛ of 18-oz. cake	215	23.8
Layer, 'n Cream	⅛ of 18-oz. cake	215	23.8
Coffee (Sara Lee):			
Almond	⅛ of 11¾-oz. cake	165	20.2
Almond ring			
Apple:			
Regular	⅛ of 15-oz. cake	175	24.1
For 2	½ of 9-oz. cake	419	58.1
Blueberry ring	⅛ of 9¾-oz. cake	134	17.6
Butter, For 2	½ of 6½-oz. cake	356	41.9
Danish, cinnamon raisin	1.3-oz. cake	146	17.4
Maple crunch ring	⅛ of 9¾-oz. cake	138	17.3
Pecan:			
Large	⅛ of 11¼-oz. cake	163	19.1
Small	¼ of 6½-oz. cake	188	22.1
Raspberry ring	⅛ of 9¾-oz. cake	133	18.5
Streusel:			
Butter	⅛ of 11½-oz. cake	164	20.3
Cinnamon	⅛ of 10.9-oz. cake	154	19.0

Food and Description	Measure or Quantity	Calories	Carbohydrates (grams)
Orange (Sara Lee)	⅛ of 13¾-oz. cake	179	25.3
Pound (Sara Lee):			
Regular	⅒ of 10¾-oz. cake	125	14.2
Banana nut	⅒ of 11-oz. cake	117	15.1
Chocolate	⅒ of 10¾-oz. cake	122	14.4
Chocolate swirl	⅒ of 11.8-oz. cake	116	16.0
Family size	⅟15 of 16½-oz. cake	127	14.8
Home style	⅒ of 9½-oz. cake	114	13.1
Raisin	⅒ of 12.9-oz. cake	126	19.6
Strawberry 'n cream (Sara Lee) layer	⅛ of 20½-oz. cake	218	29.4
Strawberry shortcake (Sara Lee)	⅛ of 21-oz. cake	193	25.9
Torte (Sara Lee):			
Apple 'n cream	⅛ of 21-oz. cake	203	26.2
Fudge & nut	⅛ of 15¾-oz. cake	200	21.0
Walnut (Sara Lee) layer	⅛ of 18-oz. cake	210	22.8

CAKE ICING:

Butter pecan (Betty Crocker) *Creamy Deluxe*	⅟12 of can	170	27.0
Caramel, home recipe (USDA)	4-oz. serving	408	86.8
Cherry (Betty Crocker) *Creamy Deluxe*	⅟12 of can	170	28.0
Chocolate:			
Home recipe (USDA)	4-oz. serving	426	76.4

(USDA): United States Department of Agriculture
(HEW/FAO): Health, Education and Welfare/Food and Agriculture Organization
* Prepared as Package Directs

Food and Description	Measure or Quantity	Calories	Carbo-hydrates (grams)
(Betty Crocker) *Creamy Deluxe*:			
Regular	1/12 of can	170	25.0
Fudge, dark dutch	1/12 of can	160	24.0
Milk	1/12 of can	170	26.0
Nut	1/12 of can	170	24.0
Sour cream	1/12 of can	170	25.0
(Pillsbury) *Frosting Supreme*:			
Fudge	1/12 of can	160	24.0
Milk	1/12 of can	160	25.0
Sour cream	1/12 of can	160	25.0
Coconut, home recipe (USDA)	4-oz. serving	413	84.9
Cream cheese:			
(Betty Crocker) *Creamy Deluxe*	1/12 of can	160	27.0
(Pillsbury) *Frosting Supreme*	1/12 of can	160	27.0
Double dutch (Pillsbury) *Frosting Supreme*	1/12 of can	160	24.0
Lemon:			
(Betty Crocker) *Sunkist, Creamy Deluxe*	1/12 of can	170	28.0
(Pillsbury) *Frosting Supreme*	1/12 of can	160	27.0
Orange (Betty Crocker) *Creamy Deluxe*	1/12 of can	170	28.0
Strawberry (Pillsbury) *Frosting Supreme*	1/12 of can	160	27.0
Vanilla:			
(Betty Crocker) *Creamy Deluxe*	1/12 of can	170	28.0
(Pillsbury) *Frosting Supreme*	1/12 of can	160	27.0
White:			
Home recipe (USDA):			
Boiled	4-oz. serving	358	91.1
Uncooked	4-oz. serving	426	92.5
(Betty Crocker) *Creamy Deluxe*	1/12 of can	160	27.0
CAKE ICING MIX:			
Regular:			
Banana (Betty Crocker) *Chiquita*, creamy	1/12 of pkg.	170	30.0
Butter Brickle (Betty Crocker) creamy	1/12 of pkg.	170	30.0

Food and Description	Measure or Quantity	Calories	Carbohydrates (grams)
Butter pecan (Betty Crocker) creamy, deluxe	½12 of pkg.	170	30.0
Caramel (Pillsbury) *Rich'n Easy*	½12 of pkg.	140	24.0
Cherry (Betty Crocker) creamy	½12 of pkg.	170	30.0
Chocolate:			
(Betty Crocker):			
Regular, creamy	½12 of pkg.	170	30.0
Dark, creamy	½12 of pkg.	170	30.0
Milk, creamy	½12 of pkg.	170	30.0
Sour cream	½12 of pkg.	170	30.0
(Pillsbury) *Rich'n Easy*:			
Regular	½12 of pkg.	150	27.0
Milk	½12 of pkg.	150	26.0
Coconut almond (Pillsbury)	½12 of pkg.	170	17.0
Coconut pecan:			
(Betty Crocker) creamy	½12 of pkg.	140	18.0
(Pillsbury)	½12 of pkg.	150	20.0
Cream cheese & nut (Betty Crocker) creamy	½12 of pkg.	150	23.0
Double dutch (Pillsbury) *Rich'n Easy*	½12 of pkg.	150	26.0
Lemon:			
(Betty Crocker) *Sunkist*, creamy	½12 of pkg.	170	30.0
(Pillsbury) *Rich'n Easy*	½12 of pkg.	140	25.0
Strawberry (Pillsbury) *Rich'n Easy*	½12 of pkg.	140	25.0
Vanilla (Pillsbury) *Rich'n Easy*	½12 of pkg.	150	25.0
White:			
(Betty Crocker):			
Fluffy	½12 of pkg.	60	16.0
Sour cream, creamy	½12 of pkg.	180	31.0
(Pillsbury) fluffy	½12 of pkg.	70	17.0

(USDA): United States Department of Agriculture
(HEW/FAO):   Health, Education and Welfare/Food and Agriculture Organization
* Prepared as Package Directs

Food and Description	Measure or Quantity	Calories	Carbo-hydrates (grams)
Dietetic or low calorie (Betty Crocker) *Lite*:			
Chocolate	¹⁄₁₂ of pkg.	100	18.0
Lemon or vanilla	¹⁄₁₂ of pkg.	100	19.0
CAKE MIX:			
Regular:			
Angel food:			
(*USDA)	¹⁄₁₂ of 10″ cake	137	31.5
(Betty Crocker):			
Chocolate	¹⁄₁₂ of pkg.	140	32.0
Confetti	¹⁄₁₂ of pkg.	150	34.0
Lemon custard	¹⁄₁₂ of pkg.	140	32.0
One-step	¹⁄₁₂ of pkg.	140	32.0
Strawberry	¹⁄₁₂ of pkg.	150	34.0
Traditional	¹⁄₁₂ of pkg.	130	30.0
(Duncan Hines)	¹⁄₁₂ of pkg.	124	28.9
*(Pillsbury) raspberry or white	¹⁄₁₂ of cake	140	33.0
Applesauce raisin (Betty Crocker) *Snackin' Cake*	¹⁄₉ of pkg.	180	33.0
*Applesauce spice, *Pillsbury Plus*	¹⁄₁₂ of cake	250	34.0
*Banana:			
(Betty Crocker) *Supermoist*	¹⁄₁₂ of cake	260	36.0
(Pillsbury):			
Pillsbury Plus	¹⁄₁₂ of cake	260	36.0
Streusel Swirl	¹⁄₁₆ of cake	260	38.0
Banana walnut (Betty Crocker) *Snackin' Cake*	¹⁄₉ of pkg.	190	31.0
*Butter (Pillsbury):			
Pillsbury Plus	¹⁄₁₂ of cake	240	35.0
Streusel Swirl	¹⁄₁₆ of cake	260	38.0
*Butter pecan (Betty Crocker) layer, *Supermoist*	¹⁄₁₂ of cake	250	35.0
*Butter yellow (Betty Crocker) *Supermoist*	¹⁄₁₂ of cake	230	36.0
*Carrot (Betty Crocker) *Supermoist*	¹⁄₁₂ of cake	260	34.0
*Carrot'n spice, *Pillsbury Plus*	¹⁄₁₂ of cake	260	35.0

Food and Description	Measure or Quantity	Calories	Carbo- hydrates (grams)
Cheesecake:			
*(Jell-O)	⅛ of 8" cake	250	33.0
*(Royal)	⅛ of cake	230	31.0
*Cherry chip (Betty Crocker) layer, *Supermoist*	¹⁄₁₂ of cake	180	36.0
Chocolate:			
(Betty Crocker):			
Almond, *Snackin' Cake*	⅑ of pkg.	190	31.0
With chocolate frosting, *Stir 'N Frost*	⅙ of pkg.	210	38.0
Fudge, *Stir 'N Frost*, with vanilla frosting	⅙ of pkg.	210	40.0
*Fudge, *Supermoist*	¹⁄₁₂ of cake	250	35.0
Fudge chip, *Snackin' Cake*	⅑ of pkg.	190	31.0
*German chocolate, layer, *Supermoist*	¹⁄₁₂ of cake	260	36.0
*Milk, layer, *Supermoist*	¹⁄₁₂ of cake	250	35.0
*Pudding recipe	⅙ of cake	230	45.0
*Sour cream, *Supermoist*	¹⁄₁₂ of cake	260	36.0
*(Pillsbury):			
Fudge, dark, *Pillsbury Plus*	¹⁄₁₂ of cake	260	35.0
Fudge marble, *Pillsbury Plus*	¹⁄₁₂ of cake	270	36.0
Fudge nut crown, *Bundt*	¹⁄₁₆ of cake	220	31.0
Fudge, triple, *Bundt*	¹⁄₁₆ of cake	210	30.0
Fudge, tunnel of, *Bundt*	¹⁄₁₆ of cake	270	37.0
German chocolate, *Pillsbury Plus*	¹⁄₁₂ of cake	250	36.0
German chocolate, *Streusel Swirl*	¹⁄₁₂ of cake	260	36.0
Macaroon, *Bundt*	¹⁄₁₆ of cake	250	35.0
Mint, *Pillsbury Plus*	¹⁄₁₂ of cake	200	33.0
*Cinnamon (Pillsbury) *Streusel Swirl*	¹⁄₁₂ of cake	260	38.0

(USDA): United States Department of Agriculture
(HEW/FAO): Health, Education and Welfare/Food and Agriculture Organization
* Prepared as Package Directs

Food and Description	Measure or Quantity	Calories	Carbo-hydrates (grams)
Coconut pecan (Betty Crocker) Snackin' Cake	⅑ of pkg.	190	30.0
Coffee cake:			
*(Aunt Jemima)	⅛ of cake	170	29.0
*(Pillsbury):			
Apple cinnamon	⅛ of cake	240	40.0
Butter pecan	⅛ of cake	310	39.0
Cinnamon streusel	⅛ of cake	250	41.0
Sour cream	⅛ of cake	270	35.0
Devil's food:			
*(Betty Crocker) layer, Supermoist	¹⁄₁₂ of cake	250	35.0
(Duncan Hines):			
Regular	¹⁄₁₂ of pkg.	190	33.0
Pudding recipe	¹⁄₁₂ of pkg.	190	33.0
*(Pillsbury):			
Pillsbury Plus	¹⁄₁₂ of cake	250	35.0
Streusel Swirl	¹⁄₁₂ of cake	260	36.0
Golden chocolate chip (Betty Crocker) Snackin' Cake	⅑ of pkg.	190	34.0
Lemon:			
*(Betty Crocker):			
Chiffon, Sunkist	¹⁄₁₂ of cake	190	35.0
Layer, Supermoist	¹⁄₁₂ of cake	260	36.0
& lemon frosting, Stir N' Frost	⅙ of cake	220	41.0
Pudding recipe	⅙ of cake	230	45.0
(Duncan Hines) pudding recipe	¹⁄₁₂ of pkg.	183	36.1
*(Pillsbury):			
Bundt, tunnel of	¹⁄₁₆ of cake	270	43.0
Pillsbury Plus	¹⁄₁₂ of cake	260	36.0
Streusel Swirl	¹⁄₁₆ of cake	260	39.0
*Lemon blueberry (Pillsbury) Bundt	¹⁄₁₆ of cake	200	28.0
Marble:			
*(Betty Crocker) layer, Supermoist	¹⁄₁₂ of cake	270	40.0
*(Pillsbury):			
Bundt, supreme	¹⁄₁₆ of cake	250	38.0
Streusel Swirl, fudge	¹⁄₁₆ of cake	260	38.0
*Orange (Betty Crocker) layer, Supermoist	¹⁄₁₂ of cake	260	36.0

Food and Description	Measure or Quantity	Calories	Carbo-hydrates (grams)
*Pound:			
(Betty Crocker) golden	1/12 of cake	200	27.0
(Dromedary)	3/4" slice (1/12 of cake)	210	29.0
(Pillsbury) *Bundt*	1/16 of cake	230	33.0
Spice (Betty Crocker):			
*Layer, *Supermoist*	1/12 of cake	260	36.0
Raisin, *Snackin' Cake*	1/9 of pkg.	180	22.0
*With vanilla frosting, *Stir N' Frost*	1/6 of cake	210	40.0
*Strawberry:			
(Betty Crocker) layer, *Supermoist*	1/12 of cake	260	36.0
Pillsbury Plus	1/12 of cake	260	37.0
*Upside down (Betty Crocker) pineapple	1/9 of cake	270	43.0
White:			
*(Betty Crocker):			
With chocolate frosting, *Stir N' Frost*	1/6 of cake	210	40.0
Layer, *Supermoist*	1/12 of cake	180	36.0
Sour cream, *Supermoist*	1/12 of cake	180	36.0
(Duncan Hines):			
Regular	1/12 of pkg.	185	34.8
Pudding recipe	1/12 of pkg.	183	36.5
Pillsbury Plus	1/12 of cake	240	35.0
Yellow:			
*(Betty Crocker):			
With chocolate frosting, *Stir N' Frost*	1/6 of cake	220	39.0
Layer, *Supermoist*	1/12 of cake	250	37.0
(Duncan Hines):			
Regular	1/12 of pkg.	186	35.6
Pudding recipe	1/12 of pkg.	183	37.0
Pillsbury Plus	1/12 of cake	260	36.0
*Dietetic or low calorie:			
Chocolate:			
(Betty Crocker) *Light Style*	1/12 of cake	150	30.0

(USDA): United States Department of Agriculture
(HEW/FAO): Health, Education and Welfare/Food and Agriculture Organization
* Prepared as Package Directs

Food and Description	Measure or Quantity	Calories	Carbo-hydrates (grams)
(Estee)	1/10 of cake	100	20.7
Devil's food (Betty Crocker)			
Light Style	1/12 of cake	160	29.0
Lemon:			
(Betty Crocker) Light			
Style	1/12 of cake	160	29.0
(Estee)	1/10 of cake	91	19.1
Yellow (Betty Crocker)			
Light Style	1/12 of cake	160	29.0
White (Estee)	1/10 of cake	85	17.9
CAMPARI, 45 proof	1 fl. oz. (1.1 oz.)	66	7.1
CANADIAN WHISKEY (See **DISTILLED LIQUOR**)			
CANDIED FRUIT (See individual kinds)			
CANDY. The following values of candies from the U.S. Department of Agriculture are representative of the types sold commercially. These values may be useful when individual brands or sizes are not known:			
Almond:			
Chocolate-coated	1 cup (6.3 oz.)	1024	71.3
Chocolate-coated	1 oz.	161	11.2
Sugar-coated or Jordan	1 oz.	129	19.9
Butterscotch	1 oz.	113	26.9
Candy corn	1 oz.	103	25.4
Caramel:			
Plain	1 oz.	113	21.7
Plain with nuts	1 oz.	121	20.0
Chocolate	1 oz.	113	21.7
Chocolate with nuts	1 oz.	121	20.0
Chocolate-flavored roll	1 oz.	112	23.4
Chocolate:			
Bittersweet	1 oz.	135	13.3
Milk:			
Plain	1 oz.	147	16.1

Food and Description	Measure or Quantity	Calories	Carbo-hydrates (grams)
With almonds	1 oz.	151	14.5
With peanuts	1 oz.	154	12.6
Semisweet	1 oz.	144	16.2
Sweet	1 oz.	150	16.4
Chocolate discs, sugar-coated	1 oz.	132	20.6
Coconut center, chocolate-coated	1 oz.	124	20.4
Fondant, plain	1 oz.	103	25.4
Fondant, chocolate-covered	1 oz.	116	23.0
Fudge:			
Chocolate fudge	1 oz.	113	21.3
Chocolate fudge, chocolate-coated	1 oz.	122	20.7
Chocolate fudge with nuts	1 oz.	121	19.6
Chocolate fudge with nuts, chocolate-coated	1 oz.	128	19.1
Vanilla fudge	1 oz.	113	21.2
Vanilla fudge with nuts	1 oz.	120	19.5
With peanuts & caramel, chocolate-coated	1 oz.	130	16.6
Gum drops	1 oz.	98	24.8
Hard	1 oz.	109	27.6
Honeycombed hard candy, with peanut butter, chocolate-covered	1 oz.	131	20.0
Jelly beans	1 oz.	104	26.4
Marshmallows	1 oz.	90	22.8
Mints, uncoated	1 oz.	103	25.4
Nougat & caramel, chocolate-covered	1 oz.	118	20.6
Peanut bar	1 oz.	146	13.4
Peanut brittle	1 oz.	119	23.0
Peanuts, chocolate-covered	1 oz.	159	11.1
Raisins, chocolate-covered	1 oz.	120	20.0
Vanilla creams, chocolate-covered	1 oz.	123	19.9

(USDA): United States Department of Agriculture
(HEW/FAO):   Health, Education and Welfare/Food and Agriculture
                        Organization
* Prepared as Package Directs

Food and Description	Measure or Quantity	Calories	Carbo-hydrates (grams)
CANDY, COMMERCIAL:			
Regular:			
Almond, chocolate covered (Hershey's) *Golden Almond*	1 oz.	163	12.4
Almond cluster (Heath)	1 oz.	142	17.0
Almond, Jordan (Banner)	1¼-oz. box	154	27.9
Apricot Delight (Sahadi)	10 oz.	100	25.0
Baby Ruth (Curtiss)	1.8-oz. bar	260	31.0
Bridge Mix (Nabisco)	1 piece (2 grams)	8	1.4
Butter brickle bar (Heath)	1 oz.	150	17.0
Butterfinger	1.6-oz. bar	220	28.0
Butterscotch Skimmers (Nabisco)	1 piece (6 grams)	25	5.7
Candy corn (Curtiss)	1 piece (2 grams)	4	1.0
Caramel:			
Caramel Flipper (Wayne)	1 oz.	128	19.0
Caramel Nip (Pearson)	1 piece	29	5.6
Pattie (Heath)	1 oz.	113	17.0
Cereal raisin bar (Heath)	2 oz.	296	37.0
Charleston Chew	1½-oz. bar	179	32.6
Cherry, chocolate-covered:			
(Nabisco) dark	1 piece (.6 oz.)	67	13.0
Welch's:			
Dark	1 piece	67	13.0
Milk	1 piece	66	13.1
Chocolate bar:			
Choco-Lite (Nestlé)	.27-oz. miniature	41	4.9
Choco-Lite (Nestlé)	1-oz. serving	150	18.0
Crunch (Nestlé)	1-oz. serving	150	18.0
Crunch (Nestlé)	1¹⁄₁₆-oz. serving	159	19.1
Krunch (Heath)	1½-oz. serving	221	28.0
Milk:			
(Heath):			
Crunch with toffee	2¼-oz. serving	334	42.0
Solids	2¼-oz. serving	339	41.0
(Hershey's)	.35-oz. miniature	55	5.7
(Hershey's)	1.2-oz. bar	187	19.4
(Hershey's)	4-oz. bar	623	64.7
(Nestlé)	.35-oz. miniature	53	6.0
(Nestlé)	1¹⁄₁₆-oz. bar	159	18.1
Special Dark (Hershey's)	1.05-oz. bar	160	18.4

Food and Description	Measure or Quantity	Calories	Carbohydrates (grams)
Special Dark (Hershey's)	4-oz. bar	611	70.2
Chocolate bar with almonds:			
(Heath)	2½-oz. serving	388	39.0
(Hershey's) milk	.35-oz. miniature	55	5.4
(Hershey's) milk	1.15-oz. bar	180	17.6
(Nestlé)	1-oz. serving	150	17.0
Chocolate Parfait (Pearson's)	1 piece	31	5.2
Chuckles	1 oz.	92	23.0
Chunky	1 oz.	131	DNA
Clark Bar	.7-oz. bar	94	14.2
Clark Bar	1.4-oz. bar	188	28.4
Clark Bar	1.65-oz. bar	222	33.4
Cluster (Nabisco):			
Crispy	1 piece (.6 oz.)	65	14.0
Royal Clusters	1 piece (.6 oz.)	78	7.5
Coco-Mello (Nabisco)	1 piece (.7 oz.)	91	13.8
Coconut:			
(Nabisco) square	1 piece (.5 oz.)	65	12.3
Welch's, bar	1 piece (1.1 oz.)	132	21.8
Coffee Nips (Pearson's)	1 piece	29	5.6
Coffioca (Pearson's)	1 piece (6.5 grams)	31	5.2
Crispy Bar (Clark)	1¼-oz. bar	187	24.2
Crispy Bar (Clark)	1.4-oz. bar	209	27.1
Crows (Mason)	1 piece	11	2.7
Dots (Mason)	1 piece	11	2.7
Dutch Treat Bar (Clark)	1¹⁄₁₆-oz. bar	160	20.3
Dutch Treat Bar (Clark)	1.3-oz. bar	196	24.9
Eggs (Nabisco) *Chuckles*	1 piece (2 grams)	10	2.3
Frappe, Welch's	1 piece (1.1 oz.)	132	23.5
Fruit Gems (Sunkist)	1 piece	31	8.2
Fruit roll (Sahadi):			
Apple, cherry or plain	1-oz. piece	90	20.0
Apricot, grape or raspberry	1-oz. piece	90	21.0
Strawberry	1-oz. piece	100	22.0

(USDA): United States Department of Agriculture
(HEW/FAO): Health, Education and Welfare/Food and Agriculture
          Organization
* Prepared as Package Directs

Food and Description	Measure or Quantity	Calories	Carbo-hydrates (grams)
Fudge:			
(Nabisco):			
Bar, *Home Style*	1 bar (.7-oz.)	90	13.9
Nut, bar or square	½-oz. serving	71	10.2
Welch's, bar	1.1-oz. piece	144	20.5
Good & Plenty	1 oz.	100	24.8
Halvah (Sahadi) plain & mashed	1 oz.	150	13.0
Hard candy:			
Cinnamon (Reed's)	1 piece	17	DNA
Cinnamon balls (Curtiss)	1 piece (7 grams)	27	7.0
Lemon drops (Curtiss)	1 piece (4 grams)	15	4.8
Root Beer Barrels	1 piece (6.5 grams)	25	5.0
Jelly (See also individual flavors and brand names in this section):			
Bean (Curtiss)	1 piece (3.5 grams)	12	3.0
Ring (Nabisco) *Chuckles*	1 piece (.4 oz.)	37	9.0
Slice, fruit (Curtiss)	1 piece (.4 oz.)	34	9.0
Jujubes, assorted (Nabisco) *Chuckles*	1 piece	13	3.3
Kisses (Hershey) milk chocolate	1 piece (5 grams)	27	2.8
Kit Kat (Hershey's)	1¼-oz. bar	179	21.0
Krackel Bar (Hershey's)	.35-oz. miniature	52	5.9
Krackel Bar (Hershey's)	1.2-oz bar	178	20.3
Licorice:			
Chuckles	1 piece (.4 oz.)	36	9.0
Licorice Nip (Pearson's)	1 piece (6.5 grams)	29	5.6
(Switzer) bars, bites or stix:			
Black	1-oz. serving	94	22.1
Cherry or strawberry	1-oz. serving	98	23.2
Lollipop (Life Savers)	.9-oz. piece	99	24.0
Mallo Cup (Boyer)	1.2-oz. cup	114	23.9
Malted milk crunch (Nabisco)	1 piece (2 grams)	9	.9
Mars Almond Bar (M&M/Mars)	1½-oz. serving	208	25.6
Marshmallow:			
(Campfire)	1 oz.	111	24.9
Chuckles, egg	1 piece	38	9.3
Mary Jane (Miller)	¼-oz. piece	18	3.2

Food and Description	Measure or Quantity	Calories	Carbohydrates (grams)
Mary Jane (Miller)	1½-oz. bar	108	19.5
Milk Duds (Clark)	¾-oz. box	89	17.8
Milk Duds (Clark)	1¼-oz. box	148	29.6
Milk Duds (Clark)	1.4-oz. box	166	33.2
Milky Way (M&M/Mars)	.8-oz. bar	102	16.3
Milky Way (M&M/Mars)	1.9-oz. bar	242	38.7
Mint or peppermint:			
Jamaica Mint (Nabisco) pattie	1 piece	24	5.8
Junior Mint (Nabisco)	1 piece	24	5.8
Liberty Mint (Nabisco)	1 piece	24	5.8
Meltaway (Heath)	1-oz. serving	156	16.0
Mint Parfait (Pearson's)	1 piece	31	5.2
Peppermint (Nabisco) pattie	1 piece	64	12 .5
Wafer (Nabisco)	1 piece	10	1.0
M&M's (M&M/Mars):			
Peanut	1½-oz. serving	219	25.0
Plain	1½-oz. serving	202	27.7
Mr. Goodbar (Hershey's)	.35-oz. miniature	54	4.9
Mr. Goodbar (Hershey's)	1½-oz. serving	233	20.8
Mr. Goodbar (Hershey's)	4-oz. bar	620	55.6
Nougat centers, *Chuckles*	1 piece (4½ grams)	17	4.2
Nutty Crunch (Nabisco)	1 piece	71	10.2
$100,000 Bar (Nestlé)	1-oz. serving	140	19.0
$100,000 Bar (Nestlé)	1½-oz. bar	175	23.8
Orange slices, *Chuckles*	1 piece (8 grams)	29	7.2
Peanut, chocolate covered (Nabisco)	1 piece (4 grams)	24	1.6
Peanut brittle (Planters)			
Jumbo Peanut Block Bar:			
Regular size	1-oz. bar	119	23.0
Fun size	1 piece (.4 oz.)	61	12.0
Peanut butter cup (Reese's)	½-oz. cup	38	3.6
Peanut Crunch (Sahadi)	¾-oz. bar	110	10.0
Pom Poms (Nabisco)	1 piece (3 grams)	14	2.3
Raisin, chocolate covered (Nabisco)	1 piece (<1 gram)	4	.6

(USDA): United States Department of Agriculture
(HEW/FAO): Health, Education and Welfare/Food and Agriculture Organization
* Prepared as Package Directs

Food and Description	Measure or Quantity	Calories	Carbo-hydrates (grams)
Reggie Bar	2-oz. bar	290	29.0
Rolo (Hershey's)	1 piece (6 grams)	30	4.1
Rolo (Hershey's)	1¾-oz. roll	245	33.5
Royals (M&M/Mars)	1½-oz. serving	202	27.9
Sesame crunch (Sahadi)	¾-oz. bar	110	7.0
Sesame crunch (Sahadi)	10 pieces from 6-oz. jar	90	6.0
Snickers (M&M/Mars)	1.8-oz. bar	247	30.2
Spearmint leaves, *Chuckles*	1 piece (8 grams)	27	6.6
Spice flavored sticks & drops, *Chuckles*	1 piece	13	3.4
Spice flavored strings, *Chuckles*	1 piece	18	4.6
Starburst (M&M/Mars)	1-oz. serving	113	26.7
Stars, chocolate (Nabisco)	1 piece (3 grams)	15	1.6
Sugar Babies (Nabisco)	1 piece (1.5 grams)	6	1.3
Sugar Daddy (Nabisco):			
Giant sucker	1 piece (1 lb.)	1809	398.6
Junior sucker	1 piece (.4 oz.)	50	11.1
Junior sucker, chocolate covered	1 piece (.4 oz.)	51	10.6
Nugget	1 piece (7 grams)	27	6.0
Sucker, caramel	1 piece (1.1 oz.)	121	26.4
Sugar Mama (Nabisco)	1 piece (.8 oz.)	101	18.6
Summit, cookie bar (M&M/Mars)	¾-oz. serving	114	11.6
Summit, cookie bar (M&M/Mars)	1.37-oz. bar	217	21.9
Taffy, turkish (Bonomo):			
Chocolate:			
Bar	10-oz. bar	108	24.4
Drop	.2-oz. drop	18	4.1
Flavored:			
Bar	1-oz. bar	109	24.7
Drop	.2-oz. drop	18	4.1
Plain:			
Bar	1-oz. bar	110	27.6
Drop	.2-oz. drop	18	4.6
3 Musketeers Bar (M&M/Mars)	.8-oz. bar	100	17.2

Food and Description	Measure or Quantity	Calories	Carbo-hydrates (grams)
3 Muskateers Bar			
(M&M/Mars)	2-oz. serving	254	43.9
Toffee brickle (Heath)	1-oz. serving	156	17.0
Tootsie Roll:			
Regular:			
Chocolate	.23-oz. midgee	26	5.3
Chocolate	.63-oz. bar	73	14.3
Chocolate	¾-oz. bar	86	17.2
Chocolate	1-oz. bar	115	22.9
Chocolate	1¼-oz. bar	144	28.6
Flavored	.16-oz. square	19	3.8
Flavored	.23-oz. midgee	27	5.4
Pop:			
Caramel	.49-oz. pop	55	12.5
Chocolate	.49-oz. pop	54	12.7
Flavored	.49-oz. pop	55	12.9
Pop drop:			
Caramel	.17-oz. piece	19	4.2
Chocolate	.17-oz. piece	18	4.3
Flavored	.17-oz. piece	19	4.4
Twix, cookie bar			
(M&M/Mars)	.85-oz. serving	118	15.6
Twix, cookie bar, peanut			
butter (M&M/Mars)	.8-oz. serving	116	12.2
Twizzler:			
Cherry	1 oz.	100	22.0
Chocolate	1 oz.	100	21.0
Licorice	1 oz.	90	20.0
Strawberry	1 oz.	100	22.0
Whatchamacallit (Hershey's)	1.15-oz. bar	176	18.7
Whirligigs (Nabisco)	1 piece (6 grams)	26	5.1
World Series Bar	1 oz. serving	128	21.3
Zagnut Bar (Clark)	.7-oz. bar	92	14.6
Zagnut Bar (Clark)	1⅜-oz. bar	180	28.7
Zagnut Bar (Clark)	1⅝-oz. bar	213	33.9
Dietetic or low calorie:			
Carob bar, *Joan's Natural*:			
Coconut	1 section of 3-oz. bar	43	2.4

(USDA): United States Department of Agriculture
(HEW/FAO): Health, Education and Welfare/Food and Agriculture Organization
* Prepared as Package Directs

Food and Description	Measure or Quantity	Calories	Carbo-hydrates (grams)
Coconut	3-oz. bar	516	28.4
Fruit & nut	1 section of 3-oz. bar	46	2.6
Fruit & nut	3-oz. bar	559	31.2
Honey bran	1 section of 3-oz. bar	40	2.8
Honey bran	3-oz. bar	487	34.0
Peanut	1 section of 3-oz. bar	43	2.3
Peanut	3-oz. bar	521	27.4
Chocolate or chocolate flavored bar:			
Bittersweet (Estee)	1 section of 2½-oz. bar	35	2.7
Bittersweet (Estee)	2½-oz. bar	417	32.0
Chocolate flavored (Featherweight)	1 piece	45	4.0
Coconut (Estee)	1 section of 2½-oz. bar	35	7.4
Coconut (Estee)	2½-oz. bar	420	88.3
Crunch (Estee)	1 section of 2½-oz. bar	34	2.7
Crunch (Estee)	2½-oz. bar	407	32.2
Fruit & nut (Estee)	1 section of 2½-oz. bar	33	2.6
Fruit & nut (Estee)	2½-oz. bar	398	31.3
Milk (Estee)	1 section of 2½-oz. bar	34	2.6
Milk (Estee)	2½-oz. bar	413	31.0
Toasted bran (Estee)	1 section of 2½-oz. bar	33	2.7
Toasted bran (Estee)	2½-oz. bar	398	32.6
Chocolate bar with almonds (Estee) milk	1 section of 2½-oz. bar	35	2.4
Chocolate bar with almonds (Estee) milk	2½-oz. bar	415	29.2
Estee-Ets, peanut	1.4-gram piece	7	.9
Gum drops (Estee) fruit and licorice	1 piece (2 grams)	3	.7

Food and Description	Measure or Quantity	Calories	Carbo-hydrates (grams)
Hard:			
(Estee):			
Assorted fruit or peppermint	1 piece (.1 oz.)	11	2.7
Tropi-mix	1 piece (.1 oz.)	10	2.7
(Featherweight) assorted	1 piece	12	3.0
Mint:			
(Estee) *Esteemint*, all flavors	1 piece	4	1.1
(Sunkist):			
Mini mint	1 piece (.23 grams)	<1	.2
Roll mint	1 piece (.89 grams)	4	.9
Peanut butter cup (Estee)	1 piece (.3 oz.)	50	3.3
Raisin, chocolate covered (Estee)	1 piece (1 gram)	6	.6
Rice crisp bar (Featherweight)	1 piece	50	4.5
TV mix (Estee)	1 piece (2 grams)	8	.6
CANNELONI FLORENTINE, frozen (Weight Watcher's) one compartment meal	13-oz. meal	450	52.0
CANTALOUPE, fresh (USDA):			
Whole, medium	1 lb. (weighed with skin & cavity contents)	68	17.0
Cubed	½ cup (2.9 oz.)	24	6.1
CAPICOLA or CAPACOLA SAUSAGE (USDA)	1-oz. serving	141	0.
***CAP'N CRUNCH*,** cereal (Quaker):			
Regular	¾ cup (1 oz.)	121	22.9

(USDA): United States Department of Agriculture
(HEW/FAO): Health, Education and Welfare/Food and Agriculture Organization
* Prepared as Package Directs

Food and Description	Measure or Quantity	Calories	Carbo-hydrates (grams)
Crunchberries	¾ cup (1 oz.)	120	22.9
Peanut butter	¾ cup (1 oz.)	127	20.9
CARAMBOLA, raw (USDA):			
Whole	1 lb. (weighed whole)	149	34.1
Flesh only	4 oz.	40	9.1
CARAWAY SEED (French's)	1 tsp.	8	.8
CARDAMOM SEED (French's)	1 tsp.	6	1.3
CARISSA or NATAL PLUM, raw (USDA):			
Whole	1 lb. (weighed whole)	273	62.4
Flesh only	4 oz.	79	18.1
*CARNATION INSTANT BREAKFAST:			
Chocolate, chocolate malt or coffee	8 fl. oz.	280	35.0
Egg nog or strawberry	8 fl. oz.	280	34.0
Vanilla	8 fl. oz.	280	33.0
CARP, raw (USDA):			
Whole	1 lb. (weighed whole)	156	0.
Meat only	4 oz.	130	0.
CARROT:			
Raw (USDA):			
Whole	1 lb. (weighed with full tops)	112	26.0
Partially trimmed	1 lb. (weighed without tops, with skins)	156	36.1
Trimmed	5½" × 1" carrot (1.8 oz.)	21	4.8
Trimmed	25 thin strips (1.8 oz.)	21	4.8
Chunks	½ cup (2.4 oz.)	29	6.7
Diced	½ cup (1½ oz.)	30	7.0

Food and Description	Measure or Quantity	Calories	Carbohydrates (grams)
Grated or shredded	½ cup (1.9 oz.)	23	5.3
Slices	½ cup (2.2 oz.)	27	6.2
Strips	½ cup (2 oz.)	24	5.6
Boiled, drained (USDA):			
Chunks	½ cup (2.9 oz.)	25	5.8
Diced	½ cup (2½ oz.)	24	5.2
Slices	½ cup (2.7 oz.)	24	5.4
Canned, regular pack:			
(Del Monte):			
Diced, drained	½ cup	35	6.8
Sliced, drained	½ cup	37	7.4
(Libby's):			
Diced, solids & liq.	½ cup	19	4.1
Sliced, solids & liq.	½ cup	24	5.3
(Stokely-Van Camp):			
Diced, solids & liq.	½ cup (4.3 oz.)	30	6.0
Sliced, solids & liq.	½ cup (4.3 oz.)	25	5.0
Canned, dietetic or low calorie, solids & liq.:			
(Blue Boy) sliced	½ of 8¼-oz. can	35	6.4
(Featherweight) sliced	½ cup	30	6.0
(S&W) *Nutridiet*, sliced	½ cup	30	7.0
Dehydrated (USDA)	1 oz.	97	23.0
Frozen:			
(Birds Eye) with brown sugar glaze	⅓ of 10-oz. pkg.	81	14.6
(Green Giant) nuggets in butter sauce	⅓ of 10-oz. pkg.	46	6.0
(McKenzie) whole	3.3-oz. serving	39	8.1
(Seabrook Farms) whole	3.3-oz. serving	39	8.1
CARROT PUREE, canned, dietetic (Featherweight)	1 cup	70	15.0
CASABA MELON, fresh (USDA):			
Whole	1 lb. (weighed whole)	61	14.7
Flesh	4 oz.	31	7.4

(USDA): United States Department of Agriculture
(HEW/FAO): Health, Education and Welfare/Food and Agriculture Organization
* Prepared as Package Directs

Food and Description	Measure or Quantity	Calories	Carbohydrates (grams)
CASHEW NUT:			
(USDA)	1 oz.	159	8.3
(USDA)	½ cup (2.5 oz.)	393	20.5
(USDA)	5 large or 8 med.	60	3.1
(Fisher):			
Dry roasted	¼ cup (1.2 oz.)	187	9.9
Oil roasted	¼ cup (1.2 oz.)	196	9.9
(Planters):			
Dry roasted, salted or unsalted	1 oz.	160	9.0
Oil roasted	1 oz.	170	8.0
CATAWBA WINE:			
(Great Western) pink, 12% alcohol	3 fl. oz.	111	11.3
(Taylor) 12% alcohol	3 fl. oz.	96	9.0
CATFISH, freshwater, raw fillet			
(USDA)	4 oz.	117	0.
CATSUP:			
Regular pack:			
(USDA)	1 T. (.6 oz.)	19	4.6
(USDA)	½ cup (5 oz.)	149	35.8
(Del Monte)	1 T. (.7 oz.)	24	5.5
(Smucker's)	1 T. (.6 oz.)	21	4.5
Dietetic or low calorie:			
(Dia-Mel)	1 T. (14 grams)	7	1.5
(Featherweight)	1 T. (.6 oz.)	6	1.0
(Tillie Lewis) *Tasti Diet*	1 T. (.5 oz.)	8	2.0
CAULIFLOWER:			
Raw (USDA):			
Whole	1 lb. (weighed untrimmed)	48	9.2
Flowerbuds	½ cup (1.8 oz.)	14	2.6
Slices	½ cup (1.5 oz.)	11	2.2
Boiled (USDA) flowerbuds, drained	½ cup (2.2 oz.)	14	2.5
Frozen:			
(Birds Eye) 5-minute style	⅓ of 10-oz. pkg.	25	3.7

Food and Description	Measure or Quantity	Calories	Carbo-hydrates (grams)
(Green Giant):			
In cheese sauce, *Bake'n Serve*	⅓ of 10-oz. pkg.	80	5.6
In cheese sauce, boil-in-bag	⅓ of 10-oz. pkg.	49	5.2
Cuts	¼ of 18-oz. pkg.	28	4.1
(Kounty Kist) cuts	⅕ of 20-oz. pkg.	25	3.6
(McKenzie)	3.3-oz. serving	27	4.5
(Mrs. Paul's) & cheese, batter fried	⅓ of 8-oz. pkg.	135	15.3
(Seabrook Farms)	3.3-oz. serving	27	4.5
(Stouffer's) au gratin	⅓ of 10-oz. pkg.	104	7.2
CAVIAR, STURGEON (USDA):			
Pressed	1 oz.	90	1.4
Whole eggs	1 T. (.6 oz.)	42	.5
CELERIAC ROOT, raw (USDA):			
Whole	1 lb. (weighed unpared)	156	39.2
Pared	4 oz.	45	9.6
CELERY, all varieties (USDA):			
Fresh:			
Whole	1 lb. (weighed untrimmed)	58	13.3
1 large outer stalk	8″ × 1½″ at root end (1.4 oz.)	7	1.6
Diced, chopped or cut in chunks	½ cup (2.1 oz.)	10	2.3
Slices	½ cup (1.9 oz.)	9	2.1
Boiled, drained solids:			
Diced or cut in chunks	½ cup (2.7 oz.)	10	2.4
Slices	½ cup (3 oz.)	12	2.6

(USDA): United States Department of Agriculture
(HEW/FAO): Health, Education and Welfare/Food and Agriculture Organization
* Prepared as Package Directs

Food and Description	Measure or Quantity	Calories	Carbo-hydrates (grams)
CELERY CABBAGE (See **CABBAGE, CHINESE**)			
CELERY SALT (French's)	1 tsp. (4.6 grams)	2	<.5
CELERY SEED (French's)	1 tsp. (2.4 grams)	11	1.1
***CELERY SOUP,** canned, cream of:			
(Campbell) condensed	10-oz. serving	120	10.0
(Rokeach) condensed:			
Prepared with milk	10-oz. serving	190	19.0
Prepared with water	10-oz. serving	90	12.0
CEREAL (see kind of cereal, such as **CORN FLAKES,** or brand names such as **KIX, CHEX,** etc.)			
CERTS (Warner-Lambert)	1 piece	6	1.5
CERVELAT (USDA):			
Dry	1 oz.	128	.5
Soft	1 oz.	87	.5
CHABLIS WINE:			
(Almaden) light, 7% alcohol	3 fl. oz.	42	DNA
(Great Western) 12% alcohol	3 fl. oz.	70	2.3
(Great Western) Diamond, 12% alcohol	3 fl. oz.	69	2.0
(Paul Masson):			
Regular, 11.8% alcohol	3 fl. oz.	71	2.7
Light, 7.1% alcohol	3 fl. oz.	45	2.7
(Taylor) 12% alcohol	3 fl. oz.	72	1.3
CHAMPAGNE:			
(Great Western):			
Regular, 12% alcohol	3 fl. oz.	71	2.4
Brut, 12% alcohol	3 fl. oz.	74	3.4
Extra dry, 12½% alcohol	3 fl. oz.	78	4.3
Pink, 12% alcohol	3 fl. oz.	81	4.9
(Lejon) 12% alcohol	3 fl. oz.	66	2.5

Food and Description	Measure or Quantity	Calories	Carbohydrates (grams)
(Taylor):			
Brut, 12½% alcohol	3 fl. oz	75	3.3
Dry, 12½% alcohol	3 fl. oz.	78	3.9
Pink, 12½% alcohol	3 fl. oz.	81	4.8
CHARD, Swiss (USDA):			
Raw, whole	1 lb. (weighed untrimmed)	104	19.2
Raw, trimmed	4 oz.	28	5.2
Boiled, drained solids	½ cup (3.4 oz.)	17	3.2
CHARLOTTE RUSSE, with ladyfingers, whipped cream filling, home recipe (USDA)	4 oz.	324	38.0
CHATEAUNEUF-DU-PAPE, French red Rhone:			
(Barton & Guestier) 13½% alcohol	3 fl. oz.	70	.5
(Chanson) 13% alcohol	3 fl. oz.	90	6.3
CHAYOTE, raw (USDA):			
Whole	1 lb. (weighed unpared)	108	27.4
Pared	4 oz.	32	8.1
***CHEDDAR CHEESE SOUP** (Campbell) condensed	11-oz. serving	180	14.0
CHEERIOS, cereal (General Mills):			
Regular	1¼ cups (1 oz.)	110	20.0
Honey-nut	1¾ cups (1 oz.)	110	23.0
CHEESE:			
American or cheddar: (USDA):			
Natural	1″ cube (.6 oz.)	68	.4
Natural, diced	1 cup (4.6 oz.)	521	2.8

(USDA): United States Department of Agriculture
(HEW/FAO): Health, Education and Welfare/Food and Agriculture Organization
* Prepared as Package Directs

Food and Description	Measure or Quantity	Calories	Carbo-hydrates (grams)
Natural, grated or shredded	1 cup (3.9 oz.)	442	2.3
Natural, grated or shredded	1 T. (.7 grams)	27	.1
Process	1″ cube (.6 oz.)	65	.3
(Borden) process	¾-oz. slice	83	1.2
Laughing Cow, baby	1 oz.	110	Tr.
(Sargento):			
Crock, sharp	1 oz.	94	2.0
Midget, midget Longhorn or shredded, regular or sharp	1 oz.	114	1.0
Shredded, non-dairy	1 oz.	90	3.0
Sliced or stick, sharp	1 oz.	114	1.0
Bleu or blue:			
(USDA) natural	1″ cube (.6 oz.)	64	.3
(Frigo)	1 oz.	100	1.0
Laughing Cow	⅙-oz. cube	12	.1
Laughing Cow	¾-oz. wedge	55	.5
Laughing Cow	1 oz.	74	.7
(Sargento) cold pack or crumbled	1 oz.	100	1.0
Bonbel, *Laughing Cow*	1 oz.	94	Tr.
Bonbino, *Laughing Cow*	1 oz.	104	Tr.
Brick:			
(USDA) natural	1 oz.	105	.5
(Sargento) sliced	1 oz.	105	1.0
Brie (Sargento) *Danish Danko*	1 oz.	80	.1
Burgercheese (Sargento)	1 oz.	106	1.0
Camembert, domestic:			
(USDA) natural	1 oz.	85	.5
(Sargento) *Danish Danko*	1 oz.	88	.1
Cheddar (see American)			
Colby:			
(Fisher)	1 oz.	110	1.0
(Frigo)	1 oz.	110	1.0
(Sargento) midget Longhorn, shredded or sliced	1 oz.	112	1.0
Cottage:			
Unflavored:			
(Bison):			
Regular	1 oz.	29	1.0
Dietetic	1 oz.	22	1.0

Food and Description	Measure or Quantity	Calories	Carbo-hydrates (grams)
(Dairylea) large or small curd	1 oz.	30	1.0
(Friendship):			
Regular	1 oz.	30	1.0
Low fat or no salt added	1 oz.	22	1.0
Low fat, pot style	1 oz.	25	1.0
(Frigo):			
Regular, creamed	1 oz.	30	.8
Part skim milk	1 oz.	24	.8
(Meadow Gold)	1 oz.	30	1.0
Viva	1 oz.	25	1.0
Flavored (Friendship):			
With dutch apple	1 oz.	31	2.5
With garden salad	1 oz.	30	1.0
With pineapple	1 oz.	35	3.8
Cream cheese:			
Plain, unwhipped:			
(Frigo)	1 oz.	100	1.0
(Kraft) *Philadelphia Brand:*			
Regular	1 oz.	104	.9
Imitation	1 oz.	52	1.9
Plain, whipped (Kraft) *Philadelphia Brand*	1 oz.	98	.6
Flavored, whipped (Kraft) *Philadelphia Brand:*			
With onion	1 oz.	86	1.9
With pimiento	1 oz.	86	1.8
Edam:			
(House of Gold)	1 oz.	100	1.0
Laughing Cow	1 oz.	100	Tr.
(Sargento)	1 oz.	101	1.0
Farmer:			
Dutch Garden Brand	1 oz.	100	1.0
(Friendship) regular or no salt added	1 oz.	40	1.0
(Sargento)	1 oz.	72	1.0
Wispride	1 oz.	100	1.0

(USDA): United States Department of Agriculture
(HEW/FAO): Health, Education and Welfare/Food and Agriculture Organization
* Prepared as Package Directs

Food and Description	Measure or Quantity	Calories	Carbo-hydrates (grams)
Feta (Sargento) Danish, cups	1 oz.	76	1.0
Fontina (Kraft) natural	1 oz.	113	.6
Frankenmuth, natural (Kraft)	1 oz.	113	.7
Gjetost (Sargento) Norwegian	1 oz.	118	13.0
Gorgonzola (Foremost Blue Moon)	1 oz.	110	Tr.
Gouda:			
(Frigo)	1 oz.	100	1.0
Laughing Cow, natural	1 oz.	110	Tr.
(Sargento) baby, caraway or smoked	1 oz.	101	1.0
Wispride	1 oz.	100	<1.0
Gruyère, *Swiss Knight*	1 oz.	101	<1.0
Havarti (Sargento):			
Creamy	1 oz.	70	.2
Creamy, 60% milk	1 oz.	117	.2
Hot pepper (Sargento) sliced	1 oz.	112	1.0
Jack—dry, natural (Kraft)	1 oz.	101	.4
Jack—fresh, natural (Kraft)	1 oz.	95	.4
Jarlsberg (Sargento) Norwegian, sliced	1 oz.	100	1.0
Kettle Moraine (Sargento) sliced	1 oz.	100	1.0
Lagerkase, natural (Kraft)	1 oz.	107	.3
Leyden, natural (Kraft)	1 oz.	80	.7
Liederkranz (Borden)	1 oz.	86	.4
Limburger (Sargento) natural	1 oz.	93	14.0
Monterey Jack:			
(Frigo)	1 oz.	100	1.0
(Sargento) shredded or sliced	1 oz.	106	1.0
Mozzarella:			
(Fisher) part skim milk, low moisture	1 oz.	90	1.0
(Frigo) part skim milk	1 oz.	80	1.0
(Sargento):			
Bar, rounds, shredded, square, sliced with spices or sliced for pizza	1 oz.	79	1.0
Whole milk	1 oz.	100	1.0
Muenster:			
(Sargento) red rind	1 oz.	104	1.0
Wispride	1 oz.	100	1.0
Neufchâtel (Kraft) loaf	1 oz.	69	.7

Food and Description	Measure or Quantity	Calories	Carbo- hydrates (grams)
Nibblin curds (Sargento)	1 oz.	114	1.0
Parmesan:			
(Frigo):			
Regular	1 oz.	110	1.0
Grated	1 T. (6 grams)	23	Tr.
(Sargento):			
Grated, non-dairy	1 T. (7 grams)	27	2.3
Wedge	1 oz.	110	1.0
Parmesan & romano, grated (Kraft)	1 oz.	130	1.0
Pimiento American, process (USDA)	1 oz.	105	.5
Pizza (Sargento) shredded or sliced, non-dairy	1 oz.	90	1.0
Port du Salut (Kraft) natural	1 oz.	100	.3
Primost (Kraft) natural	1 oz.	134	13.0
Provolone:			
(Frigo)	1 oz.	90	1.0
(Kraft) natural	1 oz.	99	.5
Laughing Cow	⅕-oz. cube	12	.1
Laughing Cow	¾-oz. wedge	55	.5
Laughing Cow		74	.7
(Sargento) sliced	1 oz.	100	1.0
Ricotta:			
(Frigo) part skim milk, moist	1 oz.	43	.9
(Sargento):			
Part skim milk	1 oz.	39	1.0
Whole milk	1 oz.	49	1.0
Romano:			
(Frigo):			
Natural	1 oz.	100	1.0
Grated	1 T. (6 grams)	21	Tr.
(Sargento) wedge	1 oz.	110	1.0
Roquefort, natural (USDA)	1 oz.	104	.6
Sage (Kraft) natural	1 oz.	113	.6
Samsoe (Sargento) Danish	1 oz.	101	.2
Sap Sago (Kraft) natural	1 oz.	76	1.7
Sardo Romano, natural (Kraft)	1 oz.	109	.8

(USDA): United States Department of Agriculture
(HEW/FAO): Health, Education and Welfare/Food and Agriculture
Organization
* Prepared as Package Directs

Food and Description	Measure or Quantity	Calories	Carbohydrates (grams)
Scamorze (Frigo)	1 oz.	79	.3
Stirred curd (Frigo)	1 oz.	110	1.0
String (Sargento)	1 oz.	90	1.0
Swiss:			
Domestic:			
(Fisher)	1 oz.	100	0.
(Frigo) natural	1 oz.	100	0.
(Sargento) sliced	1 oz.	107	1.0
Imported (Sargento) Finland, sliced	1 oz.	107	1.0
Taco (Sargento) shredded	1 oz.	105	1.0
Washed curd (Frigo)	1 oz.	110	1.0

CHEESE DIP (See **DIP**)

CHEESE FONDUE:

Home, recipe (USDA)	4 oz.	301	11.3
Swiss Knight	1-oz. serving	60	1.0

CHEESE FOOD, process:

American or cheddar:			
(Fisher)	1 oz.	90	2.0
(Pauly)	.8-oz. slice	74	1.6
(Sargento) logs with almonds & with port wine & almonds; with port wine and sharp, cold pack	1 oz.	94	2.0
(Weight Watchers) colored or white	1-oz. slice	50	1.0
Wispride, cheddar:			
Plain	1 oz.	100	7.0
& blue cheese	1 oz.	100	2.0
Hickory smoked	1 oz.	90	3.0
& port wine	1 oz.	100	<1.0
Sharp	1 oz.	90	2.0
Cheezln' Crackers, process (Kraft)	1.1-oz. piece	127	9.3
Cheez-ola (Fisher) process	1 oz.	90	.5
Colby (Pauly) low sodium	1 oz.	115	.6
Cracker snack (Sargento)	1 oz.	90	2.0
Loaf, *Count-Down* (Fisher)	1 oz.	40	3.0
Mun-chee (Pauly) chunk	1 oz.	100	2.0
Pimiento (Pauly)	.8-oz. slice	73	.8

Food and Description	Measure or Quantity	Calories	Carbo- hydrates (grams)
Sharp (Pauly)	1-oz. slice	100	.8
Swiss, *Wispride*	1 oz.	100	6.0
CHEESE PUFF, frozen			
(Durkee)	1 piece (.5 oz.)	59	3.0
CHEESE SPREAD:			
American, process:			
(USDA)	1 T. (.5 oz.)	50	1.1
(Fisher)	1 oz.	80	2.0
(Nabisco) *Snack Mate*	1 tsp. (6 grams)	16	.4
Bacon (Kraft) process	1 oz.	64	.5
Cheddar:			
(Nabisco) *Snack Mate*, regular or sharp	1 tsp. (6 grams)	16	.4
Wispride, sharp	1 oz.	80	2.0
Cheese & bacon (Nabisco) *Snack Mate*	1 tsp. (6 grams)	16	.4
Chive & green onion (Nabisco) *Snack Mate*	1 tsp. (6 grams)	16	.4
Count Down (Fisher)	1 oz.	30	3.0
Imitation (Fisher) *Chef's Delight*	1 oz.	40	3.0
Jalapeno (Kraft) *Cheez Whiz*	1 oz.	76	1.9
Pimiento:			
(Nabisco) *Snack Mate*	1 tsp. (.5 oz.)	16	.4
(Pauly)	¾-oz. serving	66	.9
(Price's)	1 oz.	80	2.0
Sharp (Pauly)	.8-oz. serving	77	.9
Swiss (Pauly) process	.8-oz. serving	76	1.2
CHEESE STRAW:			
(USDA)	5″ × ⅜″ × ⅜″ piece (6 grams)	27	2.1
(Durkee) frozen	1 piece	29	1.0
CHELOIS WINE (Great Western) 12% alcohol	3 fl. oz.	70	2.2

(USDA): United States Department of Agriculture
(HEW/FAO):   Health, Education and Welfare/Food and Agriculture
             Organization
* Prepared as Package Directs

Food and Description	Measure or Quantity	Calories	Carbo-hydrates (grams)
CHERRY:			
Sour (USDA):			
Fresh:			
Whole	1 lb. (weighed with stems)	213	52.5
Whole	1 lb. (weighed without stems)	242	59.7
Pitted	½ cup (2.7 oz.)	45	11.1
Canned, syrup pack, pitted:			
Light syrup	4 oz. (with liq.)	84	21.2
Heavy syrup	½ cup (with liq.)	116	29.5
Extra heavy syrup	4 oz. (with liq.)	127	32.4
Canned, water pack, pitted, solids & liq.	½ cup (4.3 oz.)	52	13.1
Frozen, pitted:			
Sweetened	½ cup (4.6 oz.)	146	36.1
Unsweetened	4 oz.	62	15.2
Sweet:			
Fresh (USDA):			
Whole	1 lb. (weighed with stems)	286	71.0
Whole, with stems	½ cup (2.3 oz.)	41	10.2
Pitted	½ cup (2.9 oz.)	57	14.3
Canned, syrup pack:			
(USDA):			
Light syrup, pitted	4 oz. (with liq.)	74	18.7
Heavy syrup, pitted	½ cup (with liq., 4.2 oz.)	96	24.2
Extra heavy syrup, pitted	4 oz. (with liq.)	113	29.0
(Del Monte) solids & liq.:			
Dark	½ cup (4.3 oz.)	106	25.2
Royal Anne	½ cup (4.3 oz.)	111	26.8
(Stokely-Van Camp) pitted, solids & liq.	½ cup (4.2 oz.)	50	11.0
Canned, dietetic or water pack, solids & liq.:			
(Diet Delight)	½ cup (4.4 oz.)	70	17.0
(Featherweight):			
Dark	½ cup	60	13.0
Light	½ cup	50	11.0

Food and Description	Measure or Quantity	Calories	Carbo-hydrates (grams)
CHERRY BRANDY (See **BRANDY, FLAVORED**)			
CHERRY, CANDIED (USDA)	1 oz.	96	24.6
CHERRY DRINK: Canned:			
(Hi-C)	6 fl. oz. (6.3 oz.)	93	23.0
(Lincoln) Cherry Berry	6 fl. oz.	95	23.9
*Mix (Hi-C)	6 fl. oz.	72	18.0
CHERRY EXTRACT (Ehlers) imitation	1 tsp.	16	DNA
CHERRY HEERING, Danish liqueur, 49 proof	1 fl. oz.	80	10.0
CHERRY ICE CREAM: (Good Humor) black	4 fl. oz.	130	14.0
CHERRY JELLY: Sweetened (Smucker's)	1 T. (.7 oz.)	53	13.5
Dietetic or low calorie: (Featherweight):			
Regular	1 T.	16	4.0
Artificially sweetened	1 T.	6	1.0
(Slenderella)	1 T.	24	6.0
CHERRY KIJAFA, Danish wine, 17½% alcohol	3 fl. oz.	148	15.3
CHERRY LIQUEUR:			
(DeKuyper) 50 proof	1 fl. oz.	75	8.5
(Leroux) 60 proof	1 fl. oz.	80	7.6
CHERRY, MARASCHINO (USDA)	1 oz. (with liq.)	33	8.3
CHERRY PIE (See **PIE,** Cherry)			

(USDA): United States Department of Agriculture
(HEW/FAO): Health, Education and Welfare/Food and Agriculture Organization
* Prepared as Package Directs

Food and Description	Measure or Quantity	Calories	Carbo-hydrates (grams)
CHERRY PIE FILLING (See **PIE FILLING,** Cherry)			
CHERRY PRESERVE or JAM:			
Sweetened (Smucker's)	1 T. (.7 oz.)	53	13.5
Dietetic or low calorie:			
(Dia-Mel)	1 T.	6	0.
(Featherweight) red	1 T.	16	4.0
(Smucker's)	1 T.	24	6.0
(S&W) *Nutradiet*, red, tart	1 T.	12	3.0
CHERVIL, raw (USDA)	1 oz.	16	3.3
CHESTNUT (USDA):			
Fresh:			
In shell	1 lb. (weighed in shell)	713	154.7
Shelled	4 oz.	220	47.7
Dried:			
In shell	1 lb. (weighed in shell)	1402	292.4
Shelled	4 oz.	428	89.1
CHESTNUT FLOUR (See **FLOUR,** Chestnut)			
CHEWING GUM:			
Sweetened:			
Beechies	1 tablet (2 grams)	6	1.6
Beech-Nut	1 stick	10	2.3
Beemans	1 stick	9	2.3
Big Red	1 stick	10	2.3
Black Jack	1 stick	9	2.3
Chiclets	1 piece	6	1.1
Dentyne	1 piece	4	1.2
Doublemint (Wrigley's)	1 stick	10	2.3
Freedent (Wrigley's)	1 stick	10	2.3
Juicy Fruit (Wrigley's)	1 stick	10	2.3
Peppermint (Clark)	1 piece	10	2.3
Sour lemon (Clark)	1 stick	10	2.3
Spearmint (Wrigley's)	1 stick (3 grams)	10	2.3
Teaberry	1 stick	10	2.3
Unsweetened or dietetic:			
Bazooka, bubble	1 piece	16	Tr.

Food and Description	Measure or Quantity	Calories	Carbo- hydrates (grams)
Care*Free (Beech-Nut)	1 stick (3 grams)	7	Tr.
(Estee) all flavors	1 section	5	1.4
(Featherweight) all flavors	1 piece	4	1.0
CHEX, cereal (Ralston Purina): Bran (See **BRAN BREAKFAST CEREAL**)			
Corn	1 cup (1 oz.)	110	25.0
Rice	1⅛ cups (1 oz.)	110	25.0
Wheat	⅔ cup (1 oz.)	100	23.0
Wheat & raisin	¾ cup (1⅓ oz.)	120	30.0
CHIANTI WINE (Italian Swiss Colony)			
13% alcohol	3 fl. oz.	64	1.5
CHICKEN (See also **CHICKEN, CANNED**): (USDA):			
Broiler, cooked, meat only	4 oz.	154	0.
Capon, raw, with bone	1 lb. (weighed ready-to-cook)	937	0.
Fryer: Raw:			
Ready-to-cook	1 lb. (weighed ready-to-cook)	382	0.
Breast	1 lb. (weighed with bone)	394	0.
Leg or drumstick	1 lb. (weighed with bone)	313	0.
Thigh	1 lb. (weighed with bone)	435	0.
Fried. A 2½-lb. chicken (weighed before cooking with bone) will give you:			
Back	1 back (2.2 oz.)	139	2.7
Breast	½ breast (3⅓ oz.)	154	1.1
Leg or drumstick	1 leg (2 oz.)	87	.4
Neck	1 neck (2.1 oz.)	121	1.9

(USDA): United States Department of Agriculture
(HEW/FAO):   Health, Education and Welfare/Food and Agriculture Organization
* Prepared as Package Directs

Food and Description	Measure or Quantity	Calories	Carbo-hydrates (grams)
Rib	1 rib (.7 oz.)	42	.8
Thigh	1 thigh (2¼ oz.)	118	1.2
Wing	1 wing (1¾ oz.)	78	.8
Fried skin	1 oz.	119	2.6
Hen and cock:			
Raw	1 lb. (weighed ready-to-cook)	987	0.
Stewed:			
Meat only	4 oz.	236	0.
Chopped	½ cup (2.5 oz.)	150	0.
Diced	½ cup (2.4 oz.)	139	0.
Ground	½ cup (2 oz.)	116	0.
Roaster:			
Raw:	1 lb. (weighed ready-to-cook)	791	0.
Roasted:			
Dark meat without skin	4 oz.	209	0.
Light meat without skin	4 oz.	206	0.
CHICKEN A LA KING:			
Home recipe (USDA)	1 cup (8.6 oz.)	468	12.3
Canned (Swanson)	½ of 10½-oz. can	180	9.0
Frozen:			
(Banquet) *Cookin' Bag*	5-oz. bag	138	10.4
(Green Giant) *Toast Topper*	5-oz. serving	162	7.7
(Stouffer's) with rice	9½-oz. pkg.	331	37.8
(Weight Watchers) boil-in-bag	10-oz. pkg.	233	17.0
CHICKEN & BISCUITS, frozen (Green Giant)	½ of 14-oz. pkg.	196	18.7
CHICKEN BOUILLON/BROTH, cube or powder (See also **CHICKEN SOUP**):			
(Herb-Ox):			
Cube	4-gram cube	6	.6
Powder	5-gram packet	12	2.0
(Maggi)	1 cube	7	1.0
MBT	1 packet (.2 oz.)	12	2.0
CHICKEN, CANNED, BONED: (USDA)	½ cup (3 oz.)	168	0.

Food and Description	Measure or Quantity	Calories	Carbo- hydrates (grams)
(Hormel) chunk	6¾-oz. serving	257	.8
(Swanson):			
Regular	½ of 5-oz. can	110	0.
Mixin' style	½ of 5-oz. can	140	0.
Thigh	½ of 5-oz. can	120	0.
White	½ of 5-oz. can	110	0.
CHICKEN, CREAMED, frozen			
(Stouffer's)	6½-oz. pkg.	300	5.9
CHICKEN CROQUETTE DINNER, frozen			
(Morton)	10¼-oz. dinner	413	46.5
CHICKEN DINNER or ENTREE:			
Canned (Swanson) & dumplings	2½-oz. serving	220	18.0
Frozen:			
(Banquet):			
Regular:			
& dumplings	12-oz. dinner	282	36.4
Fried	11-oz. dinner	530	48.4
Buffet Supper, & dumplings	2-lb. pkg.	1209	128.2
Man-Pleaser:			
Regular	17-oz. dinner	1026	89.2
& dressing	19-oz. dinner	713	68.4
& dumplings	19-oz. dinner	688	86.1
Fried	17-oz. dinner	942	81.7
(Morton):			
Regular:			
Boneless	10-oz. dinner	222	22.8
& dumplings	11-oz. dinner	272	31.2
Fried	11-oz. dinner	450	50.0
& noodles	10⅓-oz. dinner	252	41.0
Country Table:			
Fried	15-oz. dinner	692	94.8
Fried	12-oz. entree	583	27.3

(USDA): United States Department of Agriculture
(HEW/FAO):   Health, Education and Welfare/Food and Agriculture
            Organization
* Prepared as Package Directs

Food and Description	Measure or Quantity	Calories	Carbo-hydrates (grams)
King Size:			
Boneless	17-oz. dinner	546	53.1
Fried	17-oz. dinner	859	91.8
(Mrs. Paul's):			
Pattie, breaded & fried,			
with french fries	8½-oz. pkg.	389	51.3
Pattie, batter fried,			
with french fries	8½-oz. pkg.	426	46.3
Sticks, breaded & fried,			
with french fries	8½-oz. pkg.	424	55.3
(Stouffer's):			
Cacciatore with spaghetti	11½-oz. entree	313	28.8
Divan	8½-oz. pkg.	336	14.0
(Swanson):			
Regular:			
Fried	11½-oz. dinner	570	28.0
Fried, barbecue flavored	11¼-oz. dinner	530	47.0
Fried, crisp	10¾-oz. dinner	650	51.0
& noodle	10¼-oz. dinner	390	53.0
In white wine sauce	8¼-oz. entree	370	10.0
Hungry Man:			
Boneless	19-oz. dinner	730	74.0
Fried	15¾-oz. dinner	910	78.0
Fried, barbecue flavored	16½-oz. dinner	760	72.0
3-course, fried	15-oz. dinner	630	64.0
(Weight Watchers):			
New Orleans style	11-oz. pkg.	229	19.1
Oriental style	12-oz. pkg.	251	18.0
Parmigiana,			
2-compartment	7¾-oz. meal	220	11.0
Sliced in celery sauce,			
2-compartment	8½-oz. meal	207	13.9
Sliced with gravy &			
stuffing, 3-compartment	14¾-oz. meal	380	42.1
Southern fried patty,			
2-compartment	6¾-oz. serving	260	11.0
Sweet & sour, with			
oriental style vegetables	9½-oz. pkg.	220	27.0

CHICKEN & DUMPLINGS
  (See **CHICKEN DINNER or
  ENTREE**)

Food and Description	Measure or Quantity	Calories	Carbo-hydrates (grams)
CHICKEN FRICASSEE, home recipe (USDA)	1 cup (8½ oz.)	386	7.7
CHICKEN FRIED, frozen:			
(Banquet)	2-lb. pkg.	2591	117.3
(Morton):			
Regular	¼ of 32-oz. pkg.	298	32.7
Breast portion	¼ of 22-oz. pkg.	367	31.2
(Swanson):			
Assorted	3.2-oz. serving	260	10.0
Breast portion	3.2-oz. serving	250	8.0
Nibbler (wings)	3.2-oz. serving	290	12.0
Take-out style	4-oz. serving	260	8.0
Thighs & drumsticks	3.2-oz. serving	260	18.0
CHICKEN GIZZARD (USDA):			
Raw	2-oz. serving	64	.4
Simmered	2-oz. serving	84	.4
CHICKEN LIVER (See **LIVER**)			
CHICKEN LIVER & ONION, frozen (Weight Watchers) 2-compartment meal	9¼-oz. meal	188	10.0
CHICKEN LIVER PUFF, frozen (Durkee)	1 piece	48	3.0
CHICKEN & NOODLES:			
Home recipe (USDA)	1 cup (8½ oz.)	367	25.7
Frozen:			
(Banquet):			
Regular	12-oz. dinner	374	50.7
Buffet Supper	2-lb. pkg.	764	79.1
(Green Giant)	9-oz. pkg.	245	21.5
(Stouffer's):			
Escalloped	½ of 11½-oz. pkg.	252	15.8

(USDA): United States Department of Agriculture
(HEW/FAO): Health, Education and Welfare/Food and Agriculture Organization
* Prepared as Package Directs

Food and Description	Measure or Quantity	Calories	Carbohydrates (grams)
Paprikash, with egg noodles	10½-oz. pkg.	381	31.9
CHICKEN, PACKAGED:			
(Eckrich) sliced	1-oz. slice	47	1.3
(Louis Rich) breast, oven roasted	1-oz. slice	40	<1.0
CHICKEN PIE:			
Home recipe (USDA) baked	8-oz. pie (4¼" dia.)	533	41.5
Frozen:			
(Banquet)	8-oz. pie	427	39.0
(Morton)	8-oz. pie	345	29.5
(Stouffer's)	10-oz. pie	493	39.8
(Swanson):			
Regular	8-oz. pie	450	42.0
Hungry Man	16-oz. pie	780	66.0
(Van de Kamp's)	7½-oz. pie	520	47.0
CHICKEN PUFF, frozen (Durkee)	1 piece	49	3.0
CHICKEN SALAD, canned (Carnation) *Spreadable*	1½-oz. serving	94	2.6
CHICKEN SOUP:			
Canned, regular pack:			
(Campbell)			
Chunky:			
Regular	9½-oz. can	200	20.0
Regular	10¾-oz. can	230	22.0
& rice	9½-oz. can	140	15.0
& vegetables	9½-oz. can	170	19.0
*Condensed:			
Alphabet	10-oz. serving	110	12.0
Broth	10-oz. serving	50	4.0
Broth & noodle	10-oz. serving	80	10.0
Broth & rice	10-oz. serving	60	10.0
Broth & vegetables	10-oz. serving	40	7.0
Cream of	10-oz. serving	140	11.0
& dumplings	10-oz. serving	100	12.0

Food and Description	Measure or Quantity	Calories	Carbohydrates (grams)
Gumbo	10-oz. serving	70	10.0
& noodle	10-oz. serving	90	11.0
NoodleO's	10-oz. serving	90	11.0
With rice	10-oz. serving	80	9.0
With stars	10-oz. serving	70	9.0
& vegetables	10-oz. serving	90	10.0
Semi-condensed, Soup For One:			
& noodle	11-oz. serving	130	14.0
& vegetable, full flavored	11-oz. serving	120	13.0
(College Inn) broth	1 cup	35	0.
(Swanson) broth	7½-oz. can	35	1.0
Canned, dietetic or low calorie:			
(Campbell) *Chunky,* low sodium	7¾-oz. can	160	14.0
(Dia-Mel):			
Broth	8-oz. serving	18	1.0
& noodle	8-oz. serving	50	7.0
Mix:			
Carmel Kosher	6 fl. oz.	12	1.8
(Lipton):			
Regular:			
Giggle Noodle	1 cup (8 fl. oz.)	80	12.0
& noodle, with broth	1 cup	60	8.0
& noodle, with meat	1 cup	50	1.0
& rice	1 cup	60	8.0
Ring-O-Noodle	1 cup	60	9.0
Ripple Noodle	1 cup	80	12.0
Cup-A-Broth	6 fl. oz.	25	4.0
Cup-A-Soup:			
Cream of	6 fl. oz.	80	9.0
Giggle Noodle	6 fl. oz.	40	8.0
& noodle, with meat	6 fl. oz.	45	6.0
& rice	6 fl. oz.	45	7.0
Ring-o-Noodle	6 fl. oz.	50	9.0
& vegetable	6 fl. oz.	40	7.0

(USDA): United States Department of Agriculture
(HEW/FAO): Health, Education and Welfare/Food and Agriculture Organization
* Prepared as Package Directs

Food and Description	Measure or Quantity	Calories	Carbo-hydrates (grams)
CHICKEN SPREAD, canned:			
(Swanson)	1-oz. serving	70	1.0
(Underwood)	½ of 4¾-oz. can	150	3.0
CHICKEN STEW:			
Canned, regular pack:			
(Libby's) with dumplings	⅓ of 24-oz. can	194	20.2
(Swanson)	7⅝-oz. serving	170	16.0
Canned, dietetic or low calorie			
(Dia-Mel)	8-oz. can	150	19.0
CHICKEN STOCK BASE			
(French's)	1 tsp. (3 grams)	8	1.0
CHICK'N QUICK, frozen			
(Tyson):			
Breast pattie	¼ of 12-oz. pkg.	240	11.0
Breast fillet	¼ of 12-oz. pkg.	210	12.0
Chick'N Cheddar	¼ of 12-oz. pkg.	250	12.0
Italian Hoagie	¼ of 12-oz. pkg.	240	12.0
Turkey breast pattie	¼ of 12-oz. pkg.	210	11.0
CHICK PEAS or GARBANZOS, dry (USDA)	1 cup (7.1 oz.)	720	122.0
CHICORY GREENS, raw (USDA):			
Untrimmed	½ lb. (weighed untrimmed)	37	7.0
Trimmed	4 oz.	23	4.3
CHICORY, WITLOOF, Belgian or French endive, raw, bleached head (USDA):			
Untrimmed	½ lb. (weighed untrimmed)	30	6.4
Trimmed, cut	½ cup (1.6 oz.)	7	1.4
CHILI or CHILI CON CARNE:			
Canned, beans only:			
(Blue Boy)	1 cup	290	46.0
(Van Camp) Mexican style	1 cup	250	43.0

CHILI SAUCE [107]

Food and Description	Measure or Quantity	Calories	Carbo-hydrates (grams)
Canned, regular pack, with beans:			
(USDA)	1 cup (8.8 oz.)	330	31.1
(Bounty)	7¾-oz. can	310	29.3
(Hormel):			
Regular	7½-oz. serving	321	23.6
Short Orders, regular	7½-oz. can	300	24.0
Short Orders, hot	7½-oz. can	300	23.0
(Libby's)	½ of 15-oz. can	293	32.2
(Morton House)	7½-oz. can	340	27.0
(Nalley's) mild or hot	8-oz. serving	314	27.3
(Swanson)	½ of 15½-oz. can	310	28.0
Canned, dietetic or low calorie, with beans (Dia-Mel)	8-oz. can	360	31.0
Canned, regular pack, without beans:			
(USDA)	1 cup (9 oz.)	510	14.8
(Hormel):			
Regular	7½-oz. serving	345	7.6
Short Orders	7½-oz. cup	370	11.0
(Libby's)	½ of 15-oz. can	276	32.2
(Morton House)	½ of 15-oz. can	340	14.0
(Nalley's):			
Regular	8-oz. serving	209	15.9
Big Chunk	7½-oz. can	383	19.2
Frozen, with beans:			
(Stouffer's)	8¾-oz. pkg.	272	25.9
(Weight Watchers) one-compartment	10-oz. meal	295	32.9
CHILI BEEF SOUP, canned (Campbell):			
Chunky	9¾-oz. can	260	33.0
Chunky	11-oz. can	300	37.0
*Condensed	11-oz. serving	180	23.0
CHILI SAUCE:			
Regular:			
(USDA)	1 T. (.5 oz.)	16	3.7

(USDA): United States Department of Agriculture
(HEW/FAO): Health, Education and Welfare/Food and Agriculture Organization
* Prepared as Package Directs

Food and Description	Measure or Quantity	Calories	Carbo-hydrates (grams)
(Ortega) green	1-oz. serving	6	1.1
Dietetic:			
(USDA) low sodium	1 T. (.5 oz.)	16	3.7
(Featherweight)	1 T. (.5 oz.)	8	2.0
CHILI SEASONING MIX:			
*(Durkee)	1 cup	465	31.2
(French's) *Chili-O*	1¾-oz. pkg.	150	30.0
CHINESE DATE (See **JUJUBE**)			
CHINESE DINNER, frozen (See individual listings such as **CHOP SUEY, CHOW MEIN,** etc.)			
CHIPS (See **POTATO CHIPS** or **CRACKERS, PUFFS and CHIPS**)			
CHIVES, raw (USDA)	½ lb.	64	13.2
CHOCO-DILES (Hostess)	2.2-oz. piece	259	37.5
CHOCOLATE, BAKING:			
(Baker's):			
Bitter or unsweetened	1-oz. square	176	8.6
Bitter or unsweetened, *Redi-Blend*	1-oz. square	140	8.0
Semi-sweet:			
Regular	1-oz. square	153	16.7
Chips	2½ tsps. (1 oz.)	147	19.7
Sweetened	1-oz. square	153	16.7
(Hershey's):			
Bitter or unsweetened	1-oz. square	188	6.8
Semi-sweet, chips	1 oz.	150	17.3
Sweetened, chips:			
Dark, regular or mini	1 oz.	151	17.8
Milk	1 oz.	148	18.2
(Nestlé):			
Bitter or unsweetened, *Choco-Bake*	1-oz. packet	170	12.0

Food and Description	Measure or Quantity	Calories	Carbo-hydrates (grams)
Semi-sweet, morsels	1 oz.	150	17.0
Sweetened, milk, morsels	1 oz.	150	17.0

CHOCOLATE CAKE (See **CAKE,** Chocolate)

CHOCOLATE CANDY (See **CANDY**)

CHOCOLATE EXTRACT

(Ehlers) imitation	1 tsp.	10	DNA

CHOCOLATE, HOT, home

recipe (USDA)	1 cup (8.8 oz.)	238	26.0

CHOCOLATE ICE CREAM:

(Baskin-Robbins):			
Regular	1 scoop (2½ oz.)	165	20.4
Fudge	1 scoop (2½ oz.)	178	21.3
(Good Humor):			
Regular	4-fl. oz.	130	15.0
Chip	4-fl. oz.	150	15.0
(Meadow Gold)	¼ pt.	140	18.0
(Sealtest)	¼ pt.	140	17.0
(Swift's) sweet cream	½ cup (2.3 oz.)	129	15.8

CHOCOLATE PIE (See **PIE,** Chocolate)

CHOCOLATE PUDDING or PIE FILLING (See **PUDDING or PIE FILLING,** Chocolate)

CHOCOLATE SYRUP (See **SYRUP,** Chocolate)

CHOP SUEY:

Home recipe (USDA) with meat	1 cup (8.8 oz.)	300	12.8
Canned (USDA) with meat	1 cup (8.8 oz.)	155	10.5

(USDA): United States Department of Agriculture
(HEW/FAO): Health, Education and Welfare/Food and Agriculture Organization
* Prepared as Package Directs

Food and Description	Measure or Quantity	Calories	Carbo-hydrates (grams)
Frozen:			
(Banquet) beef:			
Buffet Supper	2-lb. pkg.	418	39.1
Cookin' Bag	7-oz. pkg.	73	9.5
Dinner	12-oz. dinner	282	38.8
(Stouffer's) beef, with rice	12-oz. pkg.	355	47.7
*Mix (Durkee)	1¾ cups	557	21.0
CHOW CHOW (USDA):			
Sour	1 oz.	8	1.2
Sweet	1 oz.	33	7.7
CHOWDER:			
Canned, regular pack:			
Beef & vegetable (Hormel)	7½-oz. can	120	15.0
Chicken & corn (Hormel)	7½-oz. can	130	15.0
Clam:			
Manhattan-style:			
(Campbell):			
Chunky	9½-oz. can	160	23.0
Chunky	10¾-oz. can	180	26.0
*Condensed	10-oz. serving	90	15.0
(Crosse & Blackwell)	½ of 13-oz. can	50	9.0
New England-style:			
*(Campbell):			
Condensed:			
Made with milk	10-oz. serving	200	20.0
Made with water	10-oz. serving	100	13.0
Semi-condensed, *Soup For One:*			
Made with milk	11-oz. serving	200	21.0
Made with water	11-oz. serving	125	16.0
(Crosse & Blackwell)	½ of 13-oz. can	90	14.0
Ham & potato (Hormel)	7½-oz. can	130	14.0
CHOW MEIN:			
Home recipe (USDA) chicken, without noodles	8-oz. serving	231	9.1
Canned, regular pack:			
(Chun King):			
Beef, *Divider-Pak*	8-oz. serving	60	5.3
Chicken	8-oz. serving	60	6.7
Chicken, *Divider-Pak*	¼ of 42-oz. can	80	9.0

Food and Description	Measure or Quantity	Calories	Carbo-hydrates (grams)
Pork, *Divider-Pak*	¼ of 42-oz. can	110	7.0
Shrimp, *Divider-Pak*	¼ of 42-oz. can	70	8.0
(Hormel) pork, *Short Orders*	7½-oz. can	140	13.0
(La Choy):			
Beef	1 cup	72	5.7
*Beef, bi-pack	1 cup	83	10.3
Chicken	1 cup	68	5.0
*Chicken, bi-pack	1 cup	101	9.3
Meatless	1 cup (1-lb. can)	47	5.9
*Mushroom, bi-pack	1 cup	85	10.7
Pepper oriental	1 cup	89	10.2
*Pepper oriental, bi-pack	1 cup	89	11.1
*Pork, bi-pack	1 cup	120	10.6
Shrimp	1 cup	61	5.7
*Shrimp, bi-pack	1 cup	110	9.7
Frozen:			
(Banquet) chicken:			
Buffet Supper	2-lb. pkg.	345	36.4
Cookin' Bag	7-oz. pkg.	89	9.7
Dinner	12-oz. dinner	282	38.8
(Chun King):			
Chicken:			
Dinner	11-oz. dinner	320	43.0
Dinner, with sweet and sour pork	13-oz. dinner	390	52.0
Pouch	½ of 12-oz. pkg.	90	12.0
Shrimp:			
Dinner	11-oz. dinner	300	43.0
Dinner, with beef pepper oriental	13-oz. dinner	350	51.0
Pouch	½ of 12-oz. pkg.	80	10.0
(Green Giant) chicken, without noodles	9-oz. entree	126	14.8
(La Choy):			
Beef, 5-compartment	11-oz. dinner	337	52.8
Chicken	11-oz. dinner	356	53.8
Pepper oriental, 5-compartment	11-oz. dinner	333	54.6

(USDA): United States Department of Agriculture
(HEW/FAO): Health, Education and Welfare/Food and Agriculture Organization
* Prepared as Package Directs

Food and Description	Measure or Quantity	Calories	Carbo-hydrates (grams)
Shrimp, 5-compartment (Stouffer's) chicken,	11-oz. dinner	324	55.4
without noodles	8-oz. pkg.	145	10.0
CHOW MEIN NOODLES (See **NOODLES, CHOW MEIN**)			
CHUB, raw (USDA):			
Whole	1 lb. (weighed whole)	217	0.
Meat only	4 oz.	164	0.
CIDER (See **APPLE CIDER**)			
CINNAMON, GROUND:			
(USDA)	1 tsp. (2.3 grams)	6	1.8
(French's)	1 tsp. (1.7 grams)	6	1.4
CINNAMON SUGAR (French's)	1 tsp.	16	4.0
CITRON, CANDIED (USDA)	1 oz.	89	22.7
CLAM:			
Raw (USDA):			
Hard or round:			
Meat & liq.	1 lb. (weighed in shell)	71	6.1
Meat only	1 cup (8 oz.)	182	13.4
Soft:			
Meat & liq.	1 lb. (weighed in shell)	142	5.3
Meat only	1 cup (8 oz.)	186	3.0
Canned (Doxsee) all kinds:			
Chopped & minced, solids & liq.	4 oz.	59	3.2
Chopped, meat only	4 oz.	111	2.1
Steamed, meat & broth	1 pt. (8 fl. oz.)	152	DNA
Steamed, meat only	1 pt. (8 fl. oz.)	66	DNA
CLAMATO COCKTAIL, canned (Mott's)	6 fl. oz.	80	19.0

Food and Description	Measure or Quantity	Calories	Carbo-hydrates (grams)
CLAM CHOWDER (See **CHOWDER,** Clam)			
CLAM JUICE, canned (USDA)	1 cup (8.3 oz.)	45	5.0
CLAM SANDWICH, frozen (Mrs. Paul's) fried	4½-oz. sandwich	419	54.3
CLARET WINE:			
(Louis M. Martini) 12½% alcohol	3 fl. oz.	90	.2
(Taylor) 12½% alcohol	3 fl. oz.	72	2.4
CLORETS:			
Chewing gum	1 piece	6	1.3
Mint	1 piece	6	1.6
CLOVE, GROUND (French's)	1 tsp. (1.7 grams)	7	1.2
CLUB SODA (See **SOFT DRINK**)			
COCOA:			
Dry:			
(USDA):			
Low fat	1 T. (5 grams)	10	3.1
Medium-low fat	1 T. (5 grams)	12	2.9
Medium-high fat	1 T. (5 grams)	14	2.8
High fat	1 T.	16	2.6
(Hershey's) unsweetened, American process	⅓ cup (1 oz.)	116	13.0
Home recipe (USDA)	1 cup (8.8 oz.)	242	27.2
Mix, regular pack:			
*(Alba '66) instant, low fat, regular and chocolate with marshmallow flavor	6 fl. oz.	60	11.0

(USDA): United States Department of Agriculture
(HEW/FAO): Health, Education and Welfare/Food and Agriculture Organization
* Prepared as Package Directs

Food and Description	Measure or Quantity	Calories	Carbo-hydrates (grams)
(Carnation) instant:			
Chocolate & artificial			
marshmallow	1-oz. pkg.	112	22.0
Milk chocolate	1-oz. pkg.	112	22.0
Rich chocolate	1-oz. pkg.	112	22.0
(Hershey's)			
Hot	1-oz. packet	115	21.0
Instant	3 T. (¾ oz.)	76	17.0
(Nestlé) hot, regular or with			
marshmallows	1-oz. packet	110	23.0
(Ovaltine) hot'n rich	1 pkg.	120	22.0
Swiss Miss, instant:			
Milk	1-oz. packet	110	21.0
With mini marshmallows	6 fl. oz.	110	22.0
Mix, dietetic or low calorie:			
(Carnation) *70 Calorie*, with			
mini marshmallows or rich			
chocolate	.73-oz. packet	70	15.0
*(Featherweight) hot	6 fl. oz.	50	8.0
(Ovaltine) reduced calorie	.45-oz. packet	50	8.0
Swiss Miss, Lite	3 T.	70	17.0
COCOA KRISPIES, cereal			
(Kellogg's)	¾ cup (1 oz.)	110	25.0
COCONUT:			
Fresh (USDA):			
Whole	1 lb. (weighed in		
	shell)	816	22.2
Meat only	4 oz.	392	10.7
Meat only	2″ × 2″ × ½″ piece		
	(1.6 oz.)	156	4.2
Grated or shredded, loosely			
packed	½ cup (1.4 oz.)	225	6.1
Dried, canned or packaged:			
(Baker's):			
Angel Flake	¼ cup (.7 oz.)	95	7.9
Cookie	¼ cup (1 oz.)	137	12.2
Premium shred	¼ cup (.8 oz.)	100	9.0
Premium shred, Southern			
style	¼ cup (.74 oz.)	99	8.2
(Durkee) shredded	¼ cup	69	2.0

Food and Description	Measure or Quantity	Calories	Carbo-hydrates (grams)
COCO WHEATS, cereal	1 T. (.42 oz.)	44	9.1
COD (USDA):			
Raw:			
Whole	1 lb. (weighed whole)	110	0.
Meat only	4 oz.	88	0.
Broiled	4 oz.	193	0.
Canned	4 oz.	96	0.
Dehydrated, lightly salted	4 oz.	425	0.
Dried, salted	5½″ × 1½″ × ½″ (2.8 oz.)	104	0.
*COFFEE:			
Ground:			
(Chase & Sanborn) drip or electric perk; *Max-Pax;* (Maxwell House) regular or *Electra-Perk;* (Yuban) regular, drip or *Electra Matic*	6 fl. oz.	2	0.
Mellow Roast	6 fl. oz.	8	2.0
Decaffeinated:			
Brim, regular, drip or electric perk; *Sanka,* regular or electric perk	6 fl. oz.	2	0.
Brim, freeze-dried; *Decaf,* instant; *Nescafé,* freeze-dried; *Sanka,* freeze-dried or instant; *Taster's Choice,* freeze-dried	6 fl. oz.	4	1.0
Freeze-dried, *Maxim* or *Taster's Choice*	6 fl. oz.	4	1.0
Instant:			
(Chase & Sanborn)	5 fl. oz.	2	0.

(USDA): United States Department of Agriculture
(HEW/FAO): Health, Education and Welfare/Food and Agriculture Organization
* Prepared as Package Directs

Food and Description	Measure or Quantity	Calories	Carbo-hydrates (grams)
(General Foods)			
International Coffee:			
Café Français; Orange			
Cappuccino or *Suisse*			
Mocha	6 fl. oz.	60	7.0
Cafe Vienna	6 fl. oz.	60	11.0
Irish Mocha Mist	6 fl. oz.	50	7.0
(Maxwell House); *Nescafé:*			
Yuban	6 fl. oz.	4	1.0
Mellow Roast	6 fl. oz.	8	2.0
COFFEE CAKE (See **CAKE,** Coffee)			
COFFEE ICE CREAM (Breyer's)	¼ pt.	140	15.0
COFFEE SOUTHERN, liqueur	1 fl. oz.	79	8.8
COGNAC (See **DISTILLED LIQUOR**)			
COLA SOFT DRINK (See **SOFT DRINK,** Cola)			
COLD DUCK WINE:			
(Great Western) pink, 12% alcohol	3 fl. oz.	92	7.7
(Taylor) 12½% alcohol	3 fl. oz.	90	6.6
COLESLAW, solids & liq. (USDA):			
Prepared with commercial French dressing	4-oz. serving	108	8.6
Prepared with homemade French dressing	4-oz. serving	146	5.8
Prepared with mayonnaise	4-oz. serving	163	5.4
Prepared with mayonnaise type salad dressing	1 cup (4.2 oz.)	119	8.5
COLLARDS:			
Raw (USDA):			
Leaves, including stems	1 lb.	181	32.7

Food and Description	Measure or Quantity	Calories	Carbo-hydrates (grams)
Leaves only	½ lb.	70	11.6
Boiled (USDA) drained:			
Leaves, cooked in large amount of water	½ cup (3.4 oz.)	29	4.6
Leaves & stems, cooked in small amount of water	½ cup (3.4 oz.)	31	4.8
Canned (Sunshine) chopped, solids & liq.	½ cup (4.1 oz.)	25	3.8
Frozen:			
(USDA):			
Not thawed	10-oz. pkg.	91	16.4
Boiled, chopped, drained	½ cup (3 oz.)	26	4.8
(Birds Eye) chopped	⅓ of 10-oz. pkg.	25	4.0
(McKenzie) chopped	3⅓-oz. serving	31	4.3
(Seabrook Farms) chopped	⅓ of 10-oz. pkg.	31	4.3
(Southland) chopped	⅓ of 16-oz. pkg.	30	5.0
COLLINS MIXER (See **SOFT DRINK,** Tom Collins)			
COMPLETE CEREAL (Elam's)	1-oz. serving	109	17.5
CONCORD WINE:			
(Gold Seal) 13-14% alcohol	3 fl. oz.	125	9.8
(Mogen David) 12% alcohol	3 fl. oz.	120	16.0
(Pleasant Valley) red, 12½% alcohol	3 fl. oz.	90	DNA
CONSOMME MADRILENE, canned (Crosse & Blackwell) clear or red	6½-oz. serving	25	4.0
COOKIE (Listed by type or brand name. See also **COOKIE, DIETETIC, COOKIE DOUGH, COOKIE, HOME RECIPE** and **COOKIE MIX**)			

(USDA): United States Department of Agriculture
(HEW/FAO): Health, Education and Welfare/Food and Agriculture Organization
* Prepared as Package Directs

Food and Description	Measure or Quantity	Calories	Carbo-hydrates (grams)
Almond Windmill (Nabisco)	1 piece	47	7.0
Animal:			
(Keebler):			
Regular	1 piece	12	1.9
100s, iced	1 piece	24	3.9
(Nabisco) *Barnum's Animals*	1 piece	12	1.9
Apple crisp (Nabisco)	1 piece	50	7.0
Assortment (Nabisco):			
Famous:			
Baronet, creme sandwich	1 piece	53	8.0
Biscos, sugar wafer	1 piece	50	6.7
Butter flavored	1 piece	28	4.2
Cameo, creme sandwich	1 piece	75	11.0
Kettle cookie	1 piece	35	5.2
Lorna Doone	1 piece	40	5.0
Oreo, chocolate sandwich	1 piece	50	7.3
Mayfair Assortment,			
English-style:			
Crown creme sandwich	1 piece	53	8.0
Fancy shortbread biscuit	1 piece	22	3.8
Filigree creme sandwich	1 piece	60	8.5
Mayfair creme sandwich	1 piece	64	9.0
Tea Rose creme sandwich	1 piece	53	7.7
Tea Time biscuit	1 piece	25	3.7
Brown edge wafer (Nabisco)	1 piece	28	4.2
Brownie:			
(Frito-Lay's) nut fudge	1.8-oz. piece	200	34.0
(Hostess):			
Large	2-oz. piece	251	38.6
Small	1¼-oz. piece	157	24.1
(Sara Lee) frozen	⅛ of 13-oz. pkg.	199	26.1
Butter (Nabisco)	1 piece	23	3.5
Buttercup (Keebler)	1 piece	24	3.7
Butterscotch chip (Nabisco)			
Bakers Bonus	1 piece	80	11.0
Caramel peanut log (Nabisco)			
Heyday	1 piece	120	13.0
Chocolate & chocolate covered:			
(Keebler) fudge covered fudge stripes	1 piece	54	7.0
(Nabisco):			
Famous chocolate wafer	1 piece	28	4.8

Food and Description	Measure or Quantity	Calories	Carbo-hydrates (grams)
Pinwheels, cake	1.1-oz. piece	140	21.0
Snaps	1 piece	16	2.8
Chocolate chip:			
(Keebler):			
C.C. Biggs	1 piece	56	7.0
Rich'n Chips	1 piece	81	10.0
(Nabisco):			
Chips Ahoy!	1 piece	53	7.0
Chocolate	1 piece	53	7.3
Coconut	1 piece	75	9.0
Cookie Little	1 piece	7	1.0
Snaps	1 piece	20	3.3
Coconut chocolate drop (Keebler)	1 piece	83	9.4
Cinnamon Treats (Nabisco)	1 piece	27	5.0
Coconut bar (Nabisco) Bakers Bonus	1 piece	43	5.3
Devil's food cake (Nabisco)	1 piece	50	10.5
Double chips fudge (Nabisco) Bakers Bonus	1 piece	80	11.0
Fig bar:			
(Keebler)	1 piece	74	14.0
(Nabisco):			
Fig Newtons	1 piece	60	11.0
Fig Wheats	1 piece	60	11.5
Gingersnap (Nabisco) old fashioned	1 piece	30	5.5
Ladyfinger (USDA)	3¼″ × 1¾″ × 1⅛″	40	7.1
Macaroon (Nabisco) soft	1 piece	95	11.5
Marshmallow (Nabisco):			
Mallomars	1 piece	60	8.5
Puffs, cocoa covered	1 piece	85	14.0
Sandwich	1 piece	30	5.7
Molasses (Nabisco) Pantry	1 piece	60	9.5
Nilla wafer (Nabisco)	1 piece	19	3.0
Oatmeal:			
(Keebler) old fashioned	1 piece	83	12.0

(USDA): United States Department of Agriculture
(HEW/FAO): Health, Education and Welfare/Food and Agriculture Organization
* Prepared as Package Directs

Food and Description	Measure or Quantity	Calories	Carbo-hydrates (grams)
(Nabisco):			
Bakers Bonus	1 piece	80	12.0
Cookie Little	1 piece	6	1.0
Party Grahams (Nabisco)	1 piece	47	6.0
Peanut or peanut butter (Nabisco):			
Biscos	1 piece	47	5.7
Cheese flavored	1 piece	35	4.3
Chocolate, Nutter	1 piece	57	7.3
Creme pattie	1 piece	35	3.8
Fudge	1 piece	50	6.7
Nutter Butter	1 piece	70	9.0
Peanut brittle (Nabisco)	1 piece	50	6.3
Pecan Sandies (Keebler)	1 piece	86	9.3
Piccolo (Nabisco)	1 piece	22	3.3
Raisin fruit biscuit (Nabisco)	1 piece	60	12.0
Raisin bar (Keebler) iced	1 piece	80	11.0
Sandwich:			
(Keebler):			
Chocolate fudge	1 piece	83	12.0
Elfwich	1 piece	55	8.1
Fudge creme	1 piece	55	8.3
Peanut butter	1 piece	64	16.0
Pitter Patter	1 piece	83	11.0
Vanilla, creme	1 piece	56	8.5
Vanilla, French	1 piece	83	12.0
(Nabisco):			
Brown edge	1 piece	80	10.0
Cameo creme	1 piece	70	10.5
Cheese flavored	1 piece	27	3.3
Gaity, fudge	1 piece	53	7.0
Malted milk peanut butter	1 piece	38	4.5
Mixed creme, Cookie Break	1 piece	53	7.3
Mystic, mint	1 piece	90	11.0
Oreo:			
Chocolate	1 piece	50	7.3
Double Stuf	1 piece	70	9.0
Vanilla, Cookie Break	1 piece	50	7.3
Shortbread (Nabisco):			
Cookie Little	1 piece	6	1.1
Lorna Doone	1 piece	40	5.0
Melt-A-Way	1 piece	70	8.0

Food and Description	Measure or Quantity	Calories	Carbo-hydrates (grams)
Pecan	1 piece	80	8.5
Striped	1 piece	50	6.3
Social Tea (Nabisco)	1 piece	22	3.5
Spiced wafers (Nabisco)	1 piece	33	5.8
Spiced Windmill (Keebler)	1 piece	60	9.2
Sugar rings (Nabisco) *Bakers Bonus*	1 piece	70	10.5
Sugar wafer:			
(Dutch Treat)	1 piece	49	6.3
(Dutch Twin)	1 piece	48	6.3
(Keebler) *Krisp Kreem*	1 piece	29	4.2
(Nabisco) *Biscos*	1 piece	19	2.6
Vanilla wafer (Keebler)	1 piece	19	2.6
Waffle creme:			
(Dutch Twin)	1 piece	45	5.7
(Nabisco) *Biscos*	1 piece	43	6.0
COOKIE, DIETETIC:			
Chocolate chip:			
(Estee)	1 piece	28	3.4
(Featherweight)	1 piece	40	4.0
Chocolate crescent			
(Featherweight)	1 piece	40	4.0
Coconut (Estee)	1 piece	25	2.7
Fudge (Estee)	1 piece	27	3.3
Lemon:			
(Estee) thin	1 piece	24	3.1
(Featherweight)	1 piece	40	4.0
Oatmeal raisin (Estee)	1 piece	23	3.3
Sandwich:			
(Estee):			
Regular	1 piece	50	8.0
Lemon	1 piece	60	8.0
(Featherweight)	1 piece	50	6.0
Vanilla:			
(Estee) thins	1 piece	24	3.1
(Featherweight)	1 piece	40	4.0

(USDA): United States Department of Agriculture
(HEW/FAO): Health, Education and Welfare/Food and Agriculture
Organization
* Prepared as Package Directs

Food and Description	Measure or Quantity	Calories	Carbo-hydrates (grams)
Wafer:			
(Estee):			
Assorted, creme	1 piece	35	4.2
Chocolate covered	1 piece	128	13.1
Chocolate creme	1 piece	24	2.8
Chocolate/strawberry	1 piece	87	10.0
Vanilla creme	1 piece	24	2.8
Vanilla, snack	1 piece	86	10.1
Wheat germ	1 piece	6	1.3
(Featherweight) creme,			
chocolate, pecan or vanilla	1 piece	40	4.0
COOKIE CRISP, cereal			
(Ralston-Purina) chocolate chip			
or vanilla	1 cup (1 oz.)	110	25.0
COOKIE DOUGH:			
Refrigerated:			
(USDA):			
Unbaked, plain	1 oz.	127	16.7
Baked, plain	1 oz.	141	18.4
*(Pillsbury) Slice'N Bake:			
Brownie, fudge	1 piece	250	39.0
Chocolate chip	1 piece	53	7.3
Oatmeal	1 piece	57	7.3
Oatmeal raisin	1 piece	53	7.3
Peanut butter	1 piece	57	6.3
Sugar	1 piece	60	7.7
*Frozen (Rich's):			
Chocolate chip	1 piece	138	20.3
Oatmeal	1 piece	125	18.3
Oatmeal with raisin	1 piece	122	19.1
Oatmeal, super jumbo	1 piece	317	46.2
Peanut butter	1 piece	128	14.6
Ranger	1 piece	130	17.0
Sugar	1 piece	118	17.4
COOKIE, HOME RECIPE			
(USDA):			
Brownie with nuts	1¾" × 1¾" × ⅞"	97	10.2
Chocolate chip	1 oz.	146	17.0
Sugar, soft, thick	1 oz.	126	19.3

Food and Description	Measure or Quantity	Calories	Carbo-hydrates (grams)
COOKIE MIX:			
Regular:			
Brownie:			
*(Betty Crocker):			
Chocolate chip butterscotch	1/16 of pkg.	130	21.0
Fudge:			
Regular size	1/16 of pkg.	150	22.0
Family size	1/24 of pkg.	130	21.0
Supreme	1/24 of pkg.	120	21.0
German chocolate	1/16 of pkg.	150	26.0
Walnut:			
Regular size	1/16 of pkg.	160	22.0
Family size	1/24 of pkg.	130	19.0
(Duncan Hines)	1/24 of pkg.	129	19.4
*(Nestlé)	1/22 of pkg.	150	22.0
*(Pillsbury):			
Fudge:			
Regular size	1/36 of pkg.	65	10.0
Family size	1/48 of pkg.	75	11.0
Walnut:			
Regular size	1/36 of pkg.	75	10.0
Family size	1/48 of pkg.	80	11.5
Chocolate:			
*(Betty Crocker) *Big Batch*, double chocolate	1 cookie	60	8.5
(Duncan Hines)	1/36 of pkg.	67	9.2
Chocolate chip:			
*(Betty Crocker) *Big Batch*	1 cookie	60	8.0
(Duncan Hines)	1/36 of pkg.	72	9.1
*(Nestlé)	1 cookie	60	7.5
*(Quaker)	1 cookie	75	8.5
Date bar (Betty Crocker)	1/32 of pkg.	60	9.0
*Macaroon, coconut (Betty Crocker)	1/24 of pkg.	80	10.0
Oatmeal:			
*(Betty Crocker) *Big Batch*	1 cookie	65	8.5

(USDA): United States Department of Agriculture
(HEW/FAO):   Health, Education and Welfare/Food and Agriculture Organization
* Prepared as Package Directs

Food and Description	Measure or Quantity	Calories	Carbo- hydrates (grams)
(Duncan Hines) raisin	⅓₆ of pkg.	68	9.1
*(Nestlé) raisin	1 cookie	60	9.0
*(Quaker)	1 cookie	66	9.4
Peanut Butter:			
*(Betty Crocker) *Big Batch:*			
Regular	1 cookie	65	7.0
With flavored chips	1 cookie	60	8.0
(Duncan Hines)	⅓₆ of pkg.	68	7.5
*(Nestlé)	1 cookie	65	7.5
*(Quaker)	1 cookie	75	8.0
Sugar:			
*(Betty Crocker) *Big Batch*	1 cookie	60	9.0
(Duncan Hines) golden	⅓₆ of pkg.	59	8.4
*(Nestlé)	1 cookie	65	8.5
Vienna Dream Bar (Betty Crocker)	¹⁄₂₄ of pkg.	90	10.0
*Dietetic (Dia-Mel) chocolate chip or oatmeal	2″ cookie	50	7.0
COOKING FATS (See **FAT**)			
COOKING SPRAY, *Mazola No Stick*	2-second spray	8	0.
CORDIAL (See individual kinds of liqueur by flavor or brand name)			
CORDON DE BORDEAUX, French Bordeaux, red or white (Chanson) 11½% alcohol	3 fl. oz.	60	6.3
CORIANDER SEED (French's)	1 tsp. (1.4 grams)	6	.8
CORN:			
Fresh, white or yellow (USDA):			
Raw:			
Untrimmed, on the cob	1 lb. (weighed in husk)	167	36.1

Food and Description	Measure or Quantity	Calories	Carbo- hydrates (grams)
Trimmed, on cob	1 lb. (husk removed)	240	55.1
Boiled:			
Kernels, cut from cob, drained	1 cup (5.8 oz.)	137	31.0
Whole	4.9-oz. ear (5″ × 1¾″)	70	16.2
Canned, regular pack:			
(USDA):			
Golden or yellow, whole kernel, solids & liq., vacuum pack	½ cup (3.7 oz.)	87	21.6
Golden or yellow, whole kernel, wet pack	½ cup (4.5 oz.)	84	20.1
Golden or yellow, whole kernel, drained solids, wet pack	½ cup (3 oz.)	72	16.4
White kernel, solids & liq.	½ cup (4.5 oz.)	84	20.1
White kernel, drained solids	½ cup (2.8 oz.)	70	16.4
White, whole kernel, drained liq., wet pack	4 oz.	29	7.8
Cream style	½ cup (4.4 oz.)	105	25.6
(Del Monte):			
Cream style:			
Golden, wet back	½ cup (4.4 oz.)	89	19.2
White, wet pack	½ cup (4.3 oz.)	97	21.3
Whole kernel:			
Golden, solids & liq.	½ cup (4 oz.)	78	16.6
Golden, drained solids	½ cup	100	21.3
Golden or yellow, vacuum pack	½ cup	101	21.6
White, solids & liq.	½ cup	78	16.6
White, drained solids	½ cup	102	21.4
(Festal):			
Cream style:			
Golden, wet pack	½ cup (4.4 oz.)	89	19.2
White, wet pack	½ cup (4.3 oz.)	97	21.3

(USDA): United States Department of Agriculture
(HEW/FAO): Health, Education and Welfare/Food and Agriculture
Organization
* Prepared as Package Directs

Food and Description	Measure or Quantity	Calories	Carbo-hydrates (grams)
Whole kernel:			
Golden or white, solids & liq.	½ cup	78	16.6
Golden or white, drained solids	½ cup	100	21.3
Golden or yellow, vacuum pack	½ cup	101	21.6
White, drained solids	½ cup	102	21.4
(Green Giant):			
Cream style, golden kernel	½ of 8½-oz. can	103	22.3
Whole kernel:			
Golden or yellow, solids & liq.	¼ of 17-oz. can	77	15.8
Golden or yellow, vacuum pack, *Niblets*	½ of 7-oz. can	82	17.1
Golden, solids & liq., *Mexicorn*	½ of 7-oz. can	85	17.8
(Kounty Kist):			
Cream style, golden kernel	½ of 8½-oz. can	106	23.2
Whole kernel:			
Golden, liquid pack, solids & liq.	½ of 7-oz. can	106	19.4
Golden, vacuum pack	½ cup	80	17.5
(Le Sueur) golden, whole kernel, solids & liq.	¼ of 17-oz. can	84	17.3
(Libby's):			
Cream style	½ cup	100	21.2
Whole kernel, solids & liq.	½ cup	92	18.8
(Lindy)			
Cream style, golden kernel	½ of 8-oz. can	106	23.2
Whole kernel:			
Golden, liquid pack, solids & liq.	½ of 7-oz. can	106	19.4
Golden, vacuum pack	½ cup	80	17.5
(Stokely-Van Camp):			
Cream style:			
Golden	½ cup	105	23.5
White	½ cup	110	24.5
Whole kernel:			
Golden or yellow, solids & liq.	½ cup (4.5 oz.)	90	19.5
Golden, vacuum pack	½ cup	120	26.5

Food and Description	Measure or Quantity	Calories	Carbo- hydrates (grams)
White, solids & liq.	½ cup	95	20.0
Canned, dietetic or low calorie: (USDA):			
Cream style	4 oz.	93	21.0
Whole kernel:			
White or yellow, solids & liq.	4 oz.	65	15.4
White or yellow, drained solids	4 oz.	86	20.4
(Diet Delight) whole kernel, solids & liq.	½ cup (4.4 oz.)	60	15.0
(Featherweight) whole kernel, solids & liq.	½ cup	80	16.0
(S&W) *Nutradiet:*			
Cream style, low sodium	½ cup	100	21.0
Whole kernel, solids & liq., low sodium	½ cup	80	15.0
Frozen:			
(USDA) boiled, drained	4 oz.	107	24.5
(Birds Eye):			
On the cob	1 ear (4.9 oz.)	130	28.0
On the cob, *Little Ears*	1 ear	70	16.0
Whole kernel, white	⅓ of 10-oz. pkg.	112	23.2
(Green Giant):			
On the cob	5½″ ear	155	32.7
On the cob, *Nibblers*	3″ ear	85	18.0
Cream style	⅓ of 10-oz. pkg.	72	15.2
Whole kernel:			
Mexicorn, in butter sauce	⅓ of 10-oz. pkg.	86	14.2
Niblets, in butter sauce	⅓ of 10-oz. pkg.	86	14.2
White	⅕ of 20-oz. pkg.	105	21.7
White, in butter sauce	⅓ of 10-oz. pkg.	89	15.2
(Kounty Kist) whole kernel, golden or white	⅕ of 20-oz. pkg.	105	21.6

(USDA): United States Department of Agriculture
(HEW/FAO): Health, Education and Welfare/Food and Agriculture Organization
* Prepared as Package Directs

Food and Description	Measure or Quantity	Calories	Carbo-hydrates (grams)
(McKenzie or Seabrook Farms):			
On the cob	5" ear	140	30.0
Whole kernel	⅓ of 10-oz. pkg.	97	19.9
CORNBREAD, HOME RECIPE (USDA):			
Corn pone, prepared with white, whole-ground cornmeal	4 oz.	231	41.1
Johnnycake, prepared with yellow, degermed cornmeal	4 oz.	303	51.6
Southern style, prepared with degermed cornmeal	2½" × 2½" × 1⅝" piece	186	28.8
Southern style, prepared with whole-ground cornmeal	4 oz.	235	33.0
Spoon bread, prepared with white, whole-ground cornmeal	4 oz.	221	19.2
CORNBREAD MIX:			
(USDA):			
Dry	1 oz.	122	20.1
*Prepared with egg and milk	2⅜" muffin (1.4 oz.)	130	20.0
*(Aunt Jemima)	⅙ of pkg.	220	34.0
*(Dromedary)	2" × 2" piece (1/16 of pkg.)	130	19.0
*(Pillsbury) *Ballard*	1/16 of pkg.	160	26.0
CORN CHEX (See **CHEX CEREAL**)			
CORN DOG, frozen:			
(Hormel):			
Regular	1 piece	230	22.0
Tater Dogs	1 piece	190	15.0
(Oscar Mayer)	1 piece	328	27.9
CORNED BEEF:			
Uncooked (USDA) boneless, medium fat	1 lb.	1329	0.

Food and Description	Measure or Quantity	Calories	Carbo-hydrates (grams)
Cooked (USDA) medium fat, boneless	4 oz.	422	0.
Canned:			
Dinty Moore (Hormel)	3-oz. serving	196	0.
(Libby's)	½ of 7-oz. can	244	1.9
Packaged:			
(Eckrich) sliced	1-oz. slice	41	.9
(Oscar Mayer) jellied loaf	1-oz. slice	44	0.
(Vienna):			
Brisket	1 oz.	88	0.
Flats	1 oz.	49	.1
CORNED BEEF HASH:			
Canned:			
(Libby's)	1 cup	454	31.1
Mary Kitchen (Hormel):			
Regular	7½-oz. serving	399	21.1
Short Orders	7½-oz. can	370	16.0
(Nalley's)	4-oz. serving	208	10.2
Frozen (Banquet)	10-oz. dinner	372	42.6
CORNED BEEF SPREAD			
(Underwood)	½ of 4½-oz. can	120	Tr.
CORN FLAKE CRUMBS			
(Kellogg's)	¼ cup	110	25.0
CORN FLAKES, cereal:			
Regular:			
(USDA):			
Regular	1 cup (1 oz.)	112	24.7
Crushed	1 cup (2.5 oz.)	270	59.7
Frosted	1 cup (1.4 oz.)	154	36.5
(Kellogg's):			
Regular	1½ cups (1 oz.)	110	25.0
Honey & Nut	¾ cup (1 oz.)	120	24.0
Sugar frosted	¾ cup (1 oz.)	110	26.0

(USDA): United States Department of Agriculture
(HEW/FAO):   Health, Education and Welfare/Food and Agriculture
               Organization
* Prepared as Package Directs

Food and Description	Measure or Quantity	Calories	Carbohydrates (grams)
King Kullen:			
Regular	1 cup (1 oz.)	107	24.3
Sugar frosted	¾ cup (1 oz.)	110	26.0
(Post) *Post Toasties*	1¼ cups (1 oz.)	107	25.4
Provigo	1 cup (1 oz.)	107	24.3
(Ralston Purina):			
Regular	1 cup (1 oz.)	110	25.0
Sugar frosted	¾ cup (1 oz.)	110	26.0
Rokeach	1 cup (1 oz.)	107	24.3
(Van Brode):			
Regular	1 cup (1 oz.)	107	24.3
Sugar toasted	¾ cup (1 oz.)	108	25.3
Low sodium:			
Nature Foods	1 cup (.8 oz.)	88	20.0
(Van Brode)	1¼ cups (1 oz.)	110	25.0

CORN FRITTER (See **FRITTER,** Corn)

CORN GRITS (See **HOMINY**)

CORNMEAL, WHITE or YELLOW:
Dry:			
Bolted:			
(USDA)	1 cup (4.3 oz.)	442	90.9
(Aunt Jemima/Quaker)	1 cup (4 oz.)	408	84.8
Degermed:			
(USDA)	1 cup (4.9 oz.)	502	108.2
(Aunt Jemima/Quaker)	1 cup (4 oz.)	404	88.8
Self-rising, degermed:			
(USDA)	1 cup (5 oz.)	491	105.9
(Aunt Jemima)	1 cup (6 oz.)	582	126.0
Self-rising, whole ground (USDA)	1 cup (5 oz.)	489	101.4
Whole ground, unbolted (USDA)	1 cup (4.3 oz.)	433	90.0
Cooked:			
(USDA)	1 cup (8.5 oz.)	120	25.7
(Albers) degermed	1 cup	119	25.5
Mix (Aunt Jemima/Quaker) bolted	1 cup (4 oz.)	392	80.4

Food and Description	Measure or Quantity	Calories	Carbo-hydrates (grams)
CORN PUDDING, home recipe (USDA)	1 cup (8.6 oz.)	255	31.9
CORN SALAD, raw (USDA):			
Untrimmed	1 lb. (weighed untrimmed)	91	15.7
Trimmed	4 oz.	24	4.1
CORNSTARCH:			
(USDA)	1 cup (4.5 oz.)	463	112.1
(Argo; Kuryea's or Kingsford's)	1 T. (9.5 grams)	34	8.3
CORN STICK (See **CORNBREAD**)			
CORN TOTAL, cereal (General Mills)	1 cup (1 oz.)	110	24.0
COTTAGE PUDDING, home recipe (USDA):			
Without sauce	2 oz.	195	30.8
With chocolate sauce	2 oz.	180	32.1
With strawberry sauce	2 oz.	166	27.4
COUGH DROP:			
(Beech-Nut)	1 drop (2 grams)	10	2.5
(H-B)	1 drop	8	1.9
(Luden's):			
Honey lemon	1 drop	8	DNA
Menthol	1 drop	9	2.1
Wild cherry	1 drop	9	DNA
(Pine Bros.)	1 drop (3 grams)	8	2.0
(Smith Brothers)	1 drop	7	2.1
COUNT CHOCULA, cereal (General Mills)	1 cup (1 oz.)	110	24.0

(USDA): United States Department of Agriculture
(HEW/FAO):   Health, Education and Welfare/Food and Agriculture
                        Organization
* Prepared as Package Directs

Food and Description	Measure or Quantity	Calories	Carbo-hydrates (grams)
COUNTRY CRISP, cereal (Post)	¾ cup (1 oz.)	114	24.4
COWPEA (USDA):			
Immature seeds:			
Raw, whole	1 lb. (weighed in pods)	317	54.4
Raw, shelled	½ cup (2.5 oz.)	92	15.8
Boiled, drained solids	½ cup (2.9 oz.)	89	15.0
Canned, solids & liq.	4 oz.	79	14.1
Frozen (See **BLACK-EYED PEAS,** frozen)			
Young pods with seeds:			
Raw, whole	1 lb. (weighed untrimmed)	182	39.2
Boiled, drained solids	4 oz.	39	7.9
Mature seeds, dry:			
Raw	1 lb.	1556	279.9
Raw	½ cup (3 oz.)	292	52.4
Boiled	½ cup (4.4 oz.)	95	17.2
CRAB, all species:			
Fresh (USDA):			
Steamed, whole	1 lb. (weighed in shell)	202	1.1
Steamed, meat only	4 oz.	105	.6
Canned (USDA) drained solids	4 oz.	115	1.2
Frozen:			
(Ship Ahoy) King crab	8-oz. pkg.	211	.6
(Wakefield's) Alaska King, thawed & drained	4 oz.	86	.7
CRAB APPLE, fresh (USDA):			
Whole	1 lb. (weighed whole)	284	74.3
Flesh only	4 oz.	77	20.2
CRABAPPLE JELLY, sweetened (Smucker's)	1 T.	53	13.5
CRABAPPLE PRESERVE or JAM, sweetened (Smucker's)	1 T.	53	13.5

Food and Description	Measure or Quantity	Calories	Carbo-hydrates (grams)
CRAB, DEVILED:			
Home recipe (USDA)	1 cup (8.5 oz.)	451	31.9
Frozen (Mrs. Paul's):			
Breaded & french-fried	3-oz. cake	154	17.0
Breaded & fried, miniatures	½ of 7-oz. pkg.	222	18.0
CRAB IMPERIAL, home recipe (USDA)	1 cup (7.8 oz.)	323	8.6
CRAB SOUP (Crosse & Blackwell)	½ of 13-oz. can	50	8.0
CRACKED WHEAT CEREAL (Elan's)	1 oz.	100	20.2
CRACKER, PUFFS and CHIPS (See also individual listings such as **POTATO CHIPS,** etc.)			
American Harvest (Nabisco)	1 piece (3 grams)	16	2.0
Arrowroot biscuit (Nabisco) *National*	1 piece (5 grams)	20	3.5
Bacon'n Dip (Nabisco)	1 piece	9	.9
Bacon flavored thins (Nabisco)	1 piece (2 grams)	11	1.2
Bacon toast (Keebler)	1 piece	16	2.0
Betcha Bacon	1 oz.	170	18.0
Biscos (Nabisco)	1 piece	19	2.6
Bugles (General Mills)	15 pieces (1 oz.)	150	17.0
Butter (USDA)	1 oz.	130	19.1
Butter thins (Nabisco)	1 piece (3 grams)	14	2.2
Cheese-flavored (See also individual brand names in this grouping):			
(USDA)	1 oz.	136	17.1
Bops (Nalley's)	1 oz.	147	13.6

(USDA): United States Department of Agriculture
(HEW/FAO): Health, Education and Welfare/Food and Agriculture Organization
* Prepared as Package Directs

Food and Description	Measure or Quantity	Calories	Carbo-hydrates (grams)
Cheddar Bitz (Frito-Lay's)	1 oz.	129	18.9
Cheddar triangles (Nabisco)	1 piece	9	.9
Cheese'n Crunch (Nabisco)	1 oz.	160	14.0
Cheese filled (Frito-Lay's)	1½ oz.	203	25.3
Chee•Tos, crunchy or puffed	1 oz.	160	15.0
Cheez Balls (Planters)	1 oz.	160	15.0
Cheez Curls (Planters)	1 oz.	160	15.0
Chip O'Cheddar (Schulze and Burch) *Flavor Kist*	1 oz.	130	17.0
Country cheddar 'n sesame (Nabisco)	1 piece	9	1.0
Dip In A Chip (Nabisco)	1 piece	10	1.1
Nacho cheese cracker (Keebler)	1 piece	11	1.1
Nips (Nabisco)	1 piece	5	.7
Swiss cheese cracker (Nabisco)	1 piece (1.9 grams)	10	1.1
Tid-Bit (Nabisco)	1 piece (< 1 gram)	5	.5
Twists:			
(Bachman):			
Baked	1 oz.	150	17.0
Fried	1 oz.	160	14.0
(Nalley's)	1 oz.	126	9.1
Cheese & peanut butter sandwich (USDA)	1 oz.	139	15.9
Chicken in a Biskit (Nabisco)	1 piece (2 grams)	11	1.1
Chipos (General Mills)	1 oz.	150	17.0
Chippers (Nabisco)	1 piece	15	1.7
Chipsters (Nabisco)	1 piece	2	.3
Club cracker (Keebler)	1 piece	15	2.1
Corn chips:			
(Bachman) regular or BBQ	1 oz.	150	15.0
Fritos:			
Regular	1 oz.	160	16.0
Barbecue-flavored	1 oz.	150	15.5
(Planters)	1 oz.	170	15.0
Corn Nuggets (Frito-Lay's)	1 oz.	128	21.2
Cornnuts	1 oz.	120	21.0
Corn nuts (Nalley's)	1 oz.	120	20.4

Food and Description	Measure or Quantity	Calories	Carbo- hydrates (grams)
Corn & Sesame Chips (Nabisco)	1 piece	10	.9
Creme wafer stocks (Nabisco)	1 piece	47	6.3
Crown Pilot (Nabisco)	1 piece (.6 oz.)	75	13.0
Diggers (Nabisco)	1 piece	4	.5
Dixies (Nabisco)	1 piece	8	.9
Doo Dads (Nabisco)	1 piece	2	.3
Escort (Nabisco)	1 piece	21	2.6
Flings (Nabisco)	1 piece (2 grams)	10	.9
Goldfish (Pepperidge Farm):			
Thins (cheese, lightly salted, rye or wheat)	1 piece (3.5 grams)	17	2.2
Tiny:			
Cheddar cheese; lightly salted, parmesan or pizza flavor	¼-oz. serving	35	4.0
Pretzel	¼-oz. serving	30	5.0
Graham:			
Flavor-Kist (Schulze and Burch) sugar-honey coated	1 double piece	57	10.0
(Keebler) chocolate or cocoa covered, deluxe	1 piece	43	5.6
(Nabisco):			
Regular	1 piece	30	5.3
Chocolate or cocoa covered:			
Regular	1 piece	57	7.0
Fancy Dip	1 piece	65	8.0
Party Grahams	1 piece	47	6.0
Sugar-honey coated, *Honey Maid*	1 piece	30	5.5
Matzo (See **MATZO**)			
Melba toast (See **MELBA TOAST**)			

(USDA): United States Department of Agriculture
(HEW/FAO): Health, Education and Welfare/Food and Agriculture Organization
* Prepared as Package Directs

Food and Description	Measure or Quantity	Calories	Carbohydrates (grams)
Meal Mates (Nabisco)	1 piece	22	3.2
Milk Lunch Biscuit (Keebler)	1 piece	27	4.5
Mucho Macho Nacho (Schulze and Burch) *Flavor Kist*	1 oz.	121	18.0
Onion flavored:			
(Keebler) onion toast	1 piece	15	2.1
(Nabisco) french	1 piece	13	1.5
Oyster:			
(USDA)	10 pieces (.4 oz.)	33	5.3
(USDA)	1 cup (1 oz.)	124	20.0
(Keebler) *Zesta*	1 piece	2	.3
(Nabisco):			
Dandy	1 piece	3	.5
Oysterettes	1 piece	3	.6
Pumpernickel toast (Keebler)	1 piece	15	2.1
Ritz (Nabisco)	1 piece (3 grams)	17	2.0
Roman Meal Wafer:			
Boxed	1 piece (2.2 grams)	11	1.3
Cellophane wrapped	1 piece (3.5 grams)	14	2.4
Royal Lunch (Nabisco)	1 piece (1.7 grams)	55	8.0
Rusk (Nabisco) *Holland*	1 piece	40	7.5
Rye toast (Keebler)	1 piece	16	2.1
Saltine:			
Flavor Kist (Schulze and Burch)	1 piece	12	2.0
(Keebler) *Zesta*, salted or unsalted	1 piece	13	3.1
(Nabisco) *Premium* salted or unsalted	1 piece	12	2.0
Sea Rounds (Nabisco)	1 piece	45	7.5
Sea Toast (Keebler)	1 piece	60	10.0
Sesame:			
Flavor Kist (Schulze and Burch)	1 oz.	134	18.0
(Keebler):			
Sticks	1 piece	6	.8
Toast	1 piece	15	2.0
(Nabisco):			
Buttery flavored	1 piece	17	1.9
Sesame Wheats!	1 piece	17	1.8

Food and Description	Measure or Quantity	Calories	Carbo- hydrates (grams)
Sesame & poppyseed (Keebler)	1 piece	12	1.5
Shindigs (Keebler)	1 piece	6	.9
Snackin' Crisp (Durkee)			
O&C	1 oz.	155	15.0
Snacks Ahoy (Nabisco)	1 piece	9	1.1
Snack Sticks (Pepperidge Farm):			
Lightly salted	1 oz.	120	18.0
Pumpernickel	1 oz.	110	17.0
Sesame	1 oz.	120	16.0
Wheat	1 oz.	110	17.0
Sociables (Nabisco)	1 piece (2 grams)	11	1.3
Soda:			
(USDA)	1 oz.	124	20.0
(USDA)	2½" sq. (6 grams)	24	3.9
Gitano (Nabisco)	1 piece	15	2.5
Table water cracker (Carr's):			
Small size	1 piece (.2 oz.)	15	2.6
Large size	1 piece (.3 oz.)	32	5.9
Tortilla chip:			
(Bachman):			
Nacho or taco cheese flavor	1 oz.	140	17.0
Toasted	1 oz.	140	16.0
Buenos (Nabisco):			
Nacho cheese flavor	1 piece	11	1.2
Sour cream & onion flavor	1 piece	11	1.3
Doritos, nacho or taco cheese flavor	1 oz.	140	18.0
(Nabisco):			
Nacho cheese flavor	1 piece (2.8 grams)	12	1.3
Toasted corn	1 piece	11	1.4
(Nalley's)	1 oz.	147	17.6
Tostitos, round	1 oz.	140	17.0

(USDA): United States Department of Agriculture
(HEW/FAO): Health, Education and Welfare/Food and Agriculture Organization
* Prepared as Package Directs

Food and Description	Measure or Quantity	Calories	Carbo-hydrates (grams)
Town House (Keebler)	1 piece	16	1.8
Triscuit (Nabisco)	1 piece	20	3.0
Twiddle Sticks (Nabisco)	1 piece	53	7.0
Twigs (Nabisco)	1 piece	14	1.6
Uneeda Biscuit (Nabisco) unsalted tops	1 piece (5 grams)	22	3.7
Vegetable thins (Nabisco)	1 piece	12	1.3
Waldorf (Keebler)	1 piece	14	2.3
Waverly Wafer (Nabisco)	1 piece (4 grams)	18	2.6
Wheat chips (Nabisco)	1 piece	4	.5
Wheat crisps (Keebler)	1 piece	13	1.7
Wheatmeal biscuit (Carr's):			
Small size	1 piece (.3 oz.)	42	5.9
Large size	1 piece (.5 oz.)	66	9.4
Wheat snacks (Schulze and Burch) *Flavor Kist:*			
Natural	1 oz.	138	16.0
Rye	1 oz.	130	17.0
Wild onion	1 oz.	125	18.0
Wheatsworth (Nabisco)	1 piece	14	1.8
Wheat Thins (Nabisco)	1 piece (2 grams)	10	1.2
Wheat Toast (Keebler)	1 piece	15	2.0
CRACKER CRUMBS, GRAHAM:			
(USDA)	1 cup (3 oz.)	330	63.0
(Nabisco)	1/8 of 9" pie shell (.6 oz.)	70	12.0
(Nabisco)	1 cup (3 oz.)	350	60.0
CRACKER MEAL:			
(USDA)	1 T. (.4 oz.)	44	7.1
(Nabisco)	1/2 cup (2 oz.)	220	47.5
CRANAPPLE juice drink (Ocean Spray):			
Canned:			
Regular pack	6 fl. oz.	129	32.1
Low calorie or dietetic	6 fl. oz.	32	7.4
*Frozen	6 fl. oz.	119	29.5

Food and Description	Measure or Quantity	Calories	Carbo-hydrates (grams)
CRANBERRY:			
Fresh:			
(USDA):			
Untrimmed	1 lb. (weighed with stems)	200	47.0
Trimmed, stems removed	1 cup (4 oz.)	52	12.2
(Ocean Spray)	½ cup (2 oz.)	25	6.1
Dehydrated (USDA)	1 oz.	104	23.9
*CRANBERRY-APPLE JUICE,			
frozen (Welch's)	6 fl. oz.	120	30.0
*CRANBERRY-GRAPE JUICE, frozen (Welch's)	6 fl. oz.	110	27.0
CRANBERRY JUICE COCKTAIL:			
Canned (Ocean Spray):			
Regular	6 fl. oz.	106	26.4
Low calorie	6 fl. oz.	36	8.3
*Frozen (Welch's)	6 fl. oz.	100	26.0
CRANBERRY-ORANGE RELISH, uncooked (USDA)	4 oz.	202	51.5
CRANBERRY-RASPBERRY SAUCE, canned (Ocean Spray)			
jellied	2-oz. serving	85	20.8
CRANBERRY SAUCE:			
Home recipe (USDA)			
sweetened, unstrained	4 oz.	202	51.6
Canned:			
(USDA) sweetened, strained	½ cup (4.8 oz.)	199	51.0
(Ocean Spray):			
Jellied	2-oz. serving	88	21.7
Whole berry	2-oz. serving	89	22.0

(USDA): United States Department of Agriculture
(HEW/FAO): Health, Education and Welfare/Food and Agriculture
Organization
* Prepared as Package Directs

Food and Description	Measure or Quantity	Calories	Carbo-hydrates (grams)
CRANGRAPE, drink (Ocean Spray)	6 fl. oz.	108	26.3
CRANICOT, drink (Ocean Spray)	6 fl. oz.	123	30.4
CRAN-ORANGE RELISH, canned (Ocean Spray)	2-oz. serving	104	25.8
CRANPRUNE JUICE DRINK (Ocean Spray)	6 fl. oz.	117	28.8
CRAN-RASPBERRY SAUCE, canned (Ocean Spray) jellied	2-oz. serving	89	20.8
CRAPPIE, white, raw, meat only (USDA)	4 oz.	90	0.
CRAYFISH, freshwater (USDA):			
Raw, in shell	1 lb. (weighed in shell)	39	.7
Raw, meat only	4 oz.	82	1.4
CRAZY COW, cereal (General Mills):			
Chocolate	1 cup (1 oz.)	110	24.0
Strawberry	1 cup (1 oz.)	110	25.0
CREAM (See also **CREAM SUBSTITUTE**):			
Half & Half (Dairylea)	1 fl. oz.	40	1.0
Light, table or coffee:			
(USDA)	1 T. (.5 oz.)	32	.6
(Sealtest) 16% fat	1 T. (.5 oz.)	26	.6
Light whipping:			
(USDA)	1 cup (8.4 oz.)	717	8.6
(USDA)	1 T. (.5 oz.)	45	.5
(Sealtest) 30% fat	1 T. (.5 oz.)	45	1.0
Heavy whipping (unwhipped):			
(USDA)	1 cup (8.4 oz.)	838	7.4
(Dairylea)	1 fl. oz.	60	1.0
Sour:			
(USDA)	1 cup (8.1 oz.)	485	9.9

Food and Description	Measure or Quantity	Calories	Carbohydrates (grams)
(Dairylea)	1 oz.	60	1.0
Sour, imitation (Pet)	1 T. (.5 oz.)	25	1.0
CREAM PUFF:			
Home recipe (USDA) with custard filling	3½″ × 2″ piece (4.6 oz.)	303	26.7
Frozen (Rich's):			
Bavarian	1⅓-oz. piece	145	17.4
Chocolate	1⅓-oz. piece	146	16.9
***CREAMSICLE*,** orange (Popsicle Industries)	2½ fl.-oz. bar	80	13.0
CREAM SUBSTITUTE:			
(USDA):			
Liquid, frozen	1 T. (.5 oz.)	20	2.0
Powdered	1 tsp. (2 grams)	10	1.0
(Alba) *Dairy Light*	2.8-oz. envelope	10	1.0
(Carnation) *Coffee-mate*	1 tsp. (1.9 grams)	11	1.1
Coffee Rich, frozen, liquid	½ oz.	22	2.1
N-Rich	1½ tsp. (3 grams)	16	1.6
(Pet) non-dairy	1 tsp. (2 grams)	10	1.0
CREAM OF WHEAT, cereal:			
*Instant	1 T. (1 oz.)	40	8.8
*Mix'n Eat:			
Regular	1-oz. packet	140	24.0
Baked apple & cinnamon	1¼-oz. packet	170	32.0
Banana & spice	1¼-oz. packet	170	32.0
Maple & brown sugar	1¼-oz. packet	170	32.0
Quick, dry	1 T.	40	8.8
Regular	1 T.	40	8.8
CREME DE BANANA LIQUEUR (Mr. Boston)	1 fl. oz.	93	12.0

(USDA): United States Department of Agriculture
(HEW/FAO):   Health, Education and Welfare/Food and Agriculture
                        Organization
* Prepared as Package Directs

Food and Description	Measure or Quantity	Calories	Carbohydrates (grams)
CREME DE CACAO			
LIQUEUR (Mr. Boston):			
Brown	1 fl. oz.	102	14.3
White	1 fl. oz.	93	12.0
CREME DE CAFE LIQUEUR			
(Leroux) 60 proof	1 fl. oz.	104	13.6
CREME DE CASSIS			
LIQUEUR (Mr. Boston)	1 fl. oz.	85	14.1
CREME DE MENTHE			
LIQUEUR, green or white:			
(Garnier)	1 fl. oz.	110	15.3
(Leroux):			
Green	1 fl. oz.	110	15.2
White	1 fl. oz.	101	12.8
(Mr. Boston):			
Green	1 fl. oz.	109	16.0
White	1 fl. oz.	97	13.0
CREME DE NOYAUX			
LIQUEUR (Mr. Boston)	1 fl. oz.	99	13.5
CREPE, frozen:			
(Mrs. Paul's):			
Crab	½ of 5½-oz. pkg.	124	12.3
Shrimp	½ of 5½-oz. pkg.	126	11.9
(Stouffer's):			
Beef burgundy	6¼-oz. pkg.	335	24.0
Chicken with mushroom sauce	8¼-oz. pkg.	390	19.0
Ham & asparagus	6¼-oz. pkg.	325	21.0
Mushroom	6¼-oz. pkg.	255	27.0
CRISP RICE, cereal:			
Regular:			
Breakfast Best:			
Regular	1 cup (1 oz.)	107	24.3
Sugar toasted	⅝ cup (1 oz.)	108	25.3
(Ralston Purina)	1 cup (1 oz.)	110	25.0
Rokeach	1 cup (1 oz.)	107	24.9

CUCUMBER [143]

Food and Description	Measure or Quantity	Calories	Carbo-hydrates (grams)
(Van Brode):			
Regular	1 cup (1 oz.)	107	24.9
Cocoa-covered	¾ cup (1 oz.)	108	25.3
Sugar toasted	⅝ cup (1 oz.)	108	25.3
Low sodium:			
Nature Foods	1 cup (1 oz.)	110	25.6
(Van Brode)	1 cup (1 oz.)	110	25.6
CRISPY WHEATS'N RAISINS, cereal (General Mills)	¾ cup (1 oz.)	110	23.0
CROAKER (USDA):			
Atlantic:			
Raw, whole	1 lb. (weighed whole)	148	0.
Raw, meat only	4 oz.	109	0.
Baked	4 oz.	151	0.
White, raw, meat only	4 oz.	95	0.
Yellowfin, raw, meat only	4 oz.	101	0.
CROUTON:			
(Arnold):			
American style	½ oz.	66	8.7
Danish style	½ oz.	67	8.8
Italian or Mexican style	½ oz.	66	9.1
(Kellogg's) *Croutettes*	⅔ cup (.7 oz.)	70	14.0
CRULLER (See **DOUGHNUT**)			
CUCUMBER, fresh (USDA):			
Eaten with skin	½ lb. (weighed whole)	32	7.4
Eaten without skin	½ lb. (weighed with skin)	23	5.3
Unpared, 10-oz. cucumber	7½″ × 2″ pared cucumber (7.3 oz.)	29	6.6

(USDA): United States Department of Agriculture
(HEW/FAO): Health, Education and Welfare/Food and Agriculture Organization
* Prepared as Package Directs

Food and Description	Measure or Quantity	Calories	Carbo-hydrates (grams)
Pared	6 slices (2″ × ⅛″)	7	1.6
Pared and diced	½ cup (2.5 oz.)	10	2.3
CUMIN SEED (French's)	1 tsp. (1.6 oz.)	7	.7
CUPCAKE:			
Home recipe (USDA):			
Without icing	1.4-oz. cupcake	146	22.4
With chocolate icing	1.8-oz. cupcake	184	29.7
With boiled white icing	1.8-oz. cupcake	176	30.9
With uncooked white icing	1.8-oz. cupcake	184	31.6
Commercial type (Hostess):			
Chocolate	1¾-oz. cupcake	166	29.8
Orange	1½-oz. cupcake	151	26.8
Frozen (Sara Lee) yellow	1¾-oz. cupcake	190	31.5
*CUPCAKE MIX (Flako)	¹⁄₁₂ of pkg.	150	25.0
CUP O'NOODLES (Nissin Foods):			
Beef:			
Regular	2½-oz. serving	343	39.2
Twin pack	1.2-oz. serving	151	18.2
Beef onion:			
Regular	2½-oz. serving	323	36.8
Twin pack	1.2-oz. serving	158	19.4
Chicken:			
Regular	2½-oz. serving	343	40.0
Twin pack	1.2-oz. serving	155	18.6
Pork	2½-oz. serving	331	40.7
Shrimp	2½-oz. serving	336	40.0
CURACAO LIQUEUR:			
(Garnier) 60 proof	1 fl. oz.	100	12.7
(Hiram Walker) 60 proof	1 fl. oz.	84	9.5
(Leroux) 60 proof	1 fl. oz.	84	9.5
CURRANT:			
Fresh (USDA):			
Black European:			
Whole	1 lb. (weighed with stems)	240	58.2
Stems removed	4 oz.	61	14.9

Food and Description	Measure or Quantity	Calories	Carbohydrates (grams)
Red and white:			
Whole	1 lb. (weighed with stems)	220	53.2
Stems removed	1 cup (3.9 oz.)	55	13.3
Dried (Del Monte) Zante	½ cup (2.4 oz.)	204	47.8
CURRANT JELLY, sweetened (Smucker's)	1 T. (.7 oz.)	53	13.5
CURRANT PRESERVE or JAM, sweetened (Smucker's)	1 T.	53	13.5
CUSTARD:			
Home recipe (USDA) baked	½ cup (4.7 oz.)	152	14.7
Chilled, *Swiss Miss:*			
Chocolate flavor	4 oz.	150	23.0
Egg flavor	4 oz.	150	22.0
*Mix, dietetic (Featherweight)	½ cup	80	15.0
CUSTARD APPLE, bullock's-heart (USDA) raw:			
Whole	1 lb. (weighed with skins & seeds)	266	66.3
Flesh only	4 oz.	115	28.6
C.W. POST, cereal:			
Family style	¼ cup (1 oz.)	131	20.3
Family style, with raisins	¼ cup (1 oz.)	128	20.4

D

DAIQUIRI COCKTAIL:			
Canned (Mr. Boston):			
Regular, 12½% alcohol	3 fl. oz.	99	9.0
Strawberry, 12½% alcohol	3 fl. oz.	111	12.0

(USDA): United States Department of Agriculture
(HEW/FAO): Health, Education and Welfare/Food and Agriculture Organization
* Prepared as Package Directs

Food and Description	Measure or Quantity	Calories	Carbo-hydrates (grams)
Mix, dry:			
(Bar-Tender's)	⅝-oz. serving	70	17.2
(Holland House) banana	.6-oz. pkg.	66	16.0
DAMSON PLUM (See **PLUM**)			
DANDELION GREENS, raw (USDA):			
Trimmed	1 lb.	204	41.7
Boiled, drained	½ cup (3.2 oz.)	30	5.8
DATE, dry:			
Domestic:			
(USDA):			
With pits	1 lb. (weighed with pits)	1081	287.7
Without pits	4 oz.	311	82.7
Without pits, chopped	1 cup (6.1 oz.)	477	126.8
(Dromedary):			
Without pits	1 date	20	4.6
Without pits, chopped	¼ cup (1¼ oz.)	130	31.0
Imported (Bordo) Iraq:			
With pits	4 average dates (.9 oz.)	73	18.2
Without pits, chopped	½ cup (2 oz.)	159	39.8
DE CHAUNAC WINE (Great Western) 12% alcohol	3 fl. oz.	71	2.4
DEWBERRY, fresh (See **BLACKBERRY,** fresh)			
DILL SEED (French's)	1 tsp. (2.1 grams)	9	1.2
DING DONG (Hostess)	1.3-oz. cake	182	21.5
DIP:			
Avocado (Nalley's)	½ oz.	57	.4
Bacon & onion (Nalley's)	½ oz.	57	.5
Barbecue (Nalley's)	½ oz.	57	.5
Blue cheese:			
(Dean) tang	1 oz.	61	2.3

Food and Description	Measure or Quantity	Calories	Carbo-hydrates (grams)
(Nalley's)	1 oz.	110	.9
Cheese-bacon (Nalley's)	1 oz.	119	.8
Clam (Nalley's)	1 oz.	101	1.1
Dill pickle (Nalley's)	1 oz.	86	.9
Enchilada, *Fritos*	1 oz.	37	3.9
Garlic:			
(Dean)	1 oz.	58	2.0
(Nalley's)	1 oz.	120	.9
Guacamole (Nalley's)	1 oz.	114	.9
Jalapeno:			
Fritos	1 oz.	34	3.7
(Hain) natural	1 T. (.6 oz.)	24	1.5
(Nalley's)	1 oz.	109	.8
Onion:			
(Breakstone)	1 T. (.5 oz.)	29	1.0
(Dean) French	1 oz.	58	2.0
(Hain) bean, natural	1 T. (.6 oz.)	25	2.1
(Nalley's) French	1 oz.	106	1.4
(Sealtest)	1 oz.	60	1.5
Ranch house (Nalley's)	1 oz.	121	.6

DISTILLED LIQUOR. The values below would apply to unflavored bourbon whiskey, brandy, Canadian whiskey, gin, Irish whiskey, rum, rye, whiskey, Scotch whiskey, tequila and vodka. The caloric content of distilled liquors depends on the percentage of alcohol. The proof is twice the alcohol percent and the following values apply to all brands (USDA):

80 proof	1 fl. oz.	65	Tr.
86 proof	1 fl. oz.	70	Tr.
90 proof	1 fl. oz.	74	Tr.

(USDA): United States Department of Agriculture
(HEW/FAO):   Health, Education and Welfare/Food and Agriculture
                        Organization
* Prepared as Package Directs

Food and Description	Measure or Quantity	Calories	Carbo-hydrates (grams)
94 proof	1 fl. oz.	77	Tr.
100 proof	1 fl. oz.	83	Tr.
DOCK, including SHEEP SORREL (USDA):			
Raw, whole	1 lb. (weighed untrimmed)	89	17.8
Boiled, drained	4 oz.	22	4.4
DOLLY VARDEN, raw (USDA) meat & skin	4 oz.	163	0.
DOUGHNUT:			
(USDA):			
Cake type	1.1-oz. piece	125	16.4
Yeast-leavened	.6-oz. piece	83	8.6
Commercial type (Hostess):			
Cinnamon	1-oz. piece	113	14.5
Enrobed	1-oz. piece	136	13.6
Krunch	1-oz. piece	105	16.5
Old fashioned	1½-oz. piece	177	19.6
Plain	1-oz. piece	120	12.8
Powdered	1-oz. piece	117	15.1
Frozen (Morton):			
Bavarian creme	2-oz. piece	180	22.1
Boston creme	2.3-oz. piece	208	28.5
Chocolate iced	1.5-oz. piece	148	19.6
Glazed	1.5-oz. piece	150	19.2
Jelly	1.8-oz. piece	175	22.9
Mini	1.1-oz. piece	122	16.0
DRAMBUIE LIQUEUR (Hiram Walker) 80 proof	1 fl. oz.	110	11.0
DRUM, raw (USDA):			
Freshwater:			
Whole	1 lb. (weighed whole)	143	0.
Meat only	4 oz.	137	0.
Red:			
Whole	1 lb. (weighed whole)	149	0.
Meat only	4 oz.	91	0.

EGG [149]

Food and Description	Measure or Quantity	Calories	Carbo-hydrates (grams)
DRUMSTICK, frozen, in a cone:			
Ice cream:			
Topped with peanuts	1 piece	181	22.7
Topped with peanuts & cone bisque	1 piece	168	23.6
Ice milk:			
Topped with peanuts	1 piece	163	24.3
Topped with peanuts & cone bisque	1 piece	150	25.2
DUCK, raw (USDA):			
Domesticated:			
Ready-to-cook	1 lb. (weighed with bone)	1213	0.
Meat only	4 oz.	187	0.
Wild:			
Dressed	1 lb. (weighed dressed)	613	0.
Meat only	4 oz.	156	0.

E

ECLAIR:			
Home recipe (USDA) with custard filling & chocolate icing	4-oz. piece	271	26.3
Frozen (Rich's) chocolate	2.6-oz. piece	234	30.0
EEL (USDA):			
Raw, meat only	4 oz.	264	0.
Smoked, meat only	4 oz.	374	0.
EGG (USDA) (See also **EGG SUBSTITUTE**):			

(USDA): United States Department of Agriculture
(HEW/FAO): Health, Education and Welfare/Food and Agriculture Organization
* Prepared as Package Directs

Food and Description	Measure or Quantity	Calories	Carbo-hydrates (grams)
Chicken:			
Raw:			
White only	1 large egg (1.2 oz.)	17	.3
White only	1 cup (9 oz.)	130	2.0
Yolk only	1 large egg (.6 oz.)	59	.1
Yolk only	1 cup (8.5 oz.)	835	1.4
Whole, small	1 egg (1.3 oz.)	60	.3
Whole, medium	1 egg (1.5 oz.)	71	.4
Whole, large	1 egg (1.8 oz.)	81	.4
Whole	1 cup (8.8 oz.)	409	2.3
Whole, extra large	1 egg (2 oz.)	94	.5
Whole, jumbo	1 egg (2.3 oz.)	105	.6
Cooked:			
Boiled	1 large egg (1.8 oz.)	81	.4
Fried in butter	1 large egg	99	.1
Omelet, mixed with milk & cooked in fat	1 large egg	107	1.5
Poached	1 large egg	78	.4
Scrambled, mixed with milk & cooked in fat	1 large egg	111	1.5
Scrambled, mixed with milk & cooked in fat	1 cup (7.8 oz.)	381	5.3
Dried:			
Whole	1 cup (3.8 oz.)	639	4.4
White, powder	1 oz.	105	1.6
Yolk	1 cup (3.4 oz.)	637	2.4
Duck, raw	1 egg (2.8 oz.)	153	.6
Goose, raw	1 egg (5.8 oz.)	303	2.1
Turkey, raw	1 egg (3.1 oz.)	150	1.5
*EGG FOO YOUNG, frozen (Chun King) stir fry	⅙ of pkg.	45	3.0
EGG MIX (Durkee):			
*Omelet:			
With bacon	½ of pkg.	210	10.0
Puffy	½ of pkg.	302	10.5
Western	½ of pkg.	302	11.0

Food and Description	Measure or Quantity	Calories	Carbo-hydrates (grams)
Scrambled:			
With bacon	1.3-oz. pkg.	181	6.0
Plain	.8-oz. pkg.	124	4.0
EGG NOG, dairy:			
(Meadow Gold)	½ cup	164	25.5
(Sealtest):			
6% fat	½ cup (4.6 oz.)	174	18.0
8% fat	½ cup (4.6 oz.)	192	17.3
EGG NOG COCKTAIL, canned			
(Mr. Boston) 15% alcohol	3 fl. oz.	180	18.9
EGGPLANT:			
Raw (USDA) whole	1 lb. (weighed untrimmed)	92	20.6
Boiled (USDA) drained, diced	1 cup (7.1 oz.)	38	8.2
Frozen:			
(Mrs. Paul's):			
Parmigiana	½ of 11-oz. pkg.	259	21.6
Slices, breaded and fried	⅓ of 9-oz. pkg.	225	22.4
Sticks, breaded and fried	½ of 7-oz. pkg.	262	27.3
(Weight Watchers) parmigiana, one-compartment meal	13-oz. meal	285	25.0
EGG ROLL, frozen:			
(Chun King):			
Chicken	½-oz. piece	23	3.0
Meat & shrimp	½-oz. piece	25	3.5
Meat & shrimp	2½-oz. piece	65	10.0
Shrimp	½-oz. piece	23	3.8
(La Choy):			
Chicken	.4-oz. piece	30	3.6
Lobster	.4-oz. piece	27	3.6
Meat & shrimp	.2-oz. piece	17	2.3
Meat & shrimp	.4-oz. piece	27	3.5

(USDA): United States Department of Agriculture
(HEW/FAO): Health, Education and Welfare/Food and Agriculture
Organization
* Prepared as Package Directs

Food and Description	Measure or Quantity	Calories	Carbo-hydrates (grams)
Shrimp	.4-oz. piece	26	3.7
Shrimp	2½-oz. piece	108	14.8
EGG, SCRAMBLED, frozen (Swanson) & sausage, with hashed brown potatoes	6¼-oz. breakfast	460	22.0
EGG SUBSTITUTE:			
Egg Beaters (Fleischmann)	¼ cup (2.1 oz.)	40	3.0
*Eggstra (Tillie Lewis)	1 large egg substitute	50	3.0
*Scramblers (Morningstar Farms)	1 egg equivalent	33	1.2
*Second Nature (Avoset)	3 T. (1½ fl. oz.)	42	2.0
ELDERBERRY, fresh (USDA):			
Whole	1 lb. (weighed with stems)	307	69.9
Stems removed	4 oz.	82	18.6
ELDERBERRY JELLY, sweetened (Smucker's)	1 T.	53	13.5
ELDERBERRY PRESERVE or JAM, sweetened (Smucker's)	1 T.	53	13.5
ENCHILADA, frozen:			
Beef:			
(Banquet):			
Buffet Supper, with cheese & chili gravy	2-lb. pkg.	1118	118.2
Cookin' Bag, with sauce	6-oz. pkg.	207	28.9
Dinner	12-oz. dinner	479	63.6
(Morton)	12-oz. dinner	351	47.7
(Swanson) *TV Brand*	15-oz. dinner	570	72.0
(Van de Kamp's):			
Dinner	12-oz. dinner	391	45.0
Entree	½ of 19-oz. entree	342	33.0
Entree, shredded	½ of 12-oz. entree	214	20.0

Food and Description	Measure or Quantity	Calories	Carbo-hydrates (grams)
Cheese:			
(Banquet) dinner:			
Regular	12-oz. dinner	459	58.8
Man-Pleaser	21¼-oz. dinner	664	82.0
(Van de Kamp's):			
Dinner	12-oz. dinner	449	44.0
Entree	7½-oz. entree	270	23.0
Entree	½ of 19-oz. entree	342	29.1
Entree, *Ranchero*	½ of 12-oz. entree	262	22.0
Chicken (Van de Kamp's)	7½-oz. pkg.	247	24.0
ENCHILADA SAUCE:			
Canned (Del Monte) hot or mild	½ cup (4 oz.)	45	11.0
*Mix (Durkee)	1 cup	57	12.5
ENCHILADA SEASONING MIX (French's)	¼ of 1⅜-oz. pkg.	30	5.0
ENDIVE, BELGIAN or FRENCH (See **CHICORY, WITLOOF**)			
ENDIVE, CURLY, raw (USDA):			
Untrimmed	1 lb. (weighed untrimmed)	80	16.4
Trimmed	½ lb.	45	9.3
Cut up or shredded	1 cup (2.5 oz.)	14	2.9
ESCAROLE, raw (USDA):			
Untrimmed	1 lb. (weighed untrimmed)	80	16.4

(USDA): United States Department of Agriculture
(HEW/FAO):   Health, Education and Welfare/Food and Agriculture
                       Organization
* Prepared as Package Directs

Food and Description	Measure or Quantity	Calories	Carbo-hydrates (grams)
Trimmed	½ lb.	46	9.2
Cut up or shredded	1 cup (2.5 oz.)	14	2.9
EULACHON or SMELT, raw (USDA) meat only	4 oz.	134	0.
EXPRESSO COFFEE LIQUEUR (Mr. Boston)	1 fl. oz.	104	15.0
EXTRACT (See individual listings)			

F

Food and Description	Measure or Quantity	Calories	Carbo-hydrates (grams)
FARINA (See also **CREAM OF WHEAT**):			
Regular:			
Dry:			
(USDA)	1 cup (6 oz.)	627	130.1
(H-O) cream, enriched	1 cup (6.1 oz.)	625	133.8
(H-O) cream, enriched	1 T.	41	8.8
Malt-O-Meal	1 oz.	97	21.0
Cooked:			
*(USDA)	1 cup (8.4 oz.)	100	20.7
*(USDA)	4 oz.	48	9.9
*(Pillsbury):			
Made with milk and salt	⅔ cup	200	26.0
Made with water and salt	⅔ cup	80	2.0
Quick-cooking:			
Dry:			
(USDA)	1 oz.	103	21.2
Malt-O-Meal	1 oz.	101	22.2
Cooked (USDA)	1 cup (8.6 oz.)	105	21.8
Instant-cooking (USDA):			
Dry	1 oz.	103	21.2
Cooked	4 oz.	62	12.9
FAT, COOKING, vegetable:			
(USDA)	1 cup (7.1 oz.)	1768	0.
(USDA)	1 T. (.4 oz.)	106	0.

FIG   [155]

Food and Description	Measure or Quantity	Calories	Carbo-hydrates (grams)
Crisco	1 T. (.4 oz.)	110	0.
Fluffo	1 T. (.4 oz.)	110	0.
Mrs. Tucker's	1 T.	120	0.
Snowdrift	1 T.	110	0.
Spry	1 T. (.4 oz.)	95	0.
FENNEL LEAVES, raw (USDA):			
Untrimmed	1 lb. (weighed untrimmed)	118	21.5
Trimmed	4 oz.	32	5.8
FENNEL SEED (French's)	1 tsp. (2.1 grams)	8	1.3
FIG:			
Fresh (USDA):			
Regular size	1 lb.	363	92.1
Small	1.3-oz. fig (1½" dia.)	30	7.7
Candied (Bama)	1 T. (.7 oz.)	37	9.6
Canned, regular pack, solids & liq.:			
(USDA):			
Light syrup	4 oz.	74	19.1
Heavy syrup	3 figs & 2 T. syrup (4 oz.)	96	24.9
Heavy syrup	½ cup (4.4 oz.)	106	27.5
Extra heavy syrup	4 oz.	117	30.3
(Del Monte) whole	½ cup (4.3 oz.)	114	28.1
Canned, unsweetened or dietetic:			
(USDA) water pack, solids & liq.	4 oz.	54	14.1
(Diet Delight) Kadota, solids & liq.	½ cup (4.4 oz.)	76	18.2
(Featherweight) Kadota, water pack, solids & liq.	½ cup	60	15.0

(USDA): United States Department of Agriculture
(HEW/FAO):   Health, Education and Welfare/Food and Agriculture
Organization
* Prepared as Package Directs

Food and Description	Measure or Quantity	Calories	Carbo-hydrates (grams)
Dried (USDA):			
Chopped	1 cup (6 oz.)	469	118.2
Whole	.7-oz. fig (2″ × 1″)	58	14.5
FIG JUICE, *Real Fig*	½ cup (4.5 oz.)	61	15.8
FIGURINES (Pillsbury) all flavors	1 bar	138	10.5
FILBERT or HAZELNUT:			
(USDA):			
Whole	4 oz. (weighed in shell)	331	8.7
Shelled	1 oz.	180	4.7
(Fisher) oil dipped, salted	½ cup (2 oz.)	360	5.4
FISH (See individual listings)			
FISH CAKE:			
Home recipe (USDA) fried	2 oz.	98	5.3
Frozen (Mrs. Paul's):			
Breaded and fried	2-oz. cake	105	11.9
Beach Haven	2-oz. cake	106	12.0
Thins, breaded and fried	½ of 10-oz. pkg.	326	30.7
FISH & CHIPS, frozen:			
(Banquet) *Man-Pleaser*	14-oz. dinner	724	86.8
(Mrs. Paul's):			
Batter fried	½ of 14-oz. pkg.	366	43.3
Batter fried, supreme light	8½-oz. pkg.	449	49.3
(Swanson):			
Dinner:			
Hungry Man	15¾-oz. dinner	820	87.0
TV Brand	10¼-oz. dinner	450	38.0
Entree, *TV Brand*	5-oz. entree	290	25.0
(Van de Kamp's) batter dipped, french-fried	8-oz. serving	500	45.0
FISH DINNER, frozen:			
(Banquet)	8¾-oz. dinner	382	43.6
(Mrs. Paul's):			
Au gratin	½ of 10-oz. pkg.	249	19.6
Parmesan	½ of 10-oz. pkg.	230	20.9

Food and Description	Measure or Quantity	Calories	Carbo-hydrates (grams)
Parmesan	¼ of 16-oz. pkg.	184	16.7
(Van de Kamp's) fillet:			
Regular	12-oz. dinner	300	25.0
Batter dipped	11-oz. dinner	540	39.0
(Weight Watchers) fillet:			
In lemon sauce, 3-compartment meal	13¼-oz. meal	250	19.1
In Newburgh sauce, 2-compartment meal	9¼-oz. meal	192	16.0
FISH FILLET, frozen:			
(Mrs. Paul's):			
Batter fried, crunchy	2¼-oz. piece	178	17.2
Batter fried, light	3.63-oz. piece	218	20.3
Buttered	2½-oz. piece	155	.9
Miniature, batter fried	⅓ of 9-oz. pkg.	181	15.3
(Van de Kamp's):			
Batter dipped, french-fried	3-oz. piece	220	12.5
Country seasoned	2.4-oz. piece	180	10.5
Light & crispy	2-oz. piece	156	16.0
FISH FLAKES, canned (USDA)	4 oz.	126	0.
FISH KABOBS, frozen:			
(Mrs. Paul's) supreme light batter	⅓ of 10-oz. pkg.	200	17.7
(Van de Kamp's) batter dipped, french fried:			
Regular	.4-oz. piece	26	1.6
Country seasoned	.4-oz. piece	29	1.9
FISH LOAF, home recipe (USDA)	4 oz.	141	8.3
FISH SANDWICH, frozen (Mrs. Paul's):			
Fillet	4⅛-oz. sandwich	200	23.2
Sticks, jumbo	½ of 6½-oz. pkg.	201	31.1

(USDA): United States Department of Agriculture
(HEW/FAO):   Health, Education and Welfare/Food and Agriculture Organization
* Prepared as Package Directs

Food and Description	Measure or Quantity	Calories	Carbo-hydrates (grams)
FISH STICK, frozen:			
(USDA) cooked, commercial, 3¾″ × 1″ × ½″ sticks	10 sticks (8-oz. pkg.)	400	14.8
(Mrs. Paul's):			
Batter-fried	1 stick (.8 oz.)	69	6.4
Breaded and fried	1 stick (¾ oz.)	43	4.1
(Van de Kamp's) batter-dipped, french-fried:			
Regular	1-oz. piece	58	5.2
Country seasoned	½ of 12-oz. pkg.	492	26.4
Light & crispy	¾-oz. piece	57	5.2
FIT'N FROSTY (Alba '77), instant milk shake mix:			
Chocolate	¾-oz. envelope	74	11.5
Chocolate and marshmallow	1 envelope	70	11.0
Strawberry	1 envelope	74	12.0
Vanilla	1 envelope	69	11.3
***FIVE ALIVE,** juice drink, chilled or frozen (Snow Crop)	6 fl. oz.	85	20.8
FLOUNDER:			
Raw (USDA):			
Whole	1 lb. (weighed whole)	118	0.
Meat only	4 oz.	90	0.
Baked (USDA)	4 oz.	229	0.
Frozen:			
(Mrs. Paul's) fillets:			
Breaded and fried	2-oz. fillet	138	11.6
With lemon butter	½ of 8½-oz. pkg.	154	9.4
(Weight Watchers):			
With lemon-flavored breadcrumbs, 2-compartment meal	6½-oz. serving	134	12.0
In Newburgh sauce, 3-compartment meal	12½-oz. meal	198	11.0
FLOUR:			
(USDA):			
Buckwheat, dark, sifted	1 cup (3.5 oz.)	326	70.6

Food and Description	Measure or Quantity	Calories	Carbo-hydrates (grams)
Buckwheat, light, sifted	1 cup (3.5 oz.)	340	77.9
Carob or St. John's-bread	1 oz.	51	22.9
Chestnut	1 oz.	103	21.6
Corn	1 cup (3.9)	405	84.5
Cottonseed	1 oz.	101	9.4
Fish, from whole fish	1 oz.	95	0.
Lima bean	1 oz.	97	17.9
Potato	1 oz.	100	22.7
Rice, stirred, spooned	1 cup (5.6 oz.)	574	125.6
Rye:			
Light:			
Unsifted, spooned	1 cup (3.6 oz.)	361	78.7
Sifted, spooned	1 cup (3.1 oz.)	314	68.6
Medium:	1 oz.	99	21.2
Dark:			
Unstirred	1 cup (4.5 oz.)	419	87.2
Stirred	1 cup (4.5 oz.)	415	86.5
Soybean, defatted, stirred	1 cup (3.6 oz.)	329	38.5
Soybean, high fat	1 oz.	108	9.4
Sunflower seed, partially defatted	1 oz.	96	10.7
Wheat:			
All-purpose:			
Unsifted, dipped	1 cup (5 oz.)	521	108.8
Unsifted, spooned	1 cup (4.4 oz.)	459	95.9
Sifted, spooned	1 cup (4.1 oz.)	422	88.3
Bread:			
Unsifted, dipped	1 cup (4.8 oz.)	496	101.6
Unsifted, spooned	1 cup (4.3 oz.)	449	91.9
Sifted, spooned	1 cup (4.1 oz.)	427	87.4
Cake:			
Unsifted, dipped	1 cup (4.2 oz.)	433	94.5
Unsifted, spooned	1 cup (3.9 oz.)	404	88.1
Sifted, spooned	1 cup (3.5 oz.)	360	78.6
Gluten:			
Unsifted, dipped	1 cup (5 oz.)	537	67.0
Unsifted, spooned	1 cup (4.8 oz.)	510	63.7
Sifted, spooned	1 cup (4.8 oz.)	514	64.2

(USDA): United States Department of Agriculture
(HEW/FAO): Health, Education and Welfare/Food and Agriculture
Organization
* Prepared as Package Directs

Food and Description	Measure or Quantity	Calories	Carbo-hydrates (grams)
Self-rising:			
Unsifted, dipped	1 cup (4.6 oz.)	458	96.5
Unsifted, spooned	1 cup (4.5 oz.)	447	94.2
Sifted, spooned	1 cup (3.7 oz.)	373	78.7
Whole wheat	1 oz.	94	20.1
(Aunt Jemima) self-rising	¼ cup (1 oz.)	109	23.6
Ballard:			
All-purpose	¼ cup	100	21.7
Self-rising	¼ cup	95	21.0
Bisquick (Betty Crocker)	¼ cup	120	19.0
Drifted Snow	¼ cup	100	21.7
Elan's:			
Brown rice, stone ground, whole grain	¼ cup	146	30.1
Buckwheat, pure	¼ cup	82	19.0
Pastry	1 oz.	102	20.7
Rye, stone ground, whole grain	¼ cup	89	18.1
Soy	1 oz.	98	8.9
3-in-1 mix	1 oz.	99	20.0
White, with wheat germ	1 oz.	101	20.7
Whole wheat, stone ground, whole grain	1 oz.	100	19.8
(Featherweight):			
Gluton	¼ cup	105	13.7
Soy	¼ cup	117	8.2
Gold Medal (Betty Crocker):			
All-purpose or unbleached	¼ cup	100	21.7
High protein	¼ cup	100	20.7
Self-rising	¼ cup	95	20.7
La Pina	¼ cup	100	21.7
(Pillsbury):			
All purpose	¼ cup	100	21.7
All purpose, unbleached	¼ cup	100	21.5
Bread	¼ cup	105	20.2
Rye, medium	¼ cup	110	22.2
Rye & wheat, bohemian style	¼ cup	100	21.5
Sauce & gravy	1 T.	25	5.5
Self-rising	¼ cup	95	21.0
Whole wheat	¼ cup	100	20.0
Presto, self-rising	¼ cup (1 oz.)	98	21.6

Food and Description	Measure or Quantity	Calories	Carbo-hydrates (grams)
Purasnow:			
Regular	¼ cup (1 oz.)	100	21.7
Self-rising	¼ cup (1 oz.)	95	20.7
Red Band:			
Regular or unbleached	¼ cup (1 oz.)	100	21.7
Self-rising	¼ cup (1 oz.)	95	20.7
Red Star, self-rising	¼ cup (1 oz.)	95	20.7
Robin Hood:			
All purpose	¼ cup (1 oz.)	100	21.2
Self-rising	¼ cup (1 oz.)	95	20.2
Softasilk	¼ cup (1 oz.)	100	23.0
Swans Down, cake:			
Regular	¼ cup	100	22.0
Self-rising	¼ cup	90	20.0
White Deer	¼ cup (1 oz.)	100	21.7
Wondra	¼ cup (1 oz.)	100	21.7
FOOD STICKS (Pillsbury) all flavors	1 stick	45	6.8
FOUR FRUIT PRESERVE, sweetened (Smucker's)	1 T.	53	13.5
FRANKEN*BERRY, cereal (General Mills)	1 cup (1 oz.)	110	24.0
FRANKFURTER, raw or cooked: (USDA):			
Raw:			
All kinds	1 frankfurter (10 per lb.)	140	.8
Meat	1 frankfurter (10 per lb.)	134	1.1
With cereal	1 frankfurter (10 per lb.)	112	<.1
Cooked, all kinds	1 frankfurter (10 per lb.)	136	.7

(USDA): United States Department of Agriculture
(HEW/FAO): Health, Education and Welfare/Food and Agriculture Organization
* Prepared as Package Directs

Food and Description	Measure or Quantity	Calories	Carbo-hydrates (grams)
(Best's Kosher):			
Regular	1.5-oz. frankfurter	133	1.5
Regular	1.6-oz. frankfurter	142	1.6
Beef	1.5-oz. frankfurter	102	1.5
Cocktail	.3-oz. frankfurter	27	.3
Dinner	2.7-oz. frankfurter	237	2.7
Jumbo	2-oz. frankfurter	178	2.1
Mild	1.5-oz. frankfurter	133	1.5
(Eckrich):			
Beef or meat	1.6-oz. frankfurter	150	3.0
Beef or meat, jumbo	2-oz. frankfurter	190	3.0
Meat	1.2-oz. frankfurter	120	2.0
(Hormel):			
Beef	1.2-oz. frankfurter	104	.5
Beef, smoked, *Range Brand Wranglers*	1 frankfurter	175	2.0
Meat	1.2-oz. frankfurter	104	.5
Smoked, *Range Brand Wranglers*	1 frankfurter	160	2.0
(Hygrade):			
Beef	1.6-oz. frankfurter	146	1.4
Beef, *Ball Park*	2-oz. frankfurter	169	<.1
Meat	1.6-oz. frankfurter	147	1.5
Meat, *Ball Park*	2-oz. frankfurter	175	<.1
(Louis Rich):			
Turkey	1.5-oz. frankfurter	95	1.0
Turkey	1.6-oz. frankfurter	100	1.0
Turkey	2-oz. frankfurter	125	1.0

Food and Description	Measure or Quantity	Calories	Carbo-hydrates (grams)
(Oscar Mayer):			
Beef	1.6-oz. frankfurter	145	.9
Beef	2-oz. frankfurter	183	1.2
Beef, *Big One*	4-oz. frankfurter	366	2.4
Little wiener	.3-oz. frankfurter	30	.2
Wiener	1.2-oz. frankfurter	109	.6
Wiener	1.6-oz. wiener	145	.8
Wiener, jumbo	2-oz. frankfurter	183	1.0
Wiener with cheese	1.6-oz. frankfurter	146	.7
(Oscherwitz):			
Regular	1.5-oz. frankfurter	133	1.5
Regular	1.6-oz. frankfurter	142	1.6
Beef	1.5-oz. frankfurter	102	1.5
Cocktail	.3-oz. frankfurter	27	.3
Dinner	2.7-oz. frankfurter	237	2.7
Jumbo	2-oz. frankfurter	178	2.1
Mild	1.5-oz. frankfurter	133	1.5
(Swift)	1.6-oz. frankfurter	150	1.2
(Vienna) beef	1 frankfurter	132	1.0
Canned (USDA)	2 oz.	125	.1

FRANKS AND BEANS (See
BEANS & FRANKFURTERS)

FRANKS-IN-BLANKETS,
frozen (Durkee)   1 piece   45   1.0

FRENCH TOAST, frozen (Aunt
Jemima):

Regular	1½-oz. slice	85	13.2

(USDA): United States Department of Agriculture
(HEW/FAO):   Health, Education and Welfare/Food and Agriculture
            Organization
* Prepared as Package Directs

Food and Description	Measure or Quantity	Calories	Carbo-hydrates (grams)
Cinnamon swirl	1½-oz. slice	97	13.6
FRENCH TOAST & SAUSAGE, frozen (Swanson)	4½-oz. breakfast	300	22.0
FRITTER:			
Home recipe, clam (USDA)	2″ × 1¼″ fritter (1.4 oz.)	124	12.4
Frozen (Mrs. Paul's):			
Apple	2-oz. fritter	125	16.1
Clam	1.9-oz. fritter	131	14.3
Corn	2-oz. fritter	73	1.1
Crab	1.9-oz. fritter	129	15.3
Shrimp	½ of 7¾-oz. pkg.	242	27.0
Tuna	½ of 7¾-oz. pkg.	272	27.5
FROG LEGS, raw (USDA):			
Bone in	1 lb. (weighed with bone)	215	0.
Meat only	4 oz.	83	0.
FROOT LOOPS, cereal (Kellogg's)	1 cup (1 oz.)	110	25.0
FROSTED RICE, cereal (Kellogg's)	¾ cup (1 oz.)	110	26.0
FROSTING (See **CAKE ICING**)			
FROZEN DESSERT, dietetic:			
(Good Humor):			
Bar, vanilla with chocolate coating	2½-fl.-oz. bar	90	12.0
Cup, vanilla & chocolate	5-fl.-oz. cup	100	17.0
(SugarLo) ice cream or ice milk, all flavors	¼ pint	135	14.0
FRUIT BITS, dried (Sun-Maid)	1-oz. serving	91	21.4
FRUIT BRUTE, cereal (General Mills)	1 cup (1 oz.)	110	24.0
FRUIT COCKTAIL:			
Canned, regular pack, solids & liq.:			

Food and Description	Measure or Quantity	Calories	Carbo-hydrates (grams)
(USDA):			
Light syrup	4 oz.	68	17.8
Heavy syrup	½ cup (4.5 oz.)	97	25.2
Extra heavy syrup	4 oz.	104	26.9
(Del Monte) heavy syrup, regular or chunky fruit	½ cup	95	23.1
(Libby's) heavy syrup	½ cup (4.5 oz.)	101	24.7
(Stokely-Van Camp)	½ cup (4.5 oz.)	95	23.0
Canned, dietetic or unsweetened, solids & liq.:			
(USDA) water pack	4 oz.	42	11.0
(Del Monte) *Lite*	½ cup	58	14.1
(Diet Delight):			
Juice pack	½ cup	70	17.0
Water pack	½ cup	40	10.0
(Featherweight):			
Juice pack	½ cup	50	12.0
Water pack	½ cup	40	10.0
(Libby's) water pack	½ cup (4.3 oz.)	44	10.4
(S&W) *Nutradiet:*			
Juice pack	½ cup	50	14.0
Water pack	½ cup	40	10.0
*FRUIT COUNTRY			
(Comstock):			
Apple	¼ of pkg.	160	36.0
Blueberry	¼ of pkg.	160	33.0
Cherry	¼ of pkg.	180	38.0
Peach	¼ of pkg.	130	28.0
FRUIT CUP (Del Monte):			
Mixed, solids & liq.	5-oz. container	110	26.7
Peaches, cling, diced, solids & liq.	5-oz. container	116	27.8
FRUIT JAM, mixed (Smucker's)	1 T.	53	13.5
FRUIT JUICE, canned (Sun-Maid) 100% real:			

(USDA): United States Department of Agriculture
(HEW/FAO): Health, Education and Welfare/Food and Agriculture Organization
* Prepared as Package Directs

Food and Description	Measure or Quantity	Calories	Carbo-hydrates (grams)
Golden	6 fl. oz.	100	23.0
Purple	6 fl. oz.	100	25.0
Red	6 fl. oz.	100	24.0
FRUIT, MIXED:			
Canned, dietetic or low calorie			
(Del Monte) *Lite,* solids & liq.	½ cup	57	13.6
Frozen (Birds Eye) quick thaw	½ of 10-oz. pkg.	143	34.5
FRUIT PUNCH:			
Canned:			
Capri Sun, natural	6¾ fl. oz.	102	25.9
(Hi-C)	6 fl. oz.	93	23.0
(Lincoln) party	8 fl. oz.	139	34.8
Chilled:			
Five Alive (Snow Crop)	6 fl. oz.	87	22.7
(Minute Maid)	6 fl. oz.	93	23.0
*Frozen, *Five Alive*			
(Snow Crop)	6 fl. oz.	87	22.7
*Mix (Hi-C)	6 fl. oz.	72	18.0
FRUIT ROLL, frozen (La Choy)			
apple cinnamon	.5-oz. roll	38	6.4
FRUIT SALAD:			
Canned, regular pack, solids & liq.:			
(USDA):			
Light syrup	4 oz.	67	17.6
Heavy syrup	½ cup (4.3 oz.)	85	22.0
Extra heavy syrup	4 oz.	102	26.5
(Del Monte):			
Fruit for salad	½ cup (4.3 oz.)	94	23.0
Tropical	½ cup (4.4 oz.)	107	26.0
(Libby's) heavy syrup	½ cup (4.4 oz.)	99	24.0
(Stokely-Van Camp)	½ cup (4.5 oz.)	95	22.0
Canned, unsweetened or dietetic pack, solids & liq.:			
(USDA) water pack	4 oz.	40	10.3
(Diet Delight) juice pack	½ cup (4.4 oz.)	60	16.0
(Featherweight):			
Juice pack	½ cup	50	12.0
Water pack	½ cup	40	10.0

Food and Description	Measure or Quantity	Calories	Carbo-hydrates (grams)
(S&W) *Nutradiet:*			
Juice pack	½ cup	60	14.0
Water pack	½ cup	35	10.0
FUDGSICLE (Popsicle Industries) chocolate	2¼-fl.-oz. bar	100	23.0

G

GARLIC, raw (USDA):			
Whole	2 oz. (weighed with skin)	68	15.4
Peeled	1 oz.	39	8.7
GARLIC FLAKES (Gilroy)	1 tsp. (1.5 grams)	13	2.6
GARLIC POWDER (Gilroy)	1 tsp.	10	2.0
GARLIC SALT (French's)	1 tsp.	4	1.0
GAZPACHO SOUP, canned (Crosse & Blackwell)	½ of 13-oz. can	30	1.0
GELATIN, unflavored, dry:			
(USDA)	7-gram envelope	24	0.
Carmel Kosher	7-gram envelope	30	0.
(Knox):			
Unflavored	1 envelope	25	0.
Orange	1 envelope	70	10.0
GELATIN DESSERT:			
Powder:			
*Regular:			
Carmel Kosher, all flavors	½ cup	80	20.0
(Jell-O) all fruit flavors	½ cup (4.9 oz.)	80	18.5
(Royal) all fruit flavors	½ cup (4.9 oz.)	80	19.0
*Dietetic or low calorie:			

(USDA): United States Department of Agriculture
(HEW/FAO): Health, Education and Welfare/Food and Agriculture Organization
* Prepared as Package Directs

Food and Description	Measure or Quantity	Calories	Carbo-hydrates (grams)
Carmel Kosher, all flavors	½ cup	8	0.
(Dia-Mel) *Gel-a-Thin*, all flavors	4-oz. serving	10	1.0
(Estee) all fruit flavors	½ cup	40	9.9
(Featherweight) all flavors, artificially sweetened	½ cup	10	0.
(Royal) *Sweet As You Please*, all flavors	½ cup	6	0.
Canned, dietetic pack:			
(Dia-Mel) *Gel-a-Thin*, all flavors	4-oz. container	1	.2
(Estee) strawberry	4-oz. serving	45	11.2
GELFILTE FISH, canned:			
(Mother's):			
Jellied, Old World	4-oz. serving	70	7.0
Jellied, whitefish & pike	4-oz. serving	60	4.0
In liquid broth	4-oz. serving	70	7.0
(Rokeach):			
Jellied	4-oz. serving	60	4.0
Jellied, whitefish & pike	4-oz. serving	50	4.0
Natural broth	4-oz. serving	60	4.0
Old Vienna	4-oz. serving	70	8.0
GERMAN DINNER, frozen (Swanson) *TV Brand*	11¾-oz. dinner	430	40.0
GIN, unflavored (see **DISTILLED LIQUOR**)			
GINGERBREAD:			
Home recipe (USDA)	1.9-oz. piece (2″ × 2″ × 2″)	174	28.6
*Mix:			
(USDA)	⅑ of 8″ sq. (2.2 oz.)	174	32.2
(Betty Crocker)	⅑ of pkg.	210	36.0
(Dromedary)	2″ × 2″ sq. (1⁄16 of pkg.)	100	20.0
(Pillsbury)	3″ sq. (⅑ of pkg.)	190	36.0
GINGER, CANDIED (USDA)	1 oz.	96	24.7

Food and Description	Measure or Quantity	Calories	Carbo-hydrates (grams)
GINGER ROOT, fresh (USDA):			
With skin	1 oz.	13	2.5
Without skin	1 oz.	14	2.7
GIN, SLOE (Mr. Boston)	1 fl. oz.	68	4.7
GOLDEN GRAHAMS, cereal (General Mills)	¾ cup (1 oz.)	110	24.0
GOOBER GRAPE (Smucker's)	1-oz. serving	125	14.0
GOOD HUMOR (See also individual flavors for bulk ice cream):			
Bullwinkle, pudding stix	2½-fl.-oz. pop	120	20.0
Chocolate eclair	3-oz. piece	220	25.0
Lite Fruit Stix	1½-fl.-oz. piece	35	8.0
Sandwich	2½-oz. piece	200	34.0
Sandwich, chocolate chip cookie	1 sandwich	480	64.0
Strawberry shortcake	3-oz. piece	200	21.0
Toasted almond bar	3-oz. piece	220	21.0
Vanilla, chocolate coated bar	3-oz. piece	170	12.0
Whammy:			
Assorted	1.6-oz. piece	100	9.0
Crunch	1.6-oz. piece	110	10.0
GOOD N' PUDDIN (Popsicle Industries) all flavors	2¼-fl.-oz. bar	170	27.0
GOOSE, domesticated (USDA):			
Raw	1 lb. (weighed ready-to-cook)	1172	0.
Roasted:			
Meat & skin	4 oz.	500	0.
Meat only	4 oz.	264	0.

(USDA): United States Department of Agriculture
(HEW/FAO): Health, Education and Welfare/Food and Agriculture Organization
* Prepared as Package Directs

Food and Description	Measure or Quantity	Calories	Carbo-hydrates (grams)
GOOSEBERRY (USDA):			
Fresh	1 lb.	177	44.0
Fresh	1 cup (5.3 oz.)	58	14.6
Canned, water pack, solids & liq.	4 oz.	29	7.5
GOOSE GIZZARD, raw (USDA)	4 oz.	158	0.
GRAHAM CRACKER (See **CRACKER**)			
GRAHAM CRAKOS, cereal (Kellogg's)	¾ cup (1 oz.)	110	24.0
GRANOLA BARS, *Nature Valley:*			
Almond, cinnamon or oats'n honey	.8-oz. bar	110	16.0
Coconut or peanut	.8-oz. bar	120	15.0
GRANOLA CEREAL:			
Heartland:			
Coconut	¼ cup (1 oz.)	130	18.0
Plain or raisin	¼ cup (1 oz.)	120	18.0
Puffs, regular or cinnamon spice	½ cup (1 oz.)	120	20.0
Nature Valley:			
Cinnamon & raisin or toasted oat	⅓ cup (1 oz.)	130	19.0
Coconut & honey	⅓ cup (1 oz.)	150	18.0
Fruit & nut	⅓ cup (1 oz.)	130	20.0
Sun Country (Kretschmer):			
Almonds	¼ cup (1 oz.)	126	17.0
Raisin	¼ cup (1 oz.)	120	13.4
GRANOLA CLUSTERS, *Nature Valley:*			
Almond	1.2-oz. roll	140	27.0
Caramel	1.2-oz. roll	150	28.0
Raisin	1.2-oz. roll	140	28.0
GRAPE:			
Fresh:			
American type (slip skin),			

Food and Description	Measure or Quantity	Calories	Carbo- hydrates (grams)
Concord, Delaware, Niagara, Catawba and Scuppernong:			
(USDA)	½ lb. (weighed with stem, skin & seeds)	98	22.4
(USDA)	½ cup (2.7 oz.)	33	7.5
(USDA)	3½″ × 3″ bunch (3.5 oz.)	43	9.9
European type (adherent skin, Malaga, Muscat, Thompson seedless, Emperor & Flame Tokay:			
(USDA)	½ lb. (weighed with stem & seeds)	139	34.9
(USDA) whole	20 grapes (¾″ dia.)	52	13.5
(USDA) whole	½ cup (.3 oz.)	56	14.5
(USDA) halves	½ cup (.3 oz.)	56	14.4
Canned, solids & liq.:			
(USDA) Thompson, seedless, heavy syrup	4 oz.	87	22.7
(USDA) Thompson, seedless, water pack	4 oz.	58	15.4
(Featherweight) water pack, seedless	½ cup	50	13.0
GRAPE DRINK:			
Canned:			
(Hi-C)	6 fl. oz.	89	22.0
(Lincoln)	6 fl. oz.	96	23.9
(Welchade)	6 fl. oz.	90	23.0
*Frozen (Welchade)	6 fl. oz.	90	23.0
*Mix (Hi-C)	6 fl. oz.	68	17.0

(USDA): United States Department of Agriculture
(HEW/FAO):   Health, Education and Welfare/Food and Agriculture
                      Organization
* Prepared as Package Directs

Food and Description	Measure or Quantity	Calories	Carbo- hydrates (grams)
GRAPEFRUIT:			
Fresh (USDA):			
White:			
Seeded type	1 lb. (weighed with seeds & skin)	86	22.4
Seedless type	1 lb. (weighed with skin)	87	22.6
Seeded type	½ med. grapefruit (3¾" dia., 8.5 oz.)	54	14.1
Pink and red:			
Seeded type	1 lb. (weighed with seeds & skin)	87	22.6
Seedless type	1 lb. (weighed with skin)	93	24.1
Seeded type	½ med. grapefruit (3¾" dia., 8.5 oz.)	46	12.0
Canned, syrup pack (Del Monte) solids & liq.	½ cup	74	17.5
Canned, unsweetened or dietetic pack, solids & liq.:			
(USDA) water pack	½ cup (4.2 oz.)	36	9.1
(Del Monte) sections	½ cup	46	10.5
(Diet Delight) sections, juice pack	½ cup (4.3 oz.)	45	11.0
(Featherweight) sections, juice pack	½ of 8-oz. can	40	9.0
(S&W) *Nutradiet,* sections	½ cup	40	9.0
GRAPEFRUIT DRINK, canned			
(Lincoln)	6 fl. oz.	104	26.1
GRAPEFRUIT JUICE:			
Fresh (USDA) pink, red or white, all varieties	½ cup (4.3 oz.)	48	11.3
Canned:			
Sweetened:			
(USDA)	½ cup (4.4 oz.)	66	16.0
(Del Monte)	6 fl. oz.	89	20.8
(Minute Maid)	6 fl. oz.	75	17.0

Food and Description	Measure or Quantity	Calories	Carbo-hydrates (grams)
Unsweetened:			
(USDA)	½ cup (4.4 oz.)	51	12.2
(Del Monte)	6 fl. oz.	72	16.6
(Ocean Spray)	6 fl. oz. (6.5 oz.)	64	14.6
(Texsun) pink	6 fl. oz.	77	18.0
Chilled (Minute Maid)	6 fl. oz.	75	18.1
*Frozen:			
Sweetened (USDA) diluted with 3 parts water	½ cup (4.4 oz.)	58	14.1
Unsweetened:			
(USDA) diluted with 3 parts water	½ cup (4.4 oz.)	51	12.2
(Minute Maid)	6 fl. oz.	75	18.3
*Dehydrated crystals (USDA) reconstituted	½ cup (4.4 oz.)	50	11.9
GRAPEFRUIT JUICE COCKTAIL, canned (Ocean Spray) pink	6 fl. oz.	84	20.0
GRAPEFRUIT-ORANGE JUICE COCKTAIL, canned, *Musselman's*	6 fl. oz.	67	17.2
GRAPEFRUIT PEEL, CANDIED (USDA)	1 oz.	90	22.9
GRAPE JAM, sweetened (Smucker's)	1 T.	53	13.7
GRAPE JELLY:			
Sweetened:			
(Smucker's)	1 T.	53	13.5
(Welch's)	1 T.	52	13.5
Dietetic (See **GRAPE SPREAD**)			

(USDA): United States Department of Agriculture
(HEW/FAO): Health, Education and Welfare/Food and Agriculture Organization
* Prepared as Package Directs

Food and Description	Measure or Quantity	Calories	Carbo-hydrates (grams)
GRAPE JUICE:			
Canned:			
(USDA)	½ cup (4.4 oz.)	83	20.9
(Seneca Foods)	6 fl. oz.	118	30.0
(Welch's) red or white,			
regular or sparkling	6 fl. oz.	120	30.0
Chilled (Welch's)	6 fl. oz.	110	27.0
*Frozen, sweetened:			
(USDA)	½ cup (4.4 oz.)	66	16.6
(Minute Maid)	6 fl. oz.	99	25.0
(Welch's)	6 fl. oz.	100	25.0
GRAPE JUICE DRINK, canned			
(USDA) approximately 30%			
grape juice	1 cup (8.8 oz.)	135	34.5
GRAPE NUT FLAKES, cereal			
(Post)	⅞ cup (1 oz.)	108	23.4
GRAPE PRESERVE or JAM,			
sweetened (Welch's)	1 T.	52	13.5
GRAPE SPREAD, low sugar:			
(Diet Delight)	1 T. (.6 oz.)	13	3.2
(Estee)	1 T. (.6 oz.)	12	3.0
(Featherweight):			
Regular	1 T.	16	4.0
Artificially sweetened	1 T.	6	1.0
(Slenderella)	1 T. (.6 oz.)	24	6.0
(Smucker's):			
Regular	1 T.	24	6.0
Artificially sweetened	1 T.	3	3.0
(S&W) *Nutradiet,* Concord	1 T.	12	3.0
(Tillie Lewis) *Tasti-Diet*	1 T.	12	3.0
(Welch's) Lite	1 T.	30	6.2
GRAVES WINE (Barton &			
Guestier) 12½% alcohol	3 fl. oz.	65	.6
GRAVY:			
Canned:			
Au jus (Franco-American)	2-oz. serving	10	2.0
Beef (Franco-American)	2-oz. serving	30	3.0

Food and Description	Measure or Quantity	Calories	Carbo- hydrates (grams)
Brown:			
(Dawn Fresh) with mushroom broth	2-oz. serving	18	3.2
(Franco-American) with onion	2-oz. serving	25	4.0
(La Choy)	½ of 5-oz. can	208	50.6
Ready Gravy	½ cup	86	15.3
Chicken (Franco-American):			
Regular	2-oz. serving	45	3.0
Giblet	2-oz. serving	35	3.0
Mushroom (Franco-American)	2-oz. serving	25	3.0
Turkey (Franco-American)	2-oz. serving	30	3.0
Mix, regular:			
Au jus:			
(Durkee):			
*Regular	1 cup	31	6.5
Roastin' Bag	1-oz. pkg.	64	14.0
*(French's) *Gravy Makins*	1 cup	32	8.0
*Brown:			
(Durkee):			
Regular	1 cup	59	10.0
With mushrooms	1 cup	59	11.0
With onions	1 cup	66	13.0
(Ehler's)	1 cup	84	14.0
(French's) *Gravy Makins*	1 cup	80	12.0
(Pillsbury)	1 cup	60	12.0
(Spatini)	1-oz. serving	8	2.0
Chicken:			
(Durkee):			
*Regular	1 cup	87	14.0
*Creamy	1 cup	156	14.0
Roastin' Bag:			
Regular	1.5-oz. pkg.	122	24.0
Creamy	2-oz. pkg.	242	22.0
Italian style	1.5-oz. pkg.	144	31.0
*(Ehler's)	1 cup	84	16.0
*(French's) *Gravy Makins*	1 cup	100	16.0
*(Pillsbury)	1 cup	100	16.0

(USDA): United States Department of Agriculture
(HEW/FAO): Health, Education and Welfare/Food and Agriculture
Organization
* Prepared as Package Directs

Food and Description	Measure or Quantity	Calories	Carbo- hydrates (grams)
*Homestyle:			
(Durkee)	1 cup	70	11.0
(French's) *Gravy Makins*	1 cup	100	16.0
Pillsbury)	1 cup	60	12.0
Meatloaf (Durkee) *Roastin' Bag*	1.5-oz. pkg.	129	18.0
*Mushroom:			
(Durkee)	1 cup	60	11.0
(French's) *Gravy Makins*	1 cup	80	12.0
*Onion:			
(Durkee)	1 cup	84	15.0
(French's) *Gravy Makins*	1 cup	100	16.0
Pork:			
(Durkee):			
Regular	1 cup	70	14.0
Roastin' Bag	1.5-oz. pkg.	130	26.0
*(French's) *Gravy Makins*	1 cup	80	12.0
Pot roast (Durkee) *Roastin' Bag:*			
·Regular	1.5-oz. pkg.	125	25.0
& onion	1.5-oz. pkg.	125	24.0
*Swiss steak (Durkee)	¾ cup	34	8.0
*Turkey:			
(Durkee)	1 cup	93	14.0
(French's) *Gravy Makins*	1 cup	100	16.0
Mix, dietetic (Weight Watchers):			
Brown:			
Regular	¼ cup	8	1.0
With mushroom	¼ cup	12	2.0
With onion	¼ cup	13	2.0
Chicken	¼ cup	10	2.0
GRAVY MASTER	1 tsp. (.2 oz.)	11	2.4
GRAVY WITH MEAT OR TURKEY:			
Canned (Morton House):			
Sliced beef	½ of 12½-oz. can	190	8.0
Sliced pork	½ of 12½-oz. can	190	9.0
Sliced turkey	½ of 12½-oz. can	140	7.0

Food and Description	Measure or Quantity	Calories	Carbohydrates (grams)
Frozen:			
(Banquet):			
Buffet Supper:			
Giblet gravy & sliced turkey	2-lb. pkg.	564	28.2
Sliced beef	2-lb. pkg.	782	34.5
Cookin' Bag:			
Giblet gravy & sliced turkey	5-oz. pkg.	98	5.3
Sliced beef	5-oz. pkg.	116	4.8
(Green Giant) *Toast Topper:*			
Sliced beef	5-oz. serving	122	5.7
Sliced turkey	5-oz. serving	92	6.7
(Swanson) *TV Brand,* with sliced beef & whipped potatoes	8-oz. entree	200	17.0
GREEN, MIXED, canned (Sunshine) solids & liq.	½ cup (4.1 oz.)	20	2.7
GREEN PEA (See **PEA, GREEN**)			
GRENADINE SYRUP:			
(Garnier) non-alcoholic	1 fl. oz.	103	26.0
(Leroux) 25 proof	1 fl. oz.	81	15.2
GRITS (See **HOMINY GRITS**)			
GROUND-CHERRY, Poha or Cape Gooseberry (USDA):			
Whole	1 lb. (weighed with husks & stems)	221	46.7
Flesh only	4 oz.	60	12.7

(USDA): United States Department of Agriculture
(HEW/FAO): Health, Education and Welfare/Food and Agriculture Organization
* Prepared as Package Directs

Food and Description	Measure or Quantity	Calories	Carbohydrates (grams)
GROUPER, raw (USDA):			
Whole	1 lb. (weighed whole)	170	0.
Meat only	4 oz.	99	0.
GUAVA, COMMON, fresh (USDA):			
Whole	1 lb. (weighed untrimmed)	273	66.0
Whole	1 guava (2.8 oz.)	48	11.7
Flesh only	4 oz.	70	17.0
GUAVA JAM (Smucker's)	1 T.	53	13.5
GUAVA JELLY (Smucker's)	1 T.	53	13.5
GUAVA, STRAWBERRY, fresh (USDA):			
Whole	1 lb. (weighed untrimmed)	289	70.2
Flesh only	4 oz.	74	17.9
GUINEA HEN, raw (USDA):			
Ready-to-cook	1 lb. (weighed ready-to-cook)	594	0.
Meat & skin	4 oz.	179	0.

H

HADDOCK:			
Raw (USDA):			
Whole	1 lb. (weighed whole)	172	0.
Meat only	4 oz.	90	0.
Fried, breaded (USDA)	4″ × 3″ × ½″ fillet (3.5 oz.)	165	5.8
Frozen:			
(Banquet)	8¾-oz. dinner	419	45.4
(Mrs. Paul's) breaded & fried	2-oz. fillet	114	11.8
(Swanson) fillet almondine	7½-oz. entree	370	9.0

Food and Description	Measure or Quantity	Calories	Carbo-hydrates (grams)
(Van de Kamp's) batter dipped, french-fried	2-oz. piece	165	8.0
(Weight Watchers) with stuffing, 2-compartment meal	7-oz. meal	205	14.1
Smoked, canned or not (USDA)	4 oz.	117	0.
HAKE, raw (USDA):			
Whole	1 lb. (weighed whole)	144	0.
Meat only	4 oz.	84	0.
HALF & HALF (milk & cream) (See **CREAM**)			
HALF & HALF WINE (Gallo)			
20% alcohol	3 fl. oz.	100	5.7
HALIBUT:			
Atlantic & Pacific (USDA):			
Raw:			
Whole	1 lb. (weighed whole)	268	0.
Meat only	4 oz.	113	0.
Broiled	4.4 oz.	214	0.
Smoked	4 oz.	254	0.
California (USDA) raw, meat only	4 oz.	110	0.
Greenland (See **TURBOT**)			
Frozen (Van de Kamp's) batter dipped, french-fried	½ of 8-oz. pkg.	270	17.0
HAM (See also **PORK**):			
Canned:			
(Hormel) *Tender Chunk*	1 oz.	49	.2
(Oscar Mayer) *Jubilee*, extra lean, cooked	¹⁄₁₂ of 3-lb. ham (4 oz.)	133	.5

(USDA): United States Department of Agriculture
(HEW/FAO): Health, Education and Welfare/Food and Agriculture Organization
* Prepared as Package Directs

Food and Description	*Measure or Quantity*	*Calories*	*Carbo-hydrates (grams)*
(Swift):			
Hostess	¼" slice (3.5 oz.)	141	.8
Premium	1¾-oz. slice (5" × 2" × ¼")	111	.3
Canned, chopped or minced:			
(USDA)	1 oz.	65	1.2
(Hormel)	1 oz. (8-lb. can)	89	.4
Canned, deviled:			
(USDA)	1 T. (.5 oz.)	46	0.
(Hormel)	1 T. (.5 oz.)	35	.1
(Libby's)	1 T. (.5 oz.)	40	.1
(Underwood)	1 T. (.5 oz.)	49	Tr.
Packaged, cooked:			
(Eckrich):			
Sliced	1.2-oz. slice	37	.9
Sliced, smoked	1-oz. slice	40	.7
(Hormel):			
Black peppered	.8-oz. slice	26	.1
Chopped	1-oz. slice	61	.3
Cooked	.8-oz. slice	26	.1
Red peppered	.8-oz. slice	26	.1
Smoked	.8-oz. slice	28	.1
(Oscar Mayer):			
Chopped	1 oz.	62	.3
Sliced, *Jubilee*	1-oz. slice	69	.5
Steak, *Jubilee*	8-oz. steak	257	0.
HAMBURGER (See **BEEF,** Ground, ***McDONALD'S*** or ***BURGER KING***)			
HAMBURGER MIX:			
(Ann Page):			
Beef noodle	⅕ of 7-oz. pkg.	146	48.2
Chili tomato	⅕ of 8-oz. pkg.	156	32.5
Hash	⅕ of 6-oz. pkg.	121	27.7
**Hamburger Helper* (General Mills):			
Beef noodle	⅕ of pkg.	320	25.0
Beef Romanoff	⅕ of pkg.	340	28.0
Cheeseburger	⅕ of pkg.	360	28.0
Chili tomato	⅕ of pkg.	320	29.0
Hash	⅕ of pkg.	300	24.0

Food and Description	Measure or Quantity	Calories	Carbo-hydrates (grams)
Lasagna	⅓ of pkg.	330	33.0
Pizza	⅓ of pkg.	340	33.0
Potato au gratin	⅓ of pkg.	320	27.0
Potato stroganoff	⅓ of pkg.	330	28.0
Rice oriental	⅓ of pkg.	320	35.0
Spaghetti	⅓ of pkg.	330	31.0
Stew	⅓ of pkg.	290	23.0
Tamale pie	⅓ of pkg.	370	39.0
Make-a-Better Burger (Lipton) mildly seasoned or onion	⅓ of pkg.	30	5.0
HAMBURGER SEASONING MIX:			
*(Durkee)	1 cup	663	7.5
(French's)	1-oz. pkg.	100	20.0
HAM & BUTTER BEAN SOUP, canned (Campbell)			
Chunky	10¾-oz. can	280	34.0
HAM & CHEESE:			
(Hormel) loaf	1-oz. slice	69	.3
(Oscar Mayer):			
Loaf	1 oz. slice	77	.6
Spread	1-oz. serving	67	.7
HAM DINNER, frozen:			
(Banquet)	10-oz. dinner	369	47.7
(Morton)	10-oz. dinner	449	56.9
(Swanson) *TV Brand*	10-oz. dinner	380	47.0
HAM SALAD SPREAD:			
(Carnation) spreadable	1½-oz. serving	78	3.4
(Oscar Mayer)	1 oz. serving	62	3.0
HAWAIIAN PUNCH:			
Canned:			
Cherry	6 fl. oz.	87	22.8

(USDA): United States Department of Agriculture
(HEW/FAO):   Health, Education and Welfare/Food and Agriculture
                        Organization
* Prepared as Package Directs

Food and Description	Measure or Quantity	Calories	Carbo-hydrates (grams)
Grape	6 fl. oz.	93	23.4
Orange	6 fl. oz.	97	24.4
Red	6 fl. oz.	84	21.3
Very Berry	6 fl. oz.	87	21.6
*Mix, red punch	8 fl. oz.	100	25.0
HAWS, SCARLET, raw (USDA):			
Whole	1 lb. (weighed with core)	316	75.5
Flesh & skin	4 oz.	99	23.6
HAZELNUT (See **FILBERT**)			
HEADCHEESE:			
(USDA)	1-oz. serving	76	.3
(Oscar Mayer)	1-oz. serving	54	0.
HERRING:			
Raw (USDA):			
Atlantic:			
Whole	1 lb. (weighed whole)	407	0.
Meat only	4 oz.	200	0.
Pacific, meat only	4 oz.	111	0.
Canned:			
(USDA) in tomato sauce, solids & liq.	4-oz. serving	200	4.2
(Vita):			
Bismarck, drained	5-oz. jar	273	6.9
In cream sauce, drained	8-oz. jar	397	18.1
Matjis, drained	8-oz. jar	304	26.2
In wine sauce, drained	8-oz. jar	401	16.6
Pickled (USDA) Bismarck type	4-oz. serving	253	0.
Salted or brined (USDA)	4-oz. serving	247	0.
Smoked (USDA):			
Bloaters	4-oz. serving	222	0.
Hard	4-oz. serving	340	0.
Kippered	4-oz. serving	239	0.

Food and Description	Measure or Quantity	Calories	Carbo-hydrates (grams)
HICKORY NUT (USDA):			
Whole	1 lb. (weighed in shell)	1068	20.3
Shelled	4 oz.	763	14.5
HO-HOS (Hostess)	1-oz. cake	124	16.5
HOMINY GRITS:			
Dry:			
(USDA):			
Degermed	1 oz.	103	22.1
Degermed	½ cup (2.8 oz.)	282	60.9
(Albers) quick, degermed	1½ oz.	150	33.0
(Aunt Jemima)	3 T. (1 oz.)	101	22.4
(Pocono) creamy	1 oz.	101	23.6
(Quaker):			
Regular or quick	1 T. (.33 oz.)	34	7.5
Instant:			
Regular	.8-oz. packet	79	17.7
With imitation bacon bits	1-oz. packet	101	21.6
With artificial cheese flavor	1-oz. packet	104	21.6
With imitation ham bits	1-oz. packet	99	21.3
(3-Minute Brand) quick, enriched	⅙ cup (1 oz.)	98	22.2
Cooked (USDA) degermed	⅔ cup (5.6 oz.)	84	18.0
HONEY, strained:			
(USDA)	½ cup (5.7 oz.)	494	134.1
(USDA)	1 T. (.7 oz.)	61	16.5
HONEYCOMB, cereal (Post)	1⅓ cups (1 oz.)	113	25.1
HONEYDEW, fresh (USDA):			
Whole	1 lb. (weighed whole)	94	22.0

(USDA): United States Department of Agriculture
(HEW/FAO):   Health, Education and Welfare/Food and Agriculture
                        Organization
* Prepared as Package Directs

Food and Description	Measure or Quantity	Calories	Carbo-hydrates (grams)
Wedge	2" × 7" wedge (5.3 oz.)	31	7.2
Flesh only	4 oz.	37	8.7
Flesh only, diced	1 cup (5.9 oz.)	55	12.9
HOPPING JOHN, frozen (Green Giant) Southern recipe	⅓ of 10-oz. pkg.	116	16.7
HORSERADISH:			
Raw (USDA):			
Whole	1 lb. (weighed unpared)	288	65.2
Pared	1 oz.	25	5.6
Prepared:			
(Gold's)	1 oz.	18	.4
(Nalley's) sauce	1 oz.	106	3.1
HYACINTH BEAN (USDA):			
Young bean, raw:			
Whole	1 lb. (weighed untrimmed)	140	29.1
Trimmed	4 oz.	40	8.3
Dry seeds	4 oz.	383	69.2

I

Food and Description	Measure or Quantity	Calories	Carbo-hydrates (grams)
ICE CREAM and FROZEN CUSTARD (See also listing by flavor or brand name, e. g., **CHOCOLATE ICE CREAM** or *GOOD HUMOR*):			
Sweetened:			
(USDA):			
10% fat	1 cup (4.7 oz.)	257	27.7
12% fat	1 cup (5 oz.)	294	29.3
12% fat, brick-type	2½-oz. slice	147	14.6
12% fat	small container (3½ fl. oz.)	128	12.8
16% fat	1 cup (5.2 oz.)	329	26.6
(Dean) fruit, 10.4% fat	1 cup (5.6 oz.)	336	41.1

Food and Description	Measure or Quantity	Calories	Carbo-hydrates (grams)
ICE CREAM CONE (Comet) cone only, any color:			
Regular	1 piece (4 grams)	20	4.0
Rolled sugar	1 piece (.4 oz.)	40	9.0
ICE CREAM CUP, cup only (Comet) any color	1 piece (5 grams)	20	4.0
ICE CREAM SANDWICH (Sealtest)	3-fl.-oz. sandwich	170	26.0
ICE MILK:			
(USDA):			
Hardened	1 cup (4.6 oz.)	199	29.3
Soft-serve	1 cup (6.3 oz.)	266	39.2
(Dean):			
Count Calorie, 2.1% fat	1 cup (4.8 oz.)	155	17.1
5% fat	1 cup (4.9 oz.)	227	35.0
(Meadow Gold):			
Chocolate, *Viva*	1 cup	200	36.0
Vanilla, *Viva*	1 cup	200	34.0
ICING (See **CAKE ICING**)			
INSTANT BREAKFAST (See individual brand name or company listings)			
IRISH WHISKEY (See **Distilled Liquors**)			
ITALIAN DINNER, frozen (Banquet)	11-oz. dinner	446	44.6

(USDA): United States Department of Agriculture
(HEW/FAO): Health, Education and Welfare/Food and Agriculture
                    Organization
* Prepared as Package Directs

Food and Description	Measure or Quantity	Calories	Carbo-hydrates (grams)

J

JACKFRUIT, fresh (USDA):
| Whole | 1 lb. (weighed with seeds & skin) | 124 | 32.3 |
| Flesh only | 4 oz. | 111 | 28.8 |

JACK MACKERAL, raw (USDA) meat only
| | 4 oz. | 162 | 0. |

JAM, sweetened (See also individual listings by flavor):
(USDA)	1 oz.	77	19.8
(USDA)	1 T. (.7 oz.)	54	14.0
(Ann Page) all flavors	1 tsp. (6.8 grams)	19	4.8

JELLY, sweetened (See also individual listings by flavor):
(USDA)	1 T. (.6 oz.)	49	12.7
(Ann Page) all flavors	1 T.	57	13.8
(Crosse & Blackwell)	1 T. (.7 oz.)	51	12.8

JERUSALEM ARTICHOKE (USDA):
| Unpared | 1 lb. (weighed with skin) | 207 | 52.3 |
| Pared | 4 oz. | 75 | 18.9 |

JOHANNISBERGER RIESLING WINE:
| (Inglenook) Estate, 12% alcohol | 3 fl. oz. | 61 | .9 |
| (Louis M. Martini) 12.5% alcohol | 3 fl. oz. | 90 | .2 |

JORDAN ALMOND (See CANDY)

JUICE (See individual flavors)

Food and Description	Measure or Quantity	Calories	Carbo- hydrates (grams)
JUJUBE or CHINESE DATE (USDA):			
Fresh, whole	1 lb. (weighed with seeds)	443	116.4
Fresh, flesh only	4 oz.	119	31.3
Dried, whole	1 lb. (weighed with seeds)	1159	297.1
Dried, flesh only	4 oz.	325	83.5
JUNIOR FOOD (See **BABY FOOD**)			

K

Food and Description	Measure or Quantity	Calories	Carbo- hydrates (grams)
KABOOM, cereal (General Mills)	1 cup (1 oz.)	110	23.0
KALE:			
Raw (USDA) leaves only	1 lb. (weighed untrimmed)	154	26.1
Boiled (USDA) leaves, including stems	½ cup (1.9 oz.)	15	2.2
Canned (Sunshine) chopped, solids & liq.	½ cup (4.1 oz.)	21	2.8
Frozen:			
(Birds Eye) chopped	⅓ of. pkg.	25	5.0
(McKenzie) chopped	3.3-oz. serving	32	4.5
(Seabrook Farms) chopped	⅓ of 10-oz. pkg.	32	4.5
(Southland) chopped	⅕ of 16-oz. pkg.	30	5.0
KEFIR (Alta-Dena Dairy):			
Plain	1 cup (8.6 oz.)	180	13.0
Flavored	1 cup (7.3 oz.)	190	24.0
KETCHUP (See **CATSUP**)			

(USDA): United States Department of Agriculture
(HEW/FAO): Health, Education and Welfare/Food and Agriculture Organization
* Prepared as Package Directs

Food and Description	Measure or Quantity	Calories	Carbo- hydrates (grams)
KIDNEY (USDA):			
Beef:			
Raw	4 oz.	147	1.0
Braised	4 oz.	286	.9
Calf, raw	4 oz.	128	.1
Hog, raw	4 oz.	120	1.2
Lamb, raw	4 oz.	119	1.0
KIELBASA:			
(Eckrich) skinless	2-oz. link	190	2.0
(Hormel) Kilbase	3-oz. serving	245	1.2
(Vienna)	2½-oz. serving	206	1.1
KINGFISH, raw (USDA):			
Whole	1 lb. (weighed whole)	210	0.
Meat only	4 oz.	119	0.
KING VITAMAN, cereal (Quaker)	1¼ cups (1 oz.)	113	23.2
KIPPERS (See **HERRING**)			
KIRSCH LIQUEUR (Garnier) 96 proof	1 fl. oz.	83	8.8
KIRSCHWASSER (Leroux) 96 proof	1 fl. oz.	80	0.
KIX, cereal (General Mills)	1½ cups (1 oz.)	110	24.0
KNOCKWURST:			
(USDA)	1 oz.	79	.6
(Best's Kosher or Oscherwitz):			
Regular	3-oz. piece	270	3.0
Beef, low fat	3-oz. piece	203	2.9
KOHLRABI (USDA):			
Raw:			
Whole	1 lb. (weighed with skin, without leaves)	96	21.9

Food and Description	Measure or Quantity	Calories	Carbo-hydrates (grams)
Diced	1 cup (4.8 oz.)	40	9.1
Boiled:			
Drained	4 oz.	27	6.0
Drained	1 cup (5.5 oz.)	37	8.2
*KOOL-AID (General Foods):			
Unsweetened package	8 fl. oz.	100	25.0
Presweetened package	8 fl. oz.	93	23.2
Presweetened package, tropical punch	8 fl. oz.	98	24.5
KUMMEL LIQUEUR:			
(Garnier) 70 proof	1 fl. oz.	75	4.3
(Leroux) 70 proof	1 fl. oz.	75	4.1
KUMQUAT, fresh (USDA):			
Whole	1 lb. (weighed with seeds)	274	72.1
Flesh & skin	4 oz.	74	19.4
Flesh only	5-6 med. kumquats	65	17.1

L

LAKE COUNTRY WINE			
(Taylor):			
Gold, 12% alcohol	3 fl. oz.	78	5.4
Pink, 12½% alcohol	3 fl. oz.	78	4.8
Red, 12½% alcohol	3 fl. oz.	81	4.8
White, 12½% alcohol	3 fl. oz.	81	4.2
LAKE HERRING, raw (USDA):			
Whole	1 lb.	226	0.
Meat only	4 oz.	109	0.

(USDA): United States Department of Agriculture
(HEW/FAO): Health, Education and Welfare/Food and Agriculture Organization
* Prepared as Package Directs

Food and Description	Measure or Quantity	Calories	Carbo-hydrates (grams)
LAKE TROUT, raw (USDA):			
Drawn	1 lb. (weighed with head, fins & bones)	282	0.
Meat only	4 oz.	191	0.
LAKE TROUT or SISCOWET, raw (USDA):			
Less than 6.5 lb.:			
Whole	1 lb. (weighed whole)	404	0.
Meat only	4 oz.	273	0.
More than 6.5 lb.:			
Whole	1 lb. (weighed whole)	856	0.
Meat only	4 oz.	594	0.
LAMB, choice grade (USDA):			
Chop, broiled:			
Loin. One 5-oz. chop (weighed before cooking with bone) will give you:			
Lean & fat	2.8 oz.	280	0.
Lean only	2.3 oz.	122	0.
Rib. One 5-oz. chop (weighed before cooking with bone) will give you:			
Lean & fat	2.9 oz.	334	0.
Lean only	2 oz.	118	0.
Fat, separable, cooked	1 oz.	201	0.
Leg:			
Raw, lean & fat	1 lb. (weighed with bone)	845	0.
Roasted, lean & fat	4 oz.	316	0.
Roasted, lean only	4 oz.	211	0.
Shoulder:			
Raw, lean & fat	1 lb. (weighed with bone)	1082	0.
Roasted, lean & fat	4 oz.	383	0.
Roasted, lean only	4 oz.	232	0.

Food and Description	Measure or Quantity	Calories	Carbo-hydrates (grams)
LAMB'S-QUARTERS (USDA):			
Raw, trimmed	1 lb.	195	33.1
Boiled, drained	4 oz.	36	5.7
LARD:			
(USDA)	1 cup (7.2 oz.)	1849	0.
(USDA)	1 T. (.5 oz.)	117	0.
LASAGANA:			
Canned:			
(Hormel) *Short Orders*	7½-oz. can	260	24.0
(Nalley's)	8-oz. serving	239	25.0
Frozen:			
(Green Giant):			
With meat sauce, boil-in-bag	9-oz. pkg.	294	32.2
With meat sauce, oven bake	⅓ of 21-oz. pkg.	295	27.8
(Hormel) beef	10-oz. serving	371	30.4
(Stouffer's)	½ of 21-oz. pkg.	380	35.8
(Swanson):			
Regular, with meat in tomato sauce	12¼-oz. entree	490	54.0
Hungry Man: with meat:			
Dinner	17¾-oz. dinner	790	91.0
Entree	12¾-oz. entree	540	51.0
TV Brand	13-oz. dinner	390	54.0
(Weight Watchers) 1-compartment meal	12¾-oz. meal	409	49.3
Mix (Golden Grain) *Stir-n-Serve*	⅕ of 7-oz. pkg.	153	25.9
LEEKS, raw (USDA):			
Whole	1 lb. (weighed untrimmed)	123	26.4
Trimmed	4 oz.	59	12.7

(USDA): United States Department of Agriculture
(HEW/FAO): Health, Education and Welfare/Food and Agriculture Organization
* Prepared as Package Directs

Food and Description	Measure or Quantity	Calories	Carbohydrates (grams)
LEMON, fresh (USDA) peeled	1 med. (2 ⅛" dia.)	20	6.1
LEMONADE:			
Canned:			
Capri Sun, natural	6 ¾ fl. oz.	63	23.3
Country Time	12-fl.-oz. can	134	33.5
(Hi-C)	6 fl. oz.	68	17.0
Chilled (Minute Maid):			
Regular	6 fl. oz.	79	18.0
Pink	6 fl. oz.	78	18.0
*Frozen:			
(USDA)	½ cup (4.4 oz.)	55	14.1
Country Time, regular or pink	8 fl. oz.	91	22.7
(Minute Maid)	6 fl. oz.	74	19.6
(Sunkist) regular or pink	6 fl. oz.	81	21.1
*Mix:			
Country Time, regular or pink	8 fl. oz.	90	22.0
(Hi-C)	6 fl. oz.	76	19.0
(Kool-Aid) unsweetened package, regular or pink	8 fl. oz.	100	25.0
(Kool-Aid) presweetened package, regular or pink	8 fl. oz.	89	22.2
Lemon Tree (Lipton)	8 fl. oz.	90	22.0
(Minute Maid) regular or pink	6 fl. oz.	80	20.0
LEMON EXTRACT:			
(Durkee) imitation	1 tsp.	17	DNA
(Virginia Dare) 78% alcohol	1 tsp.	21	0.
LEMON JUICE:			
Fresh:			
(USDA)	1 cup (8.6 oz.)	61	19.5
(USDA)	1 T. (.5 oz.)	4	1.2
Canned, unsweetened:			
(USDA)	1 cup (8.6 oz.)	56	18.6
(USDA)	1 T. (.5 oz.)	3	1.1
(Sunkist)	1 T.	3	1.2

Food and Description	Measure or Quantity	Calories	Carbo-hydrates (grams)
Plastic container:.			
(USDA)	¼ cup (2 oz.)	13	4.3
ReaLemon	1 T. (.5 oz.)	3	.8
Frozen, unsweetened:			
(USDA):			
Concentrate	½ cup (5.1 oz.)	169	54.6
Single strength	½ cup (4.3 oz.)	27	8.80
(Minute Maid) full strength, already constituted	1 fl. oz.	7	2.2
*LEMON-LIMEADE, mix (Minute Maid)	6 fl. oz.	80	20.0
LEMON PEEL, CANDIED (USDA)	1 oz.	90	22.9
LEMON & PEPPER SEASONING (French's)	1 tsp. (3.6 grams)	6	1.0
LENTIL:			
Whole:			
Dry:			
(USDA)	½ lb.	771	136.3
(USDA)	1 cup (6.7 oz.)	649	114.8
(Sinsheimer)	1 oz.	95	17.0
Cooked (USDA) drained	½ cup (3.6 oz.)	107	19.5
Split (USDA) dry	½ lb.	782	140.2
LENTIL SOUP, canned (Crosse & Blackwell) with ham	½ of 13-oz. can	80	13.0
LETTUCE (USDA):			
Bibb, untrimmed	1 lb. (weighed untrimmed)	47	8.4
Bibb, untrimmed	7.8-oz. head (4″ dia.)	23	4.1

(USDA): United States Department of Agriculture
(HEW/FAO): Health, Education and Welfare/Food and Agriculture
             Organization
* Prepared as Package Directs

Food and Description	Measure or Quantity	Calories	Carbo-hydrates (grams)
Boston, untrimmed	1 lb. (weighed untrimmed)	47	8.4
Boston, untrimmed	7.8 oz. head (4″ dia.)	23	4.1
Butterhead varieties (See Bibb & Boston)			
Cos (See Romaine)			
Dark green (See Romaine)			
Grand Rapids	1 lb. (weighed untrimmed)	52	10.2
Grand Rapids	2 large leaves (1.8 oz.)	9	1.8
Great Lakes	1 lb. (weighed untrimmed)	56	12.5
Great Lakes, trimmed	1-lb. head (4¾″ dia.)	59	13.2
Iceberg:			
Untrimmed	1 lb. (weighed untrimmed)	56	12.5
Trimmed	1 lb. head (4¾″ dia.)	59	13.2
Leaves	1 cup (2.3 oz.)	9	1.9
Chopped	1 cup (2 oz.)	8	1.7
Chunks	1 cup (2.6 oz.)	10	2.1
Looseleaf varieties (See Salad Bowl)			
New York	1 lb. (weighed untrimmed)	56	12.5
New York	1-lb. head (4¾″ dia.)	59	13.2
Romaine:			
Untrimmed	1 lb. (weighed untrimmed)	52	10.2
Trimmed, shredded & broken into pieces	½ cup (.8 oz.)	4	.8
Salad Bowl	1 lb. (weighed untrimmed)	52	10. 2
Salad Bowl	2 large leaves (1.8 oz.)	9	1.8
Simpson	1 lb. (weighed untrimmed)	52	10.2

Food and Description	Measure or Quantity	Calories	Carbo-hydrates (grams)
Simpson	2 large leaves (1.8 oz.)	9	1.8
White Paris (See Romaine)			
LIFE, cereal (Quaker) regular or cinnamon	⅔ cup (1 oz.)	105	19.7
LIMA BEAN (See BEAN, LIMA)			
LIME, fresh (USDA):			
Whole	1 lb. (weighed with skin & seeds)	107	36.2
Whole	1 med. (2" dia., 2.4 oz.)	15	4.9
***LIMEADE,** frozen, sweetened: (USDA) diluted with 4 ⅓			
parts water	½ cup (4.4 oz.)	51	13.6
(Minute Maid)	6 fl. oz.	75	20.1
LIME JUICE,:			
Fresh (USDA)	1 cup (8.7 oz.)	64	22.1
Canned or bottled, unsweetened:			
(USDA)	1 cup (8.7 oz.)	64	22.1
(USDA)	1 fl. oz. (1.1 oz.)	8	2.8
Plastic container, *ReaLime*	1 T. (.5 oz.)	2	.5
LINGCOD, raw (USDA):			
Whole	1 lb. (weighed whole)	130	0.
Meat only	4 oz.	95	0.
LINGUINI IN CLAM SAUCE, frozen (Stouffer's)	10½-oz. pkg.	284	35.8

(USDA): United States Department of Agriculture
(HEW/FAO):   Health, Education and Welfare/Food and Agriculture
                        Organization
* Prepared as Package Directs

Food and Description	Measure or Quantity	Calories	Carbo-hydrates (grams)
LIQUEUR (See individual kinds)			
LITCHI NUT (USDA):			
Fresh:			
Whole	4 oz. (weighed in shell with seeds)	44	11.2
Flesh only	4 oz.	73	18.6
Dried:			
Whole	4 oz. (weighed in shell with seeds)	145	36.9
Flesh only	2 oz.	157	40.1
LIVER:			
Beef:			
(USDA):			
Raw	1 lb.	635	24.0
Fried	4 oz.	260	6.0
(Swift) packaged, True-Tender, sliced, cooked	⅓ of 1-lb. pkg.	141	3.1
Calf (USDA):			
Raw	1 lb.	635	18.6
Fried	4 oz.	296	4.5
Chicken:			
Raw	1 lb.	585	13.2
Simmered	4 oz.	187	3.5
Goose, raw (USDA)	1 lb.	826	24.5
Hog (USDA):			
Raw	1 lb.	594	11.8
Fried	4 oz.	273	2.8
Lamb (USDA):			
Raw	1 lb.	617	13.2
Broiled	4 oz.	296	3.2
Turkey, raw (USDA)	1 lb.	626	13.2
LIVER PÂTÉ (See **PÂTÉ**)			
LIVER SAUSAGE or LIVERWURST, spread (Underwood)	1 oz.	92	1.1

Food and Description	Measure or Quantity	Calories	Carbo-hydrates (grams)
LOBSTER:			
Raw (USDA):			
Whole	1 lb. (weighed whole)	107	.6
Meat only	4 oz.	103	.6
Cooked, meat only (USDA)	4 oz.	108	.3
Canned (USDA) meat only	4 oz.	108	.3
Frozen, South African rock lobster tail	2-oz. tail	65	.1
LOBSTER NEWBURG, home recipe (USDA)	4 oz.	220	5.8
LOBSTER PASTE, canned (USDA)	1 oz.	51	.4
LOBSTER SALAD, home recipe (USDA)	4 oz.	125	2.6
LOCHON ORA, Scottish liqueur (Leroux) 70 proof	1 fl. oz	89	7.4
LOGANBERRY (USDA):			
Fresh:			
Untrimmed	1 lb. (weighed with caps)	267	64.2
Trimmed	1 cup (5.1 oz.)	89	21.5
Canned, solids & liq.:			
Extra heavy syrup	4 oz.	101	25.2
Heavy syrup	4 oz.	101	25.2
Juice pack	4 oz.	61	14.4
Light syrup	4 oz.	79	19.5
Water pack	4 oz.	45	10.7
LONGAN (USDA):			
Fresh:			
Whole	1 lb. (weighed with shell & seeds)	147	38.0

(USDA): United States Department of Agriculture
(HEW/FAO): Health, Education and Welfare/Food and Agriculture Organization
* Prepared as Package Directs

Food and Description	Measure or Quantity	Calories	Carbo-hydrates (grams)
Flesh only	4 oz.	69	17.9
Dried:			
Whole	1 lb. (weighed with shell & seeds)	467	120.8
Flesh only	4 oz.	324	83.9
LOQUAT, fresh (USDA):			
Whole	1 lb. (weighed with seeds)	168	43.3
Flesh only	4 oz.	54	14.1
LUCKY CHARMS, cereal (General Mills)	1 cup (1 oz.)	110	24.0
LUNCHEON MEAT (See also individual listings, e. g., **BOLOGNA,** etc.):			
All meat (Oscar Mayer)	1-oz. slice	98	.4
Banquet loaf (Eckrich)	1-oz. slice	75	1.5
Bar-B-Q-Loaf (Oscar Mayer) 90% fat free	1-oz. slice	49	1.4
BBQ Loaf (Hormel)	1-oz. slice	50	.5
Beef honey roll sausage (Oscar Mayer) 90% fat free	.8-oz. slice	40	.7
Beef, jellied (Hormel) loaf	1.2-oz. slice	35	0.
Buffet loaf (Hormel)	1-oz. slice	50	.5
Gourmet loaf (Eckrich)	1-oz. slice	32	1.7
Ham & cheese (See **HAM & CHEESE**)			
Ham roll sausage (Oscar Mayer)	.5-oz. slice	21	.3
Ham roll sausage (Oscar Mayer)	1-oz. slice	43	.6
Honey loaf:			
(Eckrich)	1-oz. slice	40	1.8
(Hormel)	1-oz. slice	47	.6
(Oscar Mayer) 95% fat free	1-oz. slice	37	1.1
Liver cheese (Oscar Mayer) pork fat wrapped	1.3-oz. slice	114	.6
Liver loaf (Hormel)	1-oz. slice	81	.6
Luxury loaf (Oscar Mayer) 95% fat free	1-oz. slice	39	1.5
Meat loaf (USDA)	1-oz. serving	57	.9

Food and Description	Measure or Quantity	Calories	Carbo-hydrates (grams)
New England brand sausage:			
(Hormel)	1-oz. slice	49	.2
(Oscar Mayer) 92% fat free	.8-oz. slice	34	.5
Old fashioned loaf:			
(Eckrich)	1-oz. slice	75	2.0
(Oscar Mayer)	1-oz. slice	65	2.3
Olive loaf:			
(Hormel)	1-oz. slice	59	1.5
(Oscar Mayer)	1-oz. slice	65	2.8
Peppered beef (Vienna)	1-oz. serving	50	.4
Peppered loaf:			
(Hormel)	1-oz. serving	72	.4
(Oscar Mayer) 93% fat free	1-oz. slice	42	1.3
Pickle loaf:			
(Eckrich)	1-oz. slice	85	1.5
(Hormel)	1-oz. slice	59	1.3
Pickle & pimiento loaf (Oscar Mayer)	1-oz. slice	65	3.0
Picnic loaf (Oscar Mayer)	1-oz. slice	64	1.6
Spiced (Hormel)	1-oz. serving	77	.5
LUNG, raw (USDA)			
Beef	1 lb.	435	0.
Calf	1 lb.	481	0.
Lamb	1 lb.	467	0.

M

MACADAMIA NUT:			
Whole (USDA)	1 lb. (weighed in shell)	972	22.4
Shelled (Royal Hawaiian)	¼ cup (2 oz.)	394	9.0

MACARONI. Plain macaroni products are essentially the

(USDA): United States Department of Agriculture
(HEW/FAO):   Health, Education and Welfare/Food and Agriculture
                      Organization
* Prepared as Package Directs

Food and Description	Measure or Quantity	Calories	Carbo- hydrates (grams)
same in caloric value and carbo- hydrate content on the same weight basis. The longer they are cooked, the more water is absorbed and this affects the nutritive values.			
Dry (USDA):			
Elbow-type	1 cup (4.8 oz.)	502	102.3
1-inch pieces	1 cup (3.8 oz.)	406	82.7
2-inch pieces	1 cup (3 oz.)	317	64.7
Cooked (USDA):			
8-10 minutes, firm	1 cup (4.6 oz.)	192	39.1
8-10 minutes, firm	4 oz.	168	34.1
14-20 minutes, tender	1 cup (4.9 oz.)	155	32.2
14-20 minutes, tender	4 oz.	126	26.1
Canned (Franco-American) *PizzOs*, in pizza sauce	7½-oz. can	170	34.0
MACARONI & BEEF:			
Canned:			
(Bounty) *Chili Mac*, in tomato sauce	7¾-oz. can	255	29.7
(Franco-American) *BeefyOs*, in tomato sauce	7½-oz. can	220	29.0
(Nalley's)	8-oz. serving	236	29.5
Frozen:			
(Banquet):			
Buffet Supper	2-lb. pkg.	1000	106.4
Dinner	12-oz. dinner	394	55.1
(Green Giant) with tomato sauce	9-oz. entree	233	30.7
(Morton)	10-oz. dinner	267	45.4
(Stouffer's) with tomatoes	11½-oz. pkg.	384	39.8
(Swanson) *TV Brand*	12-oz. dinner	400	55.0
MACARONI & CHEESE:			
Home recipe (USDA) baked	1 cup (7.1 oz.)	430	40.2
Canned:			
(USDA)	1 cup	228	25.7
(Franco-American):			
Regular	7 ¾ oz. can	170	24.0
CheeseOs	7½-oz. can	170	21.0

Food and Description	Measure or Quantity	Calories	Carbo-hydrates (grams)
Elbow	7⅜-oz. can	170	23.0
(Hormel) *Short Orders*	7½-oz. can	170	22.0
Frozen:			
(Banquet):			
Buffet Supper	1-lb. pkg.	1027	110.9
Cookin' Bag	8-oz. pkg.	261	28.6
Dinner	12-oz. dinner	326	45.6
Entree	8-oz. entree	279	35.9
(Green Giant):			
Bake'n Serve	12-oz. serving	432	47.4
Boil-in-bag	9-oz. serving	304	35.8
(Morton):			
Casserole	8-oz. casserole	227	36.4
Dinner	11-oz. dinner	306	53.1
(Stouffer's)	12-oz. pkg.	502	47.8
(Swanson):			
Regular	12-oz. entree	420	40.0
TV Brand	12½-oz. dinner	390	55.0
(Van de Kamp's)	10-oz. pkg.	300	46.0
Mix:			
(USDA) dry	1 oz.	113	17.8
(Golden Grain)	¼ of 7¼-oz. pkg.	202	38.1
*(Pennsylvania Dutch Brand)	½ cup serving	160	25.0
*(Prince)	¾-cup serving	268	34.6
Tuna Helper (General Mills)	¼ pkg.	310	38.0
MACARONI & CHEESE PIE, frozen (Swanson)	7-oz. pie	230	26.0
MACARONI SALAD, canned (Nalley's)	4-oz. serving	206	15.9
MACE (French's)	1 tsp. (1.8 grams)	10	.8

(USDA): United States Department of Agriculture
(HEW/FAO):   Health, Education and Welfare/Food and Agriculture
                        Organization
* Prepared as Package Directs

Food and Description	Measure or Quantity	Calories	Carbo-hydrates (grams)
MACKEREL (USDA):			
Atlantic:			
Raw:			
Whole	1 lb. (weighed whole)	468	0.
Meat only	4 oz.	217	0.
Broiled with butter	4 oz.	268	0.
Canned, solids & liq.	4 oz.	208	0.
Pacific:			
Raw:			
Dressed	1 lb. (weighed with bones & skin)	519	0.
Meat only	4 oz.	180	0.
Canned, solids & liq.	4 oz.	204	0.
Salted	4 oz.	346	0.
Smoked	4 oz.	248	0.
MACKEREL, JACK (See **JACK MACKEREL**)			
MADEIRA WINE (Leacock) 19% alcohol	3 fl. oz.	120	6.3
MAI TAI COCKTAIL, canned (Mr. Boston) 12% alcohol	3 fl. oz.	111	12.3
MALT, dry (USDA)	1 oz.	104	21.9
MALTED MILK MIX:			
(USDA) dry powder	1 oz.	116	20.1
(Carnation):			
Chocolate	3 heaping tsps. (.7 oz.)	85	18.0
Natural	3 heaping tsps. (.7 oz.)	90	15.6
(Horlicks):			
Chocolate	3 heaping tsps. (1.1 oz.)	124	26.0
Natural	3 heaping tsps. (1.1 oz.)	127	22.3

Food and Description	Measure or Quantity	Calories	Carbo-hydrates (grams)
MALT EXTRACT, dried			
(USDA)	1 oz.	104	25.3
MALT LIQUOR:			
Champale, 6¼% alcohol	12 fl. oz.	173	11.5
Country Club, 6.8% alcohol	12 fl. oz.	183	2.8
MALT-O-MEAL, cereal:			
Regular	1 T. (.3 oz.)	33	7.3
Chocolate flavored	1 T (.3 oz.)	33	7.0
MAMEY or MAMMEE APPLE,			
fresh (USDA)	1 lb. (weighed with skin & seeds)	143	35.2
MANDARIN ORANGE (See **TANGERINE**)			
MANGO, fresh (USDA):			
Whole	1 lb. (weighed with seeds & skin)	201	51.1
Whole	1 med. (7 oz.)	88	22.5
Flesh only, diced or sliced	½ cup (2.9 oz.)	54	13.8
MANHATTAN COCKTAIL,			
canned (Mr. Boston) 20% alcohol	3 fl. oz.	123	6.3
MAPLE SYRUP (See **SYRUP**)			
MARGARINE, salted or unsalted:			
Regular:			
(USDA)	1 lb.	3266	1.8

(USDA): United States Department of Agriculture
(HEW/FAO):   Health, Education and Welfare/Food and Agriculture
                         Organization
* Prepared as Package Directs

Food and Description	Measure or Quantity	Calories	Carbo-hydrates (grams)
(USDA)	1 cup (8 oz.)	1633	.9
(USDA)	1 T. (.5 oz.)	101	<.1
Autumn, soft or stick	1 T.	102	Tr.
(Blue Bonnet) soft or stick	1 T. (.5 oz.)	100	0.
Chiffon:			
Soft	1 T.	90	0.
Stick	1 T.	100	0.
(Fleishmann's) soft or stick	1 T. (.5 oz.)	100	0.
Golden Mist	1 T.	100	0.
Holiday	1 T. (.5 oz.)	102	0.
(Imperial) soft or stick	1 T. (.5 oz.)	102	.1
Mazola:			
Regular	1 T. (.5 oz.)	104	.2
Unsalted	1 T. (.5 oz.)	103	0.
(Meadowlake) soft	1 T.	90	0.
(Mother's) soft or stick	1 T. (.5 oz.)	100	0.
(Nucoa):			
Regular	1 T. (.5 oz.)	103	Tr.
Soft	1 T. (.4 oz.)	82	Tr.
(Parkay) Squeeze	1 T. (.5 oz.)	101	.2
(Promise) soft or stick	1 T. (.5 oz.)	102	.1
Imitation or dietetic:			
(Blue Bonnet)	1 T.	50	0.
(Imperial) soft	1 T. (.5 oz.)	50	Tr.
(Mazola)	1 T. (.5 oz.)	50	0.
(Weight Watchers)	1 T.	50	0.
Whipped:			
(Blue Bonnet)	1 T. (9 grams)	70	0.
Chiffon	1 T.	70	0.
Fleishmann's, soft	1 T.	70	0.
Imperial	1 T. (9 grams)	65	Tr.
(Parkay) cup	1 T.	67	**<.1**
MARGARITA COCKTAIL, canned (Mr. Boston):			
Regular, 12½% alcohol	3 fl. oz.	105	10.8
Strawberry, 12½% alcohol	3 fl. oz.	138	18.9
MARINADE MIX, MEAT:			
(Durkee)	1-oz. pkg.	47	9.0
(French's)	1-oz. pkg.	80	16.0

Food and Description	Measure or Quantity	Calories	Carbohydrates (grams)
MARJORAM (French's)	1 tsp. (1.2 grams)	4	.8
MARMALADE:			
Sweetened:			
(USDA)	1 T. (.7 oz.)	51	14.0
(Crosse & Blackwell) all flavors	1 T. (.6 oz.)	60	14.9
(Keiller) all flavors	1 T.	60	15.0
(Smucker's) English style or sweet	1 T. (.7 oz.)	53	13.5
Dietetic or low calorie:			
(Dia-Mel)	1 tsp.	6	0.
(Featherweight)	1 T.	16	4.0
(Slenderella) imitation	1 T.	24	6.0
(Smucker's) low sugar spread	1 T.	24	6.0
(S&W) *Nutradiet*	1 T.	12	3.0
MARSHMALLOW FLUFF	1 heaping tsp. (.6 oz.)	59	14.4
MARTINI COCKTAIL, canned (Mr. Boston):			
Gin, extra dry, 20% alcohol	3 fl. oz.	99	0.
Vodka, 20% alcohol	3 fl. oz.	102	.9
MASA HARINO (Quaker)	⅓ cup (1.3 oz.)	137	27.4
MASA TRIGO (Quaker)	⅓ cup (1.3 oz.)	149	24.7
MATZO:			
(Goodman's):			
Diet-10's	1 sq.	109	23.0
Unsalted	1 matzo (1 oz.)	109	23.0
(Horowitz-Margareten) unsalted	1 matzo (1.2 oz.)	135	28.2

(USDA): United States Department of Agriculture
(HEW/FAO): Health, Education and Welfare/Food and Agriculture Organization
* Prepared as Package Directs

Food and Description	Measure or Quantity	Calories	Carbo-hydrates (grams)
(Manischewitz):			
Regular	1 matzo (1.1 oz.)	114	28.1
Egg	1 matzo (1.2 oz.)	133	26.6
Thin tea	1 matzo (1 oz.)	114	24.8
Whole wheat	1 matzo (1.2 oz.)	124	24.2
MATZO MEAL (Manischewitz)	1 cup (4.1 oz.)	438	96.2
MAYONNAISE:			
Real:			
(Ann Page)	1 T. (.5 oz.)	105	.1
(Hellmann's)	1 T. (.5 oz.)	103	.1
(Hellman's)	½ cup (3.9 oz.)	802	.7
(Nalley's)	1 T. (.5 oz.)	103	.3
Dietetic or imitation:			
(Dia-Mel)	1 T. (.5 oz.)	106	.2
(Diet Delight) *Mayo-Lite*	1 T.	24	0.
(Featherweight) *Soyamaise*	1 T.	100	0.
(Tillie Lewis) *Tasti-Diet*	1 T. (.5 oz.)	25	1.0
(Weight Watchers)	1 T. (.5 oz.)	40	1.0
MAY WINE (Deinhard) 11% alcohol	3 fl. oz.	60	11.0
McDONALD'S:			
Big Mac	1 hamburger (7.2 oz.)	563	40.6
Biscuit:			
Ham	4.2-oz. biscuit	422	43.0
Sausage	4.8-oz. biscuit	582	42.5
Cheeseburger	1 cheeseburger (4 oz.)	307	29.8
Chicken McNuggets	1 serving (4.3 oz.)	332	17.6
Cookie:			
Chocolate chip	2.4-oz. pkg.	342	44.8
McDonaldland	2.4-oz. pkg.	308	48.7
Egg McMuffin	1 serving	327	31.0
Egg, scrambled	1 serving	180	2.5

Food and Description	Measure or Quantity	Calories	Carbohydrates (grams)
English muffin, buttered	2.2-oz. muffin	186	29.5
Filet-o-Fish sandwich	1 sandwich	432	37.4
Grapefruit juice	6 fl. oz.	80	17.9
Hamburger	1 hamburger	255	29.5
Hot cakes, with butter & syrup	1 serving	500	93.9
McChicken Sandwich	1 sandwich	475	39.8
McFeast Sandwich	1 sandwich	485	31.3
McRib Sandwich	1 sandwich	461	43.7
Orange juice	6 fl. oz.	85	19.6
Pie:			
Apple	3-oz. pie	253	29.3
Cherry	3.1-oz. pie	260	32.1
Potato:			
French fries	1 regular order	220	26.1
Hash browns	1 regular order	125	14.0
Quarter Pounder:			
Regular	1 burger	424	32.7
With cheese	1 burger with cheese	524	32.2
Sausage, pork	1.9-oz. serving	206	.6
Shake:			
Chocolate	10.3-oz. serving	383	65.5
Strawberry	10.3-oz. serving	362	62.1
Vanilla	10.3-oz. serving	352	59.6
Sundae:			
Caramel	5.8-oz. serving	328	52.5
Hot fudge	5.8-oz. serving	310	46.2
Strawberry	5.8-oz. serving	289	46.1
MEATBALL DINNER or ENTREE, frozen (Swanson) with brown gravy & whipped potatoes	9½-oz. entree	330	26.0
MEATBALL SEASONING MIX:			
*(Durkee) Italian	½ cup	309	2.4
(French's)	1½-oz. pkg.	140	28.0

(USDA): United States Department of Agriculture
(HEW/FAO):   Health, Education and Welfare/Food and Agriculture
                         Organization
* Prepared as Package Directs

Food and Description	Measure or Quantity	Calories	Carbo-hydrates (grams)
*MEATBALL SOUP, canned (Campbell) alphabet	10-oz. serving	140	16.0
MEATBALL STEW, canned:			
Dinty Moore (Hormel)	7½-oz. serving	245	15.1
(Libby's)	⅓ of 24-oz. can	281	24.3
(Morton House)	⅓ of 24-oz. can	290	18.0
(Nalley's)	8-oz. serving	261	18.2
MEATBALL, SWEDISH, frozen (Stouffer's) with parsley noodles	11-oz. pkg.	473	32.8
MEAT LOAF DINNER or ENTREE, frozen:			
(Banquet):			
Buffet Supper	1-lb. pkg.	1445	46.4
Cookin' Bag	5-oz. pkg.	224	13.6
Dinner:			
Regular	11-oz. dinner	412	29.0
Man Pleaser	19-oz. dinner	916	63.6
(Morton) dinner:			
Regular	11-oz. dinner	341	28.1
Country Table	15-oz. dinner	477	59.7
(Swanson) TV Brand:			
Dinner	10¾-oz. dinner	530	48.0
Entree, with tomato sauce & whipped potatoes	9-oz. entree	330	30.0
MEAT LOAF SEASONING MIX:			
(Contadina)	3¾-oz. pkg.	360	72.6
(French's)	1½-oz. pkg.	160	40.0
MEAT, POTTED (Libby's)	1-oz. serving	57	.3
MEAT TENDERIZER (French's) unseasoned or seasoned	1 tsp. (5 grams)	2	Tr.
MELBA TOAST (Old London):			
Garlic rounds	1 piece (2 grams)	10	1.8

Food and Description	Measure or Quantity	Calories	Carbo-hydrates (grams)
Pumpernickel	1 piece (5 grams)	17	3.4
Rye:			
Regular	1 piece (5 grams)	17	3.4
Unsalted	1 piece (5 grams)	18	3.5
Sesame rounds	1 piece (2 grams)	11	1.6
Wheat:			
Regular	1 piece (5 grams)	17	3.4
Unsalted	1 piece (5 grams)	18	3.5
White:			
Regular	1 piece (5 grams)	17	3.4
Rounds	1 piece (2 grams)	10	1.8
Unsalted	1 piece (5 grams)	18	3.5
MELON (See individual listings such as **CANTALOUPE, WATERMELON,** etc.)			
MELON BALLS (cantaloupe & honeydew) in syrup, frozen (USDA)	½ cup (4.1 oz.)	72	18.2
MENAHADEN, Atlantic (USDA) canned, solids & liq.	4 oz.	195	0.
MEXICAN DINNER, frozen:			
(Banquet) dinner:			
Regular	16-oz. dinner	608	73.5
Combination	12-oz. dinner	571	72.1
Man Pleaser	20-oz. dinner	721	86.9
(Swanson):			
3-course	18-oz. dinner	630	72.0
TV-Brand	16-oz. dinner	700	75.0
(Van de Kamp's):			
Regular	12-oz. dinner	521	41.0
Combination	11-oz. dinner	430	49.0
MILK, CONDENSED (USDA) sweetened, canned	1 cup (10.8 oz.)	982	166.2

(USDA): United States Department of Agriculture
(HEW/FAO):   Health, Education and Welfare/Food and Agriculture
                        Organization
* Prepared as Package Directs

Food and Description	Measure or Quantity	Calories	Carbo-hydrates (grams)
MILK, DRY:			
Whole (USDA) packed cup	1 cup (5.1 oz.)	728	55.4
*Nonfat, instant:			
(USDA)	8 fl. oz.	82	10.8
(Alba):			
Regular	8 fl. oz.	81	11.6
Chocolate flavor	8 fl. oz.	80	12.9
(Carnation)	8 fl. oz.	80	12.0
(Pet)	1 cup	80	12.0
Sanalac (Sanna)	1 cup	80	11.0
MILK, EVAPORATED, canned:			
Regular:			
(USDA) sweetened	1 cup (8.9 oz.)	345	24.4
(Carnation)	1 fl. oz.	42	3.0
(Pet)	1 fl. oz.	43	3.1
Filled:			
Dairymate	½ cup	150	12.0
(Pet)	½ cup (4 oz.)	150	12.0
Low fat (Carnation)	1 fl. oz.	28	3.0
Skimmed:			
(Carnation)	1 fl. oz.	24	3.5
Pet 99	1 fl. oz.	25	3.5
MILK, FRESH:			
Buttermilk, cultured, fresh (Friendship) no salt added	8 fl. oz.	120	12.0
Chocolate milk drink, fresh (Friendship)	8 fl. oz.	180	24.0
Low fat, *Viva*, 2% fat	1 cup	130	12.0
Skim:			
(Dairylea)	8 fl. oz.	90	11.0
(Meadow Gold)	1 cup	90	11.0
Whole:			
(Dairylea)	8 fl. oz.	150	11.0
(Dean)	1 cup (8.6 oz.)	151	11.0
(Meadow Gold) Vitamin A & D, 2% fat	1 cup	120	11.0
MILK, GOAT (USDA)	1 cup (8.6 oz.)	162	11.2
MILK, HUMAN (USDA)	1 oz. (by wt.)	22	2.7

Food and Description	Measure or Quantity	Calories	Carbo-hydrates (grams)
MILLET, whole-grain (USDA)	1 lb.	1483	330.7
MILNOT, dairy vegetable blend	1 fl. oz.	38	3.1
MINCEMEAT (See **PIE FILLING**)			
MINESTRONE SOUP:			
*(USDA) prepared with equal volume water	1 cup (8.6 oz.)	105	14.2
(Campbell):			
Chunky	9½-oz. can	140	21.0
*Condensed	10-oz. serving	90	13.0
(Crosse & Blackwell)	½ of 13-oz. can	90	18.0
MINI-WHEATS, cereal (Kellogg's) brown-sugar cinnamon or sugar frosted	1 biscuit (.25 oz.)	29	6.0
MINT LEAVES (HEW/FAO):			
Raw, untrimmed	1 lb. (weighed with tough stems & branches)	44	7.3
Raw, trimmed	½ oz.	4	.8
MOLASSES:			
(USDA):			
Barbados	1 T. (.7 oz.)	51	13.3
Blackstrap	1 T. (.7 oz.)	40	10.4
Light	1 T. (.7 oz.)	48	12.4
Dark	1 T. (.7 oz.)	48	12.4
Medium	1 T. (.7 oz.)	44	11.4
(Brer Rabbit) dark, green label	1 T.	33	10.6
(Grandma's) unsulphured	1 T.	60	15.0
MORTADELLA (USDA) sausage	1 oz.	89	.2

(USDA): United States Department of Agriculture
(HEW/FAO):   Health, Education and Welfare/Food and Agriculture
              Organization
* Prepared as Package Directs

Food and Description	Measure or Quantity	Calories	Carbohydrates (grams)
MOSELLE WINE (Great Western) Delaware, 12% alcohol	3 fl. oz.	73	2.9
MOST, cereal (Kellogg's)	½ cup (1 oz.)	100	22.0
MOUSSE, canned, dietetic (Featherweight) chocolate	½ cup (4 oz.)	100	4.0
MUFFIN (See also **MUFFIN MIX**):			
Blueberry:			
Home recipe (USDA)	3″ muffin (1.4 oz.)	112	16.8
Frozen (Morton):			
Regular	1.6-oz. muffin	125	22.9
Rounds	1.6-oz. muffin	115	20.9
Bran:			
Home recipe (USDA)	3″ muffin (1.4 oz.)	104	17.2
(Arnold) *Oroweat, Bran'nola*	2.3-oz. muffin	160	30.0
Corn:			
Home recipe (USDA) prepared with whole-ground cornmeal	1.4-oz. muffin	115	17.0
(Thomas')	2-oz. muffin	184	25.8
Frozen (Morton):			
Regular	1.7-oz. muffin	129	20.3
Rounds	1.5-oz. muffin	127	20.9
English:			
(Arnold) extra crisp	2.3-oz. muffin	150	30.0
Home Pride:			
Regular	2-oz. muffin	136	25.0
Wheat	2-oz. muffin	141	25.0
(Pepperidge Farm):			
Regular	1 muffin	140	27.0
Cinnamon raisin	1 muffin	150	28.0
Roman Meal	2⅓-oz. muffin	150	29.8
Roman Meal	2½-oz. muffin	161	31.9
(Thomas') regular or frozen	2-oz. muffin	131	25.9
(Wonder)	2-oz. muffin	131	26.1
Plain, home recipe (USDA)	1.4-oz. muffin (3″ dia.)	118	16.9

Food and Description	Measure or Quantity	Calories	Carbo-hydrates (grams)
Raisin (Arnold) *Oroweat*	2½-oz. muffin	170	35.0
Sourdough (Wonder)	2-oz. muffin	135	27.3
MUFFIN MIX:			
Blueberry:			
*(Betty Crocker) wild	1 muffin	120	19.0
(Duncan Hines)	½12 of pkg.	99	17.0
Bran (Duncan Hines)	½12 of pkg.	97	16.3
Corn:			
Home recipe (USDA) prepared with egg & milk	1.4-oz. muffin	92	14.2
Home recipe (USDA) prepared with egg and water	1.4-oz. muffin	119	20.8
*(Betty Crocker)	1 muffin	160	25.0
*(Dromedary)	1 muffin	130	20.0
*(Flako)	1 muffin	140	23.0
MUG-O-LUNCH			
(General Mills):			
Chicken flavored noodles & sauce	1 pouch	150	25.0
Macaroni & cheese	1 pouch	240	41.0
Noodles & beef flavored sauce	1 pouch	170	30.0
Spaghetti & sauce	1 pouch	150	31.0
MULLET, raw (USDA):			
Whole	1 lb. (weighed whole)	351	0.
Meat only	4 oz.	166	0.
MUNG BEAN SPROUT (See **BEAN SPROUT**)			
MUSCATEL WINE:			
(Gallo) 20% alcohol	3 fl. oz.	111	8.3
(Gold Seal) 19% alcohol	3 fl. oz.	159	9.4

(USDA): United States Department of Agriculture
(HEW/FAO): Health, Education and Welfare/Food and Agriculture Organization
* Prepared as Package Directs

Food and Description	Measure or Quantity	Calories	Carbo- hydrates (grams)
MUSHROOM:			
Raw (USDA):			
Whole	½ lb. (weighed untrimmed)	62	9.7
Trimmed, slices	½ cup (1.2 oz.)	10	1.6
Canned, solids & liq.:			
(USDA)	½ cup (4.3-oz.)	21	2.9
(Green Giant)	2-oz. serving	12	1.7
(Shady Oak)	4-oz. can	19	2.0
Dried (HEW/FAO)	1 oz.	72	10.5
Frozen:			
(Green Giant) in butter sauce	½ of 6-oz. pkg.	42	2.6
(McKenzie or Seabrook Farms) chopped	⅓ of 10-oz. pkg.	25	3.4
MUSHROOM, CHINESE (HEW/FAO):			
Dried	1 oz.	81	18.9
Dried, soaked, drained	1 oz.	12	2.4
MUSHROOM SOUP:			
Canned, regular pack:			
*(USDA) cream of, condensed:			
Prepared with equal volume milk	1 cup (8.6 oz.)	216	16.2
Prepared with equal volume water	1 cup (8.5 oz.)	134	10.1
*(Campbell):			
Condensed:			
Cream of	10-oz. serving	120	11.0
Golden	10-oz. serving	110	11.0
Semicondensed, *Soup For One,* cream of, savory	11-oz. serving	140	13.0
(Crosse & Blackwell) cream of, bisque	½ of 13-oz. can	90	8.0
*(Rokeach) condensed, cream of:			
Prepared with milk	10-oz. serving	240	20.0
Prepared with water	10-oz. serving	150	13.0

Food and Description	Measure or Quantity	Calories	Carbo-hydrates (grams)
Canned, dietetic or low calorie:			
(Campbell) cream of, low sodium	7¼-oz. can	120	10.0
*(Dia-Mel) cream of, condensed	8-oz. serving	45	9.0
*Mix:			
Carmel Kosher	6 fl. oz. (1 tsp. dry mix)	12	2.0
*(Lipton):			
Beef mushroom	8 fl. oz.	40	7.0
Cream of, Cup-A-Soup	6 fl. oz.	80	0.0
MUSKELLUNGE, raw (USDA):			
Whole	1 lb. (weighed whole)	242	0.
Meat only	4 oz.	234	0.
MUSKMELON (See CANTALOUPE, CASABA or HONEYDEW)			
MUSKRAT, roasted (USDA)	4 oz.	174	0.
MUSSEL (USDA):			
Atlantic & Pacific, raw:			
In shell	1 lb. (weighed in shell)	153	7.2
Meat only	4 oz.	108	3.7
Pacific, canned, drained	4 oz.	129	1.7
MUSTARD POWDER			
(French's)	1 tsp.	9	.3
MUSTARD, PREPARED:			
Brown:			
(USDA)	1 tsp.	8	.5
(French's) 'N Spicy	1 tsp.	5	.3

(USDA): United States Department of Agriculture
(HEW/FAO): Health, Education and Welfare/Food and Agriculture Organization
* Prepared as Package Directs

Food and Description	Measure or Quantity	Calories	Carbo-hydrates (grams)
(Gulden's)	1 scant tsp.	6	.4
Cream salad (French's)	1 tsp.	3	.3
Grey Poupon	1 tsp.	6	Tr.
Horseradish:			
(French's)	1 tsp.	5	.3
(Nalley's)	1 tsp.	6	.3
Hot, *Mr. Mustard*	1 tsp.	11	.4
Medford (French's)	1 tsp.	5	.3
Onion (French's)	1 tsp.	8	1.7
Yellow (Gulden's)	1 scant tsp.	5	.4
MUSTARD GREENS:			
Raw (USDA) whole	1 lb. (weighed untrimmed)	98	17.8
Boiled (USDA) drained	1 cup (7.8 oz.)	51	8.8
Canned (Sunshine) chopped, solids & liq.	½ cup (4.1 oz.)	22	3.2
Frozen:			
(USDA) boiled, drained	½ cup (3.8 oz.)	21	3.3
(Birds Eye) chopped	⅓ of 10-oz. pkg.	20	3.0
(Seabrook Farms) chopped	⅓ of 10-oz. pkg.	25	3.4
(Southland) chopped	⅕ of 16-oz. pkg.	20	3.0
MUSTARD SPINACH (USDA):			
Raw	1 lb.	100	17.7
Boiled, drained	4 oz.	18	3.2

N

NATURAL CEREAL:			
Heartland:			
Regular	¼ cup (1 oz.)	120	18.0
Coconut	¼ cup (1 oz.)	130	18.0
Raisin	¼ cup (1 oz.)	120	18.0
(Quaker):			
100% natural:			
Regular	¼ cup (1 oz.)	138	17.4
With apples & cinnamon	¼ cup (1 oz.)	135	18.0
With raisins & dates	¼ cup (1 oz.)	134	18.0
Whole wheat, hot	⅓ cup (1 oz.)	106	21.8

Food and Description	Measure or Quantity	Calories	Carbohydrates (grams)
NATURE SNACKS (Sun-Maid):			
Carob crunch	1-oz. serving	143	16.8
Raisin crunch	1-oz. serving	126	19.7
Rock road	1-oz. serving	126	19.1
Sesame nut crunch	1-oz. serving	154	14.6
Tahitian treat	1-oz. serving	123	19.4
Yogurt crunch	1-oz. serving	123	19.7
NEAR BEER (See **BEER, NEAR**)			
NECTARINE, fresh (USDA):			
Whole	1 lb. (weighed with pits)	267	71.4
Flesh only	4 oz.	73	19.4
NEAPOLITAN CREAM PIE, frozen (Morton)	⅙ of 16-oz. pie	192	22.7
NEW ZEALAND SPINACH (USDA):			
Raw	1 lb.	86	14.1
Boiled, drained	4 oz.	15	2.4
NOODLE. Plain noodle products are essentially the same in caloric value and carbohydrate content on the same weight basis. The longer they are cooked, the more water is absorbed and this affects the nutritive values. (USDA):			
Dry	1 oz.	110	20.4
Dry, 1½" strips	1 cup (2.6 oz.)	283	52.6
Cooked	1 oz.	35	6.6
NOODLE & BEEF:			
Canned (Hormel) *Short Orders*	7½-oz. can	230	15.0

(USDA): United States Department of Agriculture
(HEW/FAO): Health, Education and Welfare/Food and Agriculture Organization
* Prepared as Package Directs

Food and Description	*Measure or Quantity*	*Calories*	*Carbo-hydrates (grams)*
Frozen (Banquet) *Buffet Supper*	2-lb. pkg.	754	83.6
NOODLE & CHICKEN:			
Canned, *Dinty Moore* (Hormel) *Short Orders*	7½-oz. can	210	15.0
Frozen (Swanson) *TV Brand*	10¼-oz dinner	390	53.0
NOODLE, CHOW MEIN, canned:			
(USDA)	1 cup (1.6 oz.)	220	26.1
(Chun King)	⅙ of 5-oz. can	100	13.0
(La Choy)	½ cup (1 oz.)	149	16.8
NOODLE MIX:			
*(Betty Crocker):			
Almondine	¼ of pkg.	240	27.0
Romanoff	¼ of pkg.	230	23.0
Stroganoff	¼ of pkg.	240	26.0
Noodle Roni, parmesano	⅕ of 6-oz. pkg.	130	22.5
*(Pennsylvania Dutch Brand) *Noodles Plus Sauce:*			
Beef	½ cup	190	26.0
Butter	½ cup	190	24.0
Cheese	½ cup	200	24.0
Chicken	½ cup	190	25.0
**Side Quick* (General Mills):			
& beef sauce	¼ of pkg.	120	21.0
& butter sauce	¼ of pkg.	120	20.0
& cheese sauce	¼ of pkg.	120	21.0
& chicken sauce	¼ of pkg.	120	19.0
**Tuna Helper* (General Mills):			
Almondine	¼ of pkg.	240	27.0
Romanoff	¼ of pkg.	230	23.0
Stroganoff	¼ of pkg.	230	26.0
***NOODLE, RAMEN,** canned (La Choy):			
Beef	½ of 3-oz. pkg.	189	27.6
Chicken	½ of 3-oz. pkg.	187	27.6
Oriental	½ of 3-oz. pkg.	190	27.7

Food and Description	Measure or Quantity	Calories	Carbo-hydrates (grams)
NOODLE, RICE, canned			
(La Choy)	⅓ of 3-oz. can	130	20.6
NOODLE ROMANOFF, frozen			
(Stouffer's)	⅓ of 12-oz. pkg.	168	15.9
*NOODLE SOUP, canned			
(Campbell) condensed:			
Curly noodle with chicken	10-oz. serving	90	11.0
& ground beef	10-oz. serving	110	14.0
NUT, MIXED (See also			
individual kinds):			
Dry roasted:			
(A&P)	1 oz.	179	6.6
(Flavor House) salted	1 oz.	171	5.4
(Planters)	1 oz.	160	7.0
Oil roasted:			
(A&P) fancy, without			
peanuts	1 oz.	190	5.9
(Excel) with peanuts	1 oz.	187	5.4
(Planters) with or without			
peanuts	1 oz.	180	6.0
NUTMEG (French's)	1 tsp.	11	.9
NUTRI-GRAIN, cereal			
(Kellogg's):			
Barley	⅔ cup (1 oz.)	110	23.0
Corn	½ cup (1 oz.)	110	24.0
Rye or wheat	⅔ cup (1 oz.)	110	24.0
NUTRIMATO COCKTAIL,			
canned (Mott's)	6 fl. oz.	70	17.0

(USDA): United States Department of Agriculture
(HEW/FAO):   Health, Education and Welfare/Food and Agriculture
                  Organization
* Prepared as Package Directs

Food and Description	Measure or Quantity	Calories	Carbo-hydrates (grams)

O

Food and Description	Measure or Quantity	Calories	Carbo-hydrates (grams)
OAT FLAKES, cereal (Post)	⅔ cup (1 oz.)	107	20.1
OATMEAL:			
Regular, dry:			
(USDA)	1 T.	18	3.1
(H-O):			
Old fashioned	1 T. (5 grams)	17	3.0
Old fashioned	1 cup (2.6 oz.)	278	48.0
(Ralston Purina)	⅓ cup (1 oz.)	110	19.0
Regular, cooked (USDA)	1 cup (8.5 oz.)	132	23.3
Instant, dry:			
(H-O):			
Regular	1 T. (4 grams)	16	2.8
Regular	1 cup (2.4 oz.)	258	44.3
With maple & brown sugar flavor	1½-oz. packet	160	31.7
Sweet & mellow	1.4-oz. packet	150	28.9
(Quaker):			
Regular	1-oz. packet	105	18.1
Apple & cinnamon	1¼-oz. packet	134	26.0
Bran & raisins	1½-oz. packet	153	29.2
Cinnamon & spice	1⅝-oz. packet	176	34.8
Maple & brown sugar	1½-oz. packet	163	31.9
Raisins & spice	1½-oz. packet	159	31.4
(3-Minute Brand) *Stir'n Eat:*			
Dutch apple brown sugar	1⅛-oz. packet	120	23.3
Natural flavor	1-oz. packet	106	18.0
Quick, dry:			
(H-O)	1 T. (4 grams)	16	2.8
(H-O)	1 cup (2.5 oz.)	269	46.3
(Ralston Purina)	⅓ cup (1 oz.)	110	19.0
(3-Minute Brand)	⅓ cup (1 oz.)	108	18.5
OCEAN PERCH:			
Fresh (USDA):			
Atlantic:			
Raw, whole	1 lb. (weighed whole)	124	0.

Food and Description	Measure or Quantity	Calories	Carbo-hydrates (grams)
Fried	4 oz.	257	7.7
Pacific:			
Raw, whole	1 lb. (weighed whole)	116	0.
Raw, meat only	4 oz.	108	0.
Frozen:			
(USDA) Atlantic, breaded, fried, reheated	4 oz.	362	18.7
(Banquet)	8¾-oz. dinner	424	49.8
OCTOPUS, raw (USDA) meat only	4 oz.	83	0.
OIL, SALAD or COOKING:			
(USDA) all kinds, including olive	1 T. (.5 oz.)	124	0.
(USDA) all kinds, including olive	½ cup (3.9 oz.)	972	0.
Crisco	1 T.	126	0.
(Fleischmann's)	1 T. (.5 oz.)	126	0.
Golden Thistle, safflower	1 T.	130	0.
(Mazola) corn	1 T. (.5 oz.)	126	0.
(Mazola) corn	½ cup (3.9 oz.)	995	0.
Mrs. Tucker's, corn or soybean	1 T.	130	0.
(Planters) peanut	1 T.	130	0.
Puritan	1 T.	126	0.
Saffola	1 T. (.5 oz.)	124	0.
Saffola	½ cup (3.9 oz.)	972	0.
Sunlite	1 T. (.5 oz.)	120	0.
Wesson	1 T.	120	0.
OKRA:			
Raw (USDA) whole	1 lb. (weighed untrimmed)	140	29.6
Boiled (USDA) drained:			
Whole	½ cup (3.1 oz.)	26	5.3

(USDA): United States Department of Agriculture
(HEW/FAO): Health, Education and Welfare/Food and Agriculture
              Organization
* Prepared as Package Directs

Food and Description	Measure or Quantity	Calories	Carbo-hydrates (grams)
Pods	8 pods, 3" × ⅝" (3 oz.)	25	5.1
Slices	½ cup (2.8 oz.)	23	4.8
Canned (King Pharr) with tomatoes	½ cup	26	5.0
Frozen:			
(USDA) boiled, drained:			
Cut	½ cup (3.2 oz.)	35	8.1
Whole	½ cup (2.4 oz.)	26	6.1
(Birds Eye):			
Cut	⅓ of 10-oz. pkg.	25	5.0
Whole	⅓ of 10-oz. pkg.	30	7.0
(Green Giant) gumbo	⅓ of 10-oz. pkg.	83	5.2
(McKenzie or Seabrook Farms):			
Cut	⅓ of 10-oz. pkg.	31	6.1
Whole	⅓ of 10-oz. pkg.	36	6.9
(Southland):			
Cut	⅓ of 16-oz. pkg.	25	5.0
Whole	⅓ of 16-oz. pkg.	35	7.0
OLEOMARGARINE (See **MARGARINE**)			
OLIVE:			
Green style (USDA):			
With pits, drained	1 oz.	77	2.0
Pitted, drained	1 oz.	96	2.5
Green (USDA)	1 oz.	33	.4
Ripe, by variety: (USDA):			
Ascalano, any size, pitted & drained	1 oz.	37	.7
Manzanilla, any size	1 oz.	37	.7
Mission, any size	1 oz.	52	.9
Mission	3 small or 2 large	18	.3
Mission, slices	½ cup (2.2 oz.)	114	2.0
Sevillano, any size	1 oz.	26	6.1
Ripe, by size (Lindsay):			
Colassal	1 olive	13	.3

Food and Description	Measure or Quantity	Calories	Carbo-hydrates (grams)
Extra large	1 olive	5	.1
Giant	1 olive	8	.2
Jumbo	1 olive	10	.2
Large	1 olive	5	.1
Mammoth	1 olive	6	.1
Medium	1 olive	4	.1
Select	1 olive	3	.1
Supercolassal	1 olive	16	.3
Super supreme	1 olive	18	.3
ONION (See also **ONION, GREEN** and **ONION, WELCH**):			
Raw (USDA):			
Whole	1 lb. (weighed untrimmed)	157	35.9
Whole	3.9-oz. onion (2½″ dia.)	38	8.7
Chopped	½ cup (3 oz.)	33	7.5
Chopped	1 T. (.4 oz.)	4	1.0
Grated	1 T. (.5 oz.)	5	1.2
Slices	½ cup (2 oz.)	21	4.9
Boiled, drained (USDA):			
Whole	½ cup (3.7 oz.)	30	6.8
Whole, pearl onions	½ cup (3.2 oz.)	27	6.0
Halves or pieces	½ cup (3.2 oz.)	26	5.8
Canned, *O & C* (Durkee):			
Boiled	1-oz. serving	8	2.0
In cream sauce	1-oz. serving	143	17.0
Dehydrated:			
Flakes:			
(USDA)	1 tsp. (1.3 grams)	5	1.1
(Gilroy)	1 tsp.	5	1.2
Powder (Gilroy)	1 tsp.	9	2.0

(USDA): United States Department of Agriculture
(HEW/FAO): Health, Education and Welfare/Food and Agriculture
           Organization
* Prepared as Package Directs

Food and Description	Measure or Quantity	Calories	Carbohydrates (grams)
Frozen:			
(Birds Eye):			
Chopped	1 oz.	8	2.0
Small, whole	⅓ of 12-oz. pkg.	40	10.0
Small, with cream sauce	⅓ of 9-oz. pkg.	118	11.2
(Green Giant) creamed	⅓ of 10-oz. pkg.	50	5.1
(Mrs. Paul's) rings, breaded			
& fried	½ of 5-oz. pkg.	157	21.2
(Southland) chopped	⅕ of 10-oz. pkg.	20	5.0
ONION BOUILLON:			
(Herb-Ox):			
Regular	1 cube	10	1.3
Instant	1 packet	14	1.9
MBT	1 packet	16	2.0
ONION, GREEN, raw (USDA):			
Whole	1 lb. (weighed untrimmed)	157	35.7
Bulb & entire top	1 oz.	10	2.3
Bulb without green top	3 small onions (.9 oz.)	11	2.6
Slices, bulb & white portion of top	½ cup (1.8 oz.)	22	5.2
Tops only	1 oz.	8	1.6
ONION SOUP:			
Canned:			
*(USDA) condensed, prepared with equal volume water	1 cup (8.5 oz.)	65	5.3
*(Campbell) condensed:			
Regular	10-oz. serving	80	11.0
Cream of	10-oz. serving	130	15.0
Cream of, made with milk & water	10-oz. serving	180	20.0
*Mix:			
Carmel Kosher	6 fl. oz. (1 tsp. dry)	12	2.4

Food and Description	Measure or Quantity	Calories	Carbo-hydrates (grams)
*(Lipton):			
Regular	1 cup (8 oz.)	35	6.0
Beefy onion	1 cup (8 oz.)	30	4.0
Cup-A-Soup	6 fl. oz.	30	5.0
Onion mushroom	1 cup (8 oz.)	40	6.0
ONION, WELCH, raw (USDA):			
Whole	1 lb. (weighed untrimmed)	100	19.2
Trimmed	4 oz.	39	7.4
OPOSSUM (USDA) roasted, meat only	4 oz.	251	0.
ORANGE, fresh (USDA):			
California Navel:			
Whole	1 lb. (weighed with rind & seeds)	157	39.2
Whole	6.3-oz. orange (2⅘" dia.)	62	15.5
Sections	1 cup (8.5 oz.)	123	30.6
California Valencia:			
Whole	1 lb. (weighed with rind & seeds)	174	42.2
Fruit including peel	6.3-oz. orange (2⅝" dia.)	72	27.9
Sections	1 cup (8.5 oz.)	123	29.9
Florida, all varieties:			
Whole	1 lb. (weighed with rind & seeds)	158	40.3
Whole	7.4-oz. orange (3" dia.)	73	18.6
Sections	1 cup (8.5 oz.)	113	28.9

(USDA): United States Department of Agriculture
(HEW/FAO): Health, Education and Welfare/Food and Agriculture Organization
* Prepared as Package Directs

Food and Description	Measure or Quantity	Calories	Carbo-hydrates (grams)
ORANGE-APRICOT JUICE DRINK, canned (USDA) 40% fruit juices	1 cup (8.8 oz.)	123	31.6
ORANGE-APRICOT JUICE COCKTAIL, canned, *Musselman's*	8 fl. oz.	100	23.0
ORANGE DRINK:			
Canned:			
Capri Sun, natural	6¾ fl. oz.	103	26.1
(Hi-C)	6 fl. oz.	92	23.0
(Lincoln)	6 fl. oz.	96	23.9
Chilled (Sealtest)	6 fl. oz.	87	21.3
*Mix (Hi-C)	6 fl. oz.	68	17.0
ORANGE EXTRACT (Virginia Dare) 79% alcohol	1 tsp.	22	0.
ORANGE-GRAPEFRUIT JUICE:			
Canned, unsweetened:			
(USDA)	1 cup (8.7 oz.)	106	24.8
(Del Monte)	6 fl. oz.	79	18.3
Canned, sweetened:			
(USDA)	1 cup (8.9 oz.)	126	30.6
(Del Monte)	6 fl. oz. (6.5 oz.)	91	21.1
*Frozen:			
(USDA) unsweetened	½ cup (4.4 oz.)	55	13.0
(Minute Maid) unsweetened	6 fl. oz.	76	19.1
ORANGE JUICE:			
Fresh (USDA):			
California Navel	½ cup (4.4 oz.)	60	14.0
California Valencia	½ cup (4.4 oz.)	58	13.0
Florida, early or midseason	½ cup (4.4 oz.)	50	11.4
Florida Temple	½ cup (4.4 oz.)	67	16.0
Florida Valencia	½ cup (4.4 oz.)	56	13.0
Canned, unsweetened:			
(USDA)	½ cup (4.4 oz.)	60	13.9

Food and Description	Measure or Quantity	Calories	Carbo-hydrates (grams)
(Del Monte)	6 fl. oz. (6.5 oz.)	82	18.5
(Sunkist)	½ cup (4.4 oz.)	60	14.0
(Texsun)	6 fl. oz.	83	20.0
Canned, sweetened:			
(USDA)	½ cup (4.4 oz.)	66	15.4
(Del Monte)	6 fl. oz.	76	17.4
Chilled (Minute Maid)	6 fl. oz.	83	19.7
*Dehydrated crystals (USDA)	½ cup (4.4 oz.)	57	13.4
*Frozen:			
(USDA)	½ cup (4.4 oz.)	56	13.3
Bright & Early, imitation	6 fl. oz.	90	21.6
(Minute Maid)	6 fl. oz.	86	20.5
(Snow Crop)	6 fl. oz.	86	20.5
(Sunkist)	6 fl. oz.	92	21.7

ORANGE, MANDARIN (See **TANGERINE**)

ORANGE PEEL, CANDIED
(USDA) — 1 oz. — 90 — 22.9

ORANGE-PINEAPPLE DRINK, canned (Lincoln) — 6 fl. oz. — 97 — 24.3

ORANGE-PINEAPPLE JUICE, canned (Texsun) unsweetened — 6 fl. oz. — 89 — 21.0

ORANGE-PINEAPPLE JUICE COCKTAIL, canned, *Musselman's* — 8 fl. oz. — 100 — 23.0

ORANGE SPREAD, dietetic (Estee) — 1 tsp. (5.7 grams) — 8 — 1.9

OREGANO, dried (French's) — 1 tsp. — 6 — 1.0

(USDA): United States Department of Agriculture
(HEW/FAO): Health, Education and Welfare/Food and Agriculture Organization
* Prepared as Package Directs

Food and Description	Measure or Quantity	Calories	Carbo-hydrates (grams)
OVALTINE, dry:			
Chocolate flavor	4 heaping tsps. (¾ oz.)	78	17.9
Malt flavor	4 heaping tsps. (¾ oz.)	88	17.6
OYSTER:			
Raw (USDA) meat only:			
Eastern	13–19 med. oysters (1 cup, 8.5 oz.)	158	8.2
Eastern	4 oz.	75	3.9
Pacific	4 oz.	103	7.3
Canned, solids & liq.:			
(USDA)	4 oz.	86	5.6
(Bumble Bee) whole	½ of 8-oz. can	86	5.5
Fried (USDA) dipped in egg, milk & breadcrumbs	4 oz.	271	21.1
OYSTER CRACKER (See **CRACKER**)			
OYSTER STEW (USDA):			
Home recipe:			
1 part oysters to 1 part milk by volume	1 cup (8.5 oz., 6–8 oysters)	245	14.2
1 part oysters to 2 parts milk by volume	1 cup (8.5 oz.)	233	10.8
1 part oysters to 3 parts milk by volume	1 cup (8.5 oz.)	206	11.3
Frozen:			
Prepared with equal volume milk	1 cup (8.5 oz.)	201	14.2
Prepared with equal volume water	1 cup (8.5 oz.)	122	8.2

Food and Description	Measure or Quantity	Calories	Carbo-hydrates (grams)
*OYSTER STEW SOUP, canned (Campbell):			
Prepared with milk	10-oz. serving	170	12.0
Prepared with water	10-oz. serving	70	5.0

P

Food and Description	Measure or Quantity	Calories	Carbo-hydrates (grams)
PAISANO WINE (Gallo) 13% alcohol	3 fl. oz.	53	1.3
PANCAKE, home recipe (USDA)	4" pancake (1 oz.)	62	9.2
PANCAKE & SAUSAGE, frozen (Swanson)	6-oz. breakfast	500	50.0
PANCAKE & WAFFLE BATTER, frozen (Aunt Jemima):			
Plain	4" pancake	70	14.1
Blueberry	4" pancake	68	13.8
Buttermilk	4" pancake	71	14.2
PANCAKE & WAFFLE MIX:			
Plain:			
(USDA)	1 oz.	101	21.5
(USDA)	1 cup (4.8 oz.)	481	102.2
*(USDA) prepared with milk	4" pancake (1 oz.)	55	8.6
*(USDA) prepared with egg & milk	4" pancake	61	8.7
(Aunt Jemima):			
Complete	⅓ cup (1.9 oz.)	198	38.2
*Complete	4" pancake	80	15.7

(USDA): United States Department of Agriculture
(HEW/FAO):   Health, Education and Welfare/Food and Agriculture
                        Organization
* Prepared as Package Directs

Food and Description	Measure or Quantity	Calories	Carbo-hydrates (grams)
Original	¾ cup (.6 oz.)	54	11.2
*Original	4″ pancake	73	8.7
*(Log Cabin) complete	4″ pancake	58	11.2
*(Pillsbury) *Hungry Jack:*			
Complete:			
Bulk	4″ pancake	63	12.3
Packets	4″ pancake	60	11.6
Extra Lights	4″ pancake	67	9.3
Panshakes	4″ panckae	83	13.3
*Blueberry (Pillsbury) *Hungry Jack*	4″ pancake	110	14.0
Buckwheat:			
(USDA)	1 cup (4.8 oz.)	443	94.9
*(USDA) prepared with egg & milk	4″ pancake	54	6.4
*(Aunt Jemima)	4″ pancake	67	8.3
Buttermilk:			
(USDA)	1 cup (4.8 oz.)	481	102.2
*(USDA) prepared with egg & milk	4″ pancake	61	8.7
(Aunt Jemima):			
*Regular	4″ pancake	100	13.3
Complete	⅓ cup (2.3 oz.)	236	46.2
*Complete	4″ pancake	80	15.3
*(Betty Crocker):			
Regular	4″ pancake	93	13.0
Complete	4″ pancake	70	13.7
*(Log Cabin)	4″ pancake	77	11.3
*(Pillsbury) *Hungry Jack*	4″ pancake	80	9.7
*Whole wheat (Aunt Jamima)	4″ pancake	83	10.7
*Dietetic or low calorie (Tillie Lewis) *Tasti-Diet*	4″ pancake (.5 oz. dry)	47	8.7

PANCAKE & WAFFLE SYRUP
  (See **SYRUP**)

PANCREAS, raw (USDA):
  Beef, lean only · 4 oz. · 160 · 0.

Food and Description	Measure or Quantity	Calories	Carbo-hydrates (grams)
Calf	4 oz.	183	0.
Hog or hog sweetbread	4 oz.	274	0.
PAPAW, fresh (USDA):			
Whole	1 lb. (weighed with rind & seeds)	289	57.2
Flesh only	4 oz.	96	19.1
PAPAYA, fresh (USDA):			
Whole	1 lb. (weighed with skin & seeds)	119	30.4
Cubed	1 cup (6.4 oz.)	71	18.2
PAPAYA JUICE, canned (HEW/FAO)	4 oz.	77	19.6
PAPRIKA, domestic (French's)	1 tsp.	7	1.1
PARSLEY, fresh (USDA):			
Whole	½ lb.	100	19.3
Chopped	1 T. (4 grams)	2	.3
PARSLEY FLAKES, dehydrated (French's)	1 tsp. (1.1 grams)	4	.6
PARSNIP (USDA):			
Raw, whole	1 lb. (weighed unprepared)	293	67.5
Boiled, drained, cut in pieces	½ cup (3.7 oz.)	70	15.8
PASSION FRUIT, fresh (USDA):			
Whole	1 lb. (weighed with shell)	212	50.0
Pulp & seeds	4 oz.	102	24.0

(USDA): United States Department of Agriculture
(HEW/FAO): Health, Education and Welfare/Food and Agriculture Organization
* Prepared as Package Directs

Food and Description	Measure or Quantity	Calories	Carbo-hydrates (grams)
PASSION FRUIT JUICE, fresh (HEW/FAO)	4 oz.	50	11.5
PASTINA, DRY (USDA):			
Carrot	1 oz.	105	21.5
Egg	1 oz.	109	20.4
Spinach	1 oz.	104	21.2
PASTOSO (Petri) 12% alcohol	3 fl. oz.	71	1.2
PASTRAMI, packaged:			
(Eckrich) sliced	1-oz. slice	47	1.3
(Vienna)	1 oz.	86	0.
PASTRY SHELL (See also **PIE CRUST**):			
Home recipe (USDA) baked	1 shell (1.5 oz.)	212	18.6
Frozen (Pepperidge Farm)	1 shell	240	15.0
PÂTÉ, canned:			
(USDA) de foie gras	1 T. (.5 oz.)	69	.7
(USDA) de foie gras	1 oz.	131	1.4
(Hormel) liver	1 T. (.5 oz.)	35	.3
PDQ:			
Chocolate flavor	1 T. (.6 oz.)	66	15.1
Egg nog flavor	2 heaping T. (.9 oz.)	113	27.5
Strawberry flavor	1 T. (.5 oz.)	60	15.0
PEA, GREEN:			
Raw (USDA):			
In pod	1 lb. (weighed in pod)	145	24.8
Shelled	1 lb.	381	65.3
Shelled	½ cup (2.4 oz.)	58	9.9
Boiled (USDA) drained	½ cup (2.9 oz.)	58	9.9
Canned, regular pack: (USDA):			
Alaska, early or June: Solids & liq.	½ cup (4.4 oz.)	82	15.5

Food and Description	Measure or Quantity	Calories	Carbo-hydrates (grams)
Solids only	½ cup (3 oz.)	76	14.4
Sweet:			
Solids & liq.	½ cup (4.4 oz.)	71	12.9
Solids only	½ cup (3 oz.)	69	12.9
Drained liquid	4 oz.	25	4.9
(April Showers) early, solids & liq.	½ of 8½-oz. can	61	10.6
(Del Monte):			
Early garden:			
Solids & liq.	½ cup (4 oz.)	52	9.9
Solids only	½ cup (4 oz.)	72	12.5
Seasoned:			
Solids & liq.	½ cup	54	9.8
Solids only	½ cup	53	9.2
Sweet, tiny size:			
Solids & liq.	½ cup	50	9.0
Solids only	½ cup	62	10.7
(Festal):			
Early garden, solids & liq.	½ cup	52	9.9
Seasoned, solids only	½ cup	53	9.2
Sweet, tiny size, solids only	½ cup	62	10.7
(Green Giant) solids & liq.:			
Early, with onion	¼ of 17-oz. can	61	10.6
Sweet:			
Regular	½ of 8½-oz. can	52	8.5
Small, *Sweetlets*	½ of 8½-oz. can	49	8.2
With onion	¼ of 17-oz. can	52	8.5
(Kounty Kist) solids & liq.:			
Early	½ of 8½-oz. can	71	12.8
Sweet	½ of 8½-oz. can	64	10.5
(Le Sueur) early, small, solids & liq.	½ of 8½-oz. can	52	9.2
(Libby's) sweet, solids & liq.	½ cup (4.2 oz.)	66	11.6
(Lindy) solids & liq.:			
Early	½ of 8½-oz. can	71	12.8

(USDA): United States Department of Agriculture
(HEW/FAO): Health, Education and Welfare/Food and Agriculture
Organization
* Prepared as Package Directs

Food and Description	Measure or Quantity	Calories	Carbo-hydrates (grams)
Sweet	½ of 8½-oz. can	64	10.5
(Minnesota Valley) early, small, solids & liq.	½ of 8½-oz. can	53	9.4
(Stokely-Van Camp) solids & liq.:			
Early	½ cup (4.4 oz.)	65	12.5
Sweet	½ cup (4.4 oz.)	65	12.0
Canned, dietetic or low calorie:			
(USDA):			
Alaska, early or June:			
Solids & liq.	4 oz.	62	11.1
Solids only	4 oz.	88	16.2
Sweet:			
Solids & liq.	4 oz.	53	9.5
Solids only	4 oz.	82	14.7
(Blue Boy) sweet, solids & liq.	½ cup	80	15.0
(Diet Delight) solids & liq.	½ cup (4.3 oz.)	50	8.0
(Featherweight) sweet, solids & liq.	½ cup	70	12.0
(S&W) Nutradiet, sweet, solids & liq.	½ cup	40	8.0
Frozen:			
(USDA) boiled, drained	½ cup (3 oz.)	57	9.9
(Birds Eye):			
With cream sauce	⅓ of 8-oz. pkg.	134	13.7
With sliced mushrooms	⅓ of 10-oz. pkg.	65	10.7
Sweet, 5-minute style	⅓ of 10-oz. pkg.	70	12.0
Tender tiny, deluxe	⅓ of 10-oz. pkg.	55	8.6
(Green Giant):			
Creamed, with bread crumb topping, Bake'n Serve	⅓ of 10-oz. pkg.	106	11.2
Early, small	¼ of 16-oz. pkg.	76	12.5
Sweet	½ of 18-oz. pkg.	85	14.1
Sweet, in butter sauce	⅓ of 10-oz. pkg.	74	8.6
(Le Sueur) early, in butter sauce	⅓ of 10-oz. pkg.	71	9.7
(McKenzie or Seabrook Farms):			
Regular	⅓ of 10-oz. pkg.	77	13.1
Petite	⅓ of 10-oz. pkg.	62	10.3

Food and Description	Measure or Quantity	Calories	Carbo-hydrates (grams)
PEA & CARROTS:			
Canned, regular pack:			
(Del Monte):			
Solids & liq.	½ cup (4 oz.)	49	9.4
Solids only	½ cup (2.8 oz.)	44	8.2
(Libby's) solids & liq.	½ cup (4.2 oz.)	52	10.3
Canned, dietetic or low calorie, solids & liq.:			
(Blue Boy)	½ cup	60	11.0
(Diet Delight)	½ cup (4.3 oz.)	40	6.0
(S&W) *Nutradiet*	½ cup	35	7.0
Frozen:			
(USDA) boiled, without salt, drained	½ cup (3.1 oz.)	46	8.8
(Birds Eye)	⅓ pkg.	50	9.0
PEA & CAULIFLOWER, frozen (Birds Eye) with cream sauce	½ of 10-oz. pkg.	111	11.9
PEA, CROWDER, frozen (Southland)	⅕ of 16-oz. pkg.	120	21.0
PEA, MATURE SEED, dry (USDA):			
Whole	1 lb.	1542	272.5
Whole	1 cup	680	120.6
Split	1 lb.	1579	284.4
Split	1 cup (7.2 oz.)	706	127.3
Cooked, split, drained solids	½ cup (3.4 oz.)	112	20.2
PEA & ONION, frozen (Birds Eye)	⅓ of 10-oz. pkg.	67	11.7
PEA POD:			
Raw (USDA) edible podded or Chinese	1 lb. (weighed untrimmed)	228	51.7

(USDA): United States Department of Agriculture
(HEW/FAO): Health, Education and Welfare/Food and Agriculture Organization
* Prepared as Package Directs

Food and Description	Measure or Quantity	Calories	Carbo-hydrates (grams)
Boiled (USDA) drained	4 oz.	49	10.8
Frozen (La Choy)	6-oz. pkg.	90	20.4
PEA & POTATO, frozen (Birds Eye) with cream sauce	⅓ of 8-oz. pkg.	145	16.3
PEA SOUP, GREEN (See also, **PEA SOUP, SPLIT**):			
Canned, regular pack:			
(USDA) condensed	8 oz. (by wt.)	240	41.7
*(USDA) condensed:			
Prepared with equal volume milk	1 cup (8.6 oz.)	208	28.7
Prepared with equal volume water	1 cup (8.6 oz.)	130	22.5
*(Campbell) condensed	11-oz. serving	210	34.0
Canned, dietetic or low calorie:			
(Campbell) low sodium	7½-oz. can	160	23.0
*(Dia-Mel) condensed	8-oz. serving	110	18.0
*Mix:			
(USDA)	1 cup (8.5 oz.)	121	20.3
(Lipton) *Cup-a-Soup*	6 fl. oz.	120	16.0
*Frozen (USDA) condensed, with ham, prepared with equal volume water	8-oz. serving	129	18.1
PEA SOUP, SPLIT:			
Canned, regular pack:			
*(USDA) condensed, prepared with equal volume water	1 cup (8.6 oz.)	145	20.6
(Campbell):			
Chunky, with ham	10¾-oz. can	240	33.0
*Condensed, with ham & bacon	11-oz. serving	230	32.0
*(Grandma Brown's)	8-oz. serving	184	28.2
*Frozen (Mother's Own)	8-oz. serving	130	20.0

Food and Description	Measure or Quantity	Calories	Carbo-hydrates (grams)
PEACH:			
Fresh (USDA):			
Whole, without skin	1 lb. (weighed unpeeled)	150	38.3
Whole	4-oz. peach (2″ dia.)	38	9.6
Diced	½ cup (4.7 oz.)	51	12.9
Sliced	½ cup (3 oz.)	31	8.2
Canned, regular pack, solids & liq.:			
(USDA):			
Extra heavy syrup	4 oz.	110	28.5
Heavy syrup	2 med. halves & 2 T. syrup (4.1 oz.)	91	23.5
Juice pack	4 oz.	51	13.2
Light syrup	4 oz.	66	17.1
(Del Monte):			
Chunky	½ cup	95	22.8
Cling halves or slices	½ cup	95	22.8
Freestone, halves or slices	½ cup	93	22.4
Spiced	½ of 7¼-oz. can	85	20.6
(Libby's) heavy syrup:			
Halves	½ cup (4.5 oz.)	105	25.4
Slices	½ cup (4.5 oz.)	102	24.7
(Stokely-Van Camp):			
Halves	½ cup (4.4 oz.)	95	24.5
Slices	½ cup (4.5 oz.)	90	24.0
Canned, dietetic or low calorie, solids & liq.:			
(USDA) water pack	½ cup (4.3 oz.)	38	9.9
(Del Monte) *Lite*	½ cup	53	12.6
(Diet Delight):			
Cling or Freestone, juice pack	½ cup (4.4 oz.)	50	14.0
Cling, water pack	½ cup (4.3 oz.)	30	2.0

(USDA): United States Department of Agriculture
(HEW/FAO): Health, Education and Welfare/Food and Agriculture Organization
* Prepared as Package Directs

Food and Description	Measure or Quantity	Calories	Carbo-hydrates (grams)
(Featherweight):			
Cling or Freestone, halves or slices, juice pack	½ cup	50	12.0
Cling, halves or slices, water pack	½ cup	30	8.0
(Libby's) water pack, sliced	½ cup (4.3 oz.)	33	7.5
(S&W) *Nutradiet*, halves or slices:			
Cling:			
Juice pack	½ cup	60	14.0
Water pack	½ cup	30	8.0
Freestone, juice pack	½ cup	50	14.0
Dehydrated (USDA):			
Uncooked	1 oz.	96	24.9
Cooked, with added sugar, solids & liq.	½ cup (5.4 oz.)	184	47.6
Dried (USDA):			
Uncooked	½ cup	231	60.1
Cooked:			
Unsweetened	½ cup	111	28.9
Sweetened	½ cup (5.4 oz.)	181	46.8
Frozen:			
(USDA) unthawed, slices, sweetened	½ cup	104	26.7
(Birds Eye) quick thaw	½ of 10-oz. pkg.	141	34.1
PEACH BUTTER (Smucker's)	1 T. (.7 oz.)	45	16.0
PEACH CREEK (Annie Green Springs) 8% alcohol	3 fl. oz.	63	6.8
PEACH DRINK (Hi-C):			
Canned	6 fl. oz.	90	23.0
*Mix	6 fl. oz.	72	18.0
PEACH ICE CREAM:			
(Breyer's)	¼ pt.	130	18.0
(Sealtest) old fashioned	¼ pt.	130	19.0
PEACH LIQUEUR:			
(Bols) 60 proof	1 fl. oz.	93	8.9
(Hiram Walker) 60 proof	1 fl. oz.	81	8.0

Food and Description	Measure or Quantity	Calories	Carbo-hydrates (grams)
PEACH NECTAR, canned			
(USDA) 40% fruit juice	1 cup (8.8 oz.)	120	31.0
PEACH PRESERVE or JAM:			
Sweetened (Smucker's)	1 T. (.7 oz.)	53	13.5
Dietetic:			
(Dia-Mel)	1 T.	2	0.
(Featherweight):			
Regular	1 T.	16	4.0
Artificially sweetened	1 T.	6	1.0
(Louis Sherry)	1 T.	6	0.
(Tillie Lewis) *Tasti Diet*	1 T.	12	3.0
PEANUT:			
Raw (USDA):			
In shell	1 lb. (weighed in shell)	1868	61.6
With skins	1 oz.	160	5.3
Without skins	1 oz.	161	5.0
Roasted:			
(USDA):			
Whole	1 lb. (weighed in shell)	1769	62.6
Chopped	½ cup	404	13.0
Halves	½ cup	421	13.5
(Fisher):			
In shell, salted	1 oz.	105	3.7
Shelled			
Dry roasted, salted or unsalted	1 oz.	163	5.0
Oil roasted, salted	1 oz.	166	5.3
(Frito-Lay's):			
In shell, salted	1-oz. shelled	163	5.7
Shelled	1 oz.	172	6.2
(Planters):			
Dry roasted	1 oz. (jar)	170	5.4
Oil roasted	¾-oz. bag	133	3.7

(USDA): United States Department of Agriculture
(HEW/FAO): Health, Education and Welfare/Food and Agriculture Organization
* Prepared as Package Directs

Food and Description	Measure or Quantity	Calories	Carbo- hydrates (grams)
Spanish, roasted:			
(Frito-Lay's)	1 oz.	168	6.6
(Planter's):			
Dry roasted	1 oz. (jar)	175	3.4
Oil roasted	1 oz. (can)	182	3.4
PEANUT BUTTER:			
(Elam's) natural, with defatted wheat germ	1 T. (.6 oz.)	109	2.1
(Jif) creamy	1 T.	93	2.7
(Kitchen King) creamy or crunchy	1 T.	95	4.0
(Peter Pan):			
Crunchy	1 T.	101	3.0
Smooth	1 T. (.6 oz.)	94	3.1
Low sodium	1 T.	106	2.3
(Planters) creamy or crunchy	1 T. (.6 oz.)	95	3.0
(Skippy):			
Creamy	1 T. (.6 oz.)	108	3.0
Old fashioned, creamy or super chunk	1 T.	107	2.8
Super chunk	1 T. (.6 oz.)	109	2.9
(Smucker's):			
Creamy or crunchy	1 T.	90	3.0
Natural	1 T.	100	3.0
PEANUT BUTTER BAKING CHIPS (Reese's)	3 T. (1 oz.)	151	12.8
PEA PUREE, canned, dietetic (Featherweight)	½ cup	80	14.5
PEAR:			
Fresh (USDA):			
Whole	1 lb. (weighed with stems & core)	252	63.2
Whole	6.4-oz. pear (3" × 2½" × 2½" dia.)	101	25.4
Quartered	1 cup (6. 8 oz.)	117	29.4
Slices	½ cup (6.8 oz.)	50	12.5

Food and Description	Measure or Quantity	Calories	Carbo-hydrates (grams)
Canned, regular pack, solids & liq.:			
(USDA):			
Extra heavy syrup	4 oz.	104	26.8
Heavy syrup	½ cup	87	22.3
Juice pack	4 oz.	52	13.4
Light syrup	4 oz.	69	17.7
(Del Monte) Bartlett halves or slices, regular or chunky	½ cup (4 oz.)	88	21.3
(Libby's) halves, heavy syrup	½ cup (4.5 oz.)	102	25.1
(Stokely-Van Camp):			
Halves	½ cup (4.5 oz.)	105	25.0
Slices	½ cup (4.5 oz.)	100	23.5
Canned, unsweetened or dietetic, solids & liq.:			
(USDA) water pack	½ cup (4.3 oz.)	39	10.1
(Del Monte) *Lite,* Bartlett:			
Halves	½ cup	58	13.8
Slices	½ cup	* 59	14.1
(Diet Delight):			
Juice pack	½ cup (4.4 oz.)	60	16.0
Water pack	½ cup (4.3 oz.)	35	9.0
(Featherweight) Bartlett halves:			
Juice pack	½ cup	60	15.0
Water pack	½ cup	40	10.0
(Libby's) halves, water pack	½ cup (4.3 oz.)	40	9.8
(S&W) *Nutradiet,* halves, quarters or slices:			
Juice pack	½ cup	60	15.0
Water pack	½ cup	35	10.0
Dried (USDA):			
Uncooked	1 lb.	1216	305.3
Cooked:			
Without added sugar	4 oz.	143	36.0
With added sugar, solids & liq.	4 oz.	171	43.1

(USDA): United States Department of Agriculture
(HEW/FAO): Health, Education and Welfare/Food and Agriculture Organization
* Prepared as Package Directs

Food and Description	Measure or Quantity	Calories	Carbo-hydrates (grams)
PEAR, CANDIED (USDA)	1 oz.	86	21.5
PEAR NECTAR, canned (Del Monte)	6 fl. oz.	122	30.3
PEBBLES cereal (Post):			
Cocoa	⅞ cup (1 oz.)	117	24.2
Fruity	⅞ cup (1 oz.)	116	24.4
PECAN:			
In shell (USDA)	1 lb. (weighed in shell)	1652	35.1
Shelled (USDA):			
Whole	1 lb.	3116	66.2
Chopped	½ cup (1.8 oz.)	357	7.6
Chopped	1 T. (7 grams)	48	1.0
Halves	12–14 halves (.5 oz.)	96	2.0
Halves	½ cup (1.9 oz.)	371	7.9
Oil dipped (Fisher) salted	¼ cup	410	8.9
Roasted, dry:			
(Fisher) salted	¼ cup (1.1 oz.)	220	4.5
(Flavor House)	1 oz.	195	4.1
(Planters)	1 oz.	206	3.5
PEP, cereal (Kellogg's)	¾ cup (1 oz.)	100	24.0
PEPPER, BLACK (French's):			
Regular	1 tsp. (2.3 grams)	9	1.5
Seasoned	1 tsp. (2.9 grams)	8	1.0
PEPPER, HOT CHILI:			
Green:			
Raw (USDA):			
Whole	4 oz.	31	7.5
Without seeds	4 oz.	42	10.3
Canned:			
(USDA) with chili sauce	1 oz.	6	1.4
(Del Monte) whole	1 oz.	5	1.2
Old El Paso, chopped or whole	1 oz.	7	1.4

Food and Description	Measure or Quantity	Calories	Carbohydrates (grams)
Ortega, diced, strips or whole	1 oz.	6	1.1
Jalapeno, canned:			
(*Del Monte*) whole	1 oz.	7	1.5
(Ortega) diced or whole	1 oz.	9	1.7
Yellow, canned (Del Monte) whole	½ cup (3.9 oz.)	30	4.0
PEPPERONI:			
(Hormel) sliced	1 oz.	142	.3
(Swift)	1 oz.	152	1.0
***PEPPER POT SOUP,** canned (Campbell) condensed	10-oz. serving	120	11.0
PEPPER & ONION, frozen (Southland):			
Diced	2-oz. serving	15	3.0
Red & green	2-oz. serving	20	4.0
PEPPER STEAK, frozen:			
*(Chun King) stir fry	⅓ of pkg.	70	3.0
(Stouffer's) green pepper with rice	10½-oz. pkg.	354	34.9
PEPPER, STUFFED:			
Home recipe (USDA) with beef & crumbs	2¾″ × 2½″ pepper with 1⅛ cups stuffing (6.5 oz.)	314	31.1
Frozen:			
(Green Giant) with beef, in creole sauce	7-oz. serving	201	18.1
(Stouffer's) green pepper & beef in tomato sauce	½ of 15½-oz. pkg.	210	17.8
(Weight Watchers) with veal stuffing, one-compartment	11¾-oz. meal	238	22.0

(USDA): United States Department of Agriculture
(HEW/FAO):   Health, Education and Welfare/Food and Agriculture Organization
* Prepared as Package Directs

Food and Description	Measure or Quantity	Calories	Carbo-hydrates (grams)
PEPPER, SWEET:			
Green:			
Raw (USDA):			
Whole	1 lb. (weighed untrimmed)	82	17.9
Without stems & seeds	1 med. pepper (2.6 oz.)	13	2.9
Chopped	½ cup (2.6 oz.)	16	3.6
Slices	½ cup (1.4 oz.)	9	2.0
Strips	½ cup (1.7 oz.)	11	2.4
Boiled (USDA) strips, drained	½ cup (2.4 oz.)	12	2.6
Boiled (USDA) whole, drained	1 med. pepper (2.6 oz.)	13	2.8
Frozen (Southland)	2-oz. serving	10	3.0
Red (USDA):			
Raw, whole	1 lb. (weighed with stems & seeds)	112	25.8
Raw, without stems & seeds	1 med. pepper (2.2 oz.)	19	2.4
Red & green, frozen (Southland)	2-oz. serving	15	3.0
PERCH, raw (USDA):			
White, whole	1 lb. (weighed whole)	193	0.
White, meat only	4 oz.	134	0.
Yellow, whole	1 lb. (weighed whole)	161	0.
Yellow, meat only	4 oz.	103	0.
PERCH DINNER or ENTREE, frozen:			
(Banquet) ocean	8¾-oz. dinner	434	49.8
(Mrs. Paul's) fillets, breaded & fried	2-oz. fillet	127	8.8
(Van de Kamp's) batter dipped, french fried	2-oz. piece	145	10.0
(Weight Watchers) with lemon-flavored bread crumbs, 2-compartment	6½-oz. serving	160	11.0

Food and Description	Measure or Quantity	Calories	Carbo-hydrates (grams)
PERNOD (Julius Wile) 90 proof	1 fl. oz.	79	1.1
PERSIMMON (USDA):			
Japanese or Kaki, fresh:			
With seeds	1 lb. (weighed with skin, calyx & seeds)	286	78.3
With seeds	4.4-oz. persimmon	79	20.1
Seedless	1 lb. (weighed with skin & calyx)	293	75.1
Seedless	4.4-oz. persimmon 2½″ dia.)	81	20.7
Native, fresh:			
Whole	1 lb. (weighed with seeds & calyx)	472	124.6
Flesh only	4 oz.	144	38.0
PHEASANT, raw (USDA):			
Ready-to-cook	1 lb. (weighed ready-to-cook)	595	0.
Meat & skin	4 oz.	172	0.
Meat only	4 oz.	184	0.
PICKEREL, chain, raw (USDA):			
Whole	1 lb. (weighed whole)	194	0.
Meat only	4 oz.	95	0.
PICKLE:			
Chowchow (See **CHOWCHOW**)			
Cucumber, fresh or bread & butter:			
(USDA)	3 slices (¼″ × 1½″)	15	3.8
(Bond's)	3 pieces	23	5.0
(Fanning's)	1 fl. oz.	17	3.9

(USDA): United States Department of Agriculture
(HEW/FAO): Health, Education and Welfare/Food and Agriculture
Organization
* Prepared as Package Directs

Food and Description	Measure or Quantity	Calories	Carbohydrates (grams)
(Featherweight) dietetic, sliced	1 oz.	12	3.0
(Nalley's) chips	1 oz.	27	6.5
Dill:			
(USDA)	4.8-oz. pickle	15	3.0
(Bond's)	1 pickle	1	.2
(Bond's) fresh pack	1 spear	2	.2
(Featherweight) low sodium	1 oz.	5	.9
L&S	1 large pickle	15	2.0
(Nalley's) regular and Polish style	1 oz.	3	.6
(Smucker's):			
Candied stick	4″ pickle (.8 oz.)	45	11.0
Hamburger	1 slice (.13 oz.)	<1	0.
Polish, whole	3½″ pickle (1.8 oz.)	8	1.0
Spears	3½″ spear (1.4 oz.)	6	1.0
Hamburger (Nalley's) chips	1 oz.	3	.6
Kosher dill:			
(Bond's)	1 pickle	2	.2
(Claussen):			
Halves	2 oz.	7	1.3
Whole	2 oz.	7	1.1
(Featherweight) low sodium	1 oz.	4	1.0
(Nalley's)	2 oz.	12	1.7
(Smucker's):			
Baby	2¾″ pickle (.8 oz.)	4	.5
Slices	1 slice (.1 oz.)	<1	0.
Sour:			
(USDA) cucumber	1¾″ × 4″ (4.8 oz.)	14	2.7
(Aunt Jane's)	2-oz. pickle	6	1.1
Sweet:			
(USDA):			
Cucumber, whole	1 oz.	41	10.3
Cucumber, chopped	1 T. (9 grams)	13	3.3
(Aunt Jane's)	1.5-oz. pickle	62	15.5
(Nalley's):			
Regular	1 oz.	37	10.5
Chips	1 oz.	34	9.7
Nubbins	1 oz.	28	7.9

Food and Description	Measure or Quantity	Calories	Carbo-hydrates (grams)
(Smucker's):			
Candied mix	1 piece (.3 oz.)	14	3.3
Gherkins	2″ long pickle (.32 oz.)	15	3.5
Slices	1 slice (.2 oz.)	11	2.3
Sticks	4″ long stick	30	7.0
Whole	2½″ long pickle (.4 oz.)	18	4.0
PIE:			
Commercial type:			
Apple:			
Home recipe (USDA) 2-crust	⅙ of 9″ pie (5.6 oz.)	404	60.2
(Hostess)	4½-oz. pie	409	53.7
(Tastykake)	4-oz. pie	348	DNA
Banana, home recipe (USDA) cream or custard unenriched or enriched	⅙ of 9″ pie (5.4 oz.)	336	46.7
Berry (Hostess)	4½-oz. pie	404	51.1
Blackberry, home recipe (USDA) 2-crust, made with vegetable shortening	⅙ of 9″ pie (5.6 oz.)	384	54.4
Blueberry:			
Home recipe (USDA) 2-crust, made with lard	⅙ of 9″ pie (5.6 oz.)	382	55.1
(Hostess)	4½-oz. pie	394	49.9
Boston cream, home recipe (USDA)	1/12 of 8″ pie (2.4 oz.)	208	34.4
Butterscotch, home recipe (USDA)	⅙ of 9″ pie (5.4 oz.)	406	58.2

(USDA): United States Department of Agriculture
(HEW/FAO): Health, Education and Welfare/Food and Agriculture Organization
* Prepared as Package Directs

Food and Description	Measure or Quantity	Calories	Carbo-hydrates (grams)
Cherry:			
Home recipe (USDA)			
2-crust	⅙ of 9″ pie		
	(5.6 oz.)	412	60.7
(Hostess)	4½-oz. pie	435	58.8
(Tastykake)	4-oz. pie	381	DNA
Chocolate chiffon, home recipe (USDA) made with lard	⅙ of 9″ pie		
	(3.8 oz.)	354	47.2
Chocolate meringue, home recipe (USDA) made with vegetable shortening	⅙ of 9″ pie		
	(4.9 oz.)	353	46.9
Coconut custard, home recipe (USDA)	⅙ of 9″ pie		
	(5.4 oz.)	357	37.8
Custard, home recipe (USDA) enriched or unenriched	⅙ of 9″ pie		
	(5.4 oz.)	331	35.6
Lemon:			
Chiffon, home recipe (USDA) made with lard or vegetable shortening	⅙ of 9″ pie	338	47.3
Meringue, home recipe, (USDA) 1-crust	⅙ of 9″ pie		
	(4.9 oz.)	357	52.8
(Hostess)	4½-oz. pie	415	52.4
(Tastykake)	4-oz. pie	370	DNA
Mince, home recipe (USDA) 2-crust, enriched or unenriched	⅙ of 9″ pie		
	(5.6 oz.)	428	65.1
Peach:			
Home recipe (USDA)			
2-crust	⅙ of 9″ pie		
	(5.6 oz.)	405	60.4
(Hostess)	4½-oz. pie	409	52.4
(Tastykake)	4-oz. pie	349	DNA
Pecan:			
Home recipe (USDA) 1-crust, made with lard or vegetable shortening	⅙ of 9″ pie	577	70.8

Food and Description	Measure or Quantity	Calories	Carbohydrates (grams)
(Frito-Lay's)	3-oz. serving	353	53.5
Pineapple, home recipe (USDA) 2-crust, made with lard or vegetable shortening	⅙ of 9″ pie (5.6 oz.)	400	60.2
Pineapple custard, home recipe (USDA) made with lard or vegetable shortening	⅙ of 9″ pie (5.4 oz.)	334	48.8
Pumpkin, home recipe (USDA) 1 crust, made with lard or vegetable shortening	⅙ of 9″ pie (5.4 oz.)	321	37.2
Raisin, home recipe (USDA) 2-crust, made with lard or vegetable shortening	⅙ of 9″ pie (5.6 oz.)	427	67.9
Rhubarb, home recipe (USDA) 2-crust, made with lard or vegetable shortening	⅙ of 9″ pie (5.6 oz.)	400	60.4
Strawberry, home recipe (USDA) made with lard or vegetable shortening	⅙ of 9″ pie (5.6 oz.)	313	48.8
Frozen:			
Apple:			
(USDA) baked	5-oz. serving	361	56.8
(Banquet)	⅙ of 20-oz. pie	240	35.5
(Morton):			
Regular	⅙ of 24-oz. pie	295	40.9
Great Little Desserts:			
Regular	8-oz. pie	598	88.6
Dutch apple	7.8-oz. pie	607	95.3

(USDA): United States Department of Agriculture
(HEW/FAO): Health, Education and Welfare/Food and Agriculture Organization
* Prepared as Package Directs

Food and Description	Measure or Quantity	Calories	Carbohydrates (grams)
(Sara Lee):			
Regular	⅙ of 31-oz. pie	376	43.2
Dutch apple	⅙ of 30-oz. pie	354	50.6
Banana:			
(Banquet) cream	⅙ of 14-oz. pie	172	19.9
(Morton) cream:			
Regular	⅙ of 16-oz. pie	174	19.7
Great Little Desserts	3½-oz. pie	237	25.8
Blueberry:			
(Banquet)	⅙ of 20-oz. pie	253	37.5
(Morton):			
Regular	⅙ of 24-oz. pie	285	38.6
Great Little Desserts	8-oz. pie	589	86.4
(Sara Lee)	⅙ of 31-oz. pie	449	44.8
Cherry:			
(Banquet)	⅙ of 20-oz. pie	228	33.8
(Morton):			
Regular	⅙ of 24-oz. pie	300	42.0
Great Little Desserts	8-oz. pie	589	86.4
(Sara Lee)	⅙ of 31-oz. pie	397	48.0
Chocolate cream:			
(Banquet)	⅙ of 14-oz. pie	177	21.8
(Morton):			
Regular	⅙ of 16-oz. pie	199	22.8
Great Little Desserts	3½-oz. pie	266	28.8
Coconut:			
Cream:			
(Banquet)	⅙ of 14-oz. pie	174	19.1
(Morton):			
Regular	⅙ of 16-oz. pie	197	22.0
Great Little Desserts	2½-oz. pie	266	28.8
Custard:			
(Banquet)	⅙ of 20-oz. pie	203	28.2
(Morton) *Great Little Desserts*	6½-oz. pie	369	53.5
Custard (Banquet)	⅙ of 20-oz. pie	206	31.9
Lemon, cream:			
(Banquet)	⅙ of 14-oz. pie	168	21.8
(Morton):			
Regular	⅙ of 16-oz. pie	182	22.0
Great Little Desserts	3½-oz. pie	245	27.8
Mince:			
(Banquet)	⅙ of 20-oz. pie	252	38.5

Food and Description	Measure or Quantity	Calories	Carbo-hydrates (grams)
(Morton)	⅙ of 24-oz. pie	314	45.4
Neapolitan (Morton)	⅙ of 16-oz. pie	195	23.0
Peach:			
(Banquet)	⅙ of 20-oz. pie	219	29.9
(Morton)	⅕ of 24-oz. pie	286	38.7
(Sara Lee)	⅙ of 31-oz. pie	458	56.2
Pumpkin:			
(Banquet)	⅙ of 20-oz. pie	206	32.3
(Morton)	⅙ of 24-oz. pie	235	36.4
(Sara Lee)	⅛ of 45-oz. pie	354	49.4
Strawberry cream:			
(Banquet)	⅙ of 14-oz. pie	169	22.5
(Morton)	⅙ of 16-oz. pie	182	22.0

PIE CRUST (See also **PASTRY SHELL**):

Food and Description	Measure or Quantity	Calories	Carbo-hydrates (grams)
Home recipe (USDA) baked	9" pie crust (6.3 oz.)	900	76.8
Frozen (Banquet):			
Regular	9" pie shell (5 oz.)	614	61.9
Deep dish	9" pie shell (6 oz.)	751	78.8
Mix:			
(USDA) dry	10-oz. pkg.	1482	140.6
(USDA) prepared with water, baked	4 oz.	526	49.9
(Betty Crocker):			
Regular	1/16 of pkg.	120	10.0
Stick	⅛ of stick	120	10.0
*(Flako)	⅙ of 9" pie shell	245	25.2
*(Pillsbury) mix or stick	⅙ of 2-crust pie	290	27.0

PIE FILLING (See also **PUDDING or PIE FILLING**) (Comstock):

Food and Description	Measure or Quantity	Calories	Carbo-hydrates (grams)
Apple:			
Regular	21-oz. can	780	174.0
Pie-sliced	21-oz. can	270	60.0
Apricot	21-oz. can	660	144.0

(USDA): United States Department of Agriculture
(HEW/FAO): Health, Education and Welfare/Food and Agriculture Organization
* Prepared as Package Directs

Food and Description	Measure or Quantity	Calories	Carbo-hydrates (grams)
Banana cream	21-oz. can	660	132.0
Blueberry	21-oz. can	720	156.0
Cherry	21-oz. can	720	156.0
Chocolate cream	21-oz. can	840	162.0
Coconut cream	21-oz. can	720	144.0
Lemon	21-oz. can	960	198.0
Mincemeat	21-oz. can	1020	216.0
Peach	21-oz. can	660	150.0
Pineapple	21-oz. can	660	150.0
Pumpkin (See also **PUMPKIN,** canned)	4½-oz. serving	170	38.0
Raisin	21-oz. can	840	180.0
Strawberry	21-oz. can	780	168.0
*PIE MIX (Betty Crocker)			
Boston cream	⅛ of pie	260	48.0
PIEROGIES, frozen (Mrs. Paul's):			
Cabbage	5-oz. serving	333	64.0
Potato & cheese	5-oz. serving	304	56.6
Sauerkraut, Polish-style	5-oz. serving	312	60.2
PIGEON (See **SQUAB**)			
PIGEON PEA (USDA):			
Raw, immature seeds in pods	1 lb.	207	37.7
Dry seeds	1 lb.	1551	288.9
PIGNOLIA (See **PINE NUT**)			
PIGS FEET, pickled (*SDA)	4 oz.	226	0.
PIKE, raw (USDA):			
Blue:			
Whole	1 lb. (weighed whole)	180	0.
Meat only	4 oz.	102	0.
Northern:			
Whole	1 lb. (weighed whole)	104	0.
Meat only	4 oz.	100	0.

Food and Description	Measure or Quantity	Calories	Carbo-hydrates (grams)
Walleye:			
Whole	1 lb. (weighed whole)	240	0.
Meat only	4 oz.	105	0.
PILI NUT (USDA):			
In shell	1 lb. (weighed in shell)	546	6.9
Shelled	4 oz.	759	9.5
PIMIENTO, canned:			
(USDA) solids & liq.	4 oz.	31	6.6
(Dromedary) diced, sliced or whole, drained solids	1 oz.	10	2.0
(Sunshine) diced or sliced, drained	1 T. (.6 oz.)	4	.9
PIÑA COLADA, canned (Mr. Boston) 12% alcohol	3 fl. oz.	240	34.2
PINEAPPLE:			
Fresh (USDA):			
Whole	1 lb. (weighed untrimmed)	123	32.3
Diced	½ cup (2.8 oz.)	41	10.7
Sliced	¾" × 3½" slice (3 oz.)	44	11.5
Canned, regular pack, solids & liq.:			
(USDA):			
Heavy syrup:			
Crushed	½ cup (5.6 oz.)	97	25.4
Slices	1 large slice & 2 T. syrup (4.3 oz.)	90	23.7
Tidbits	½ cup (4.6 oz.)	95	25.0
Juice pack	4 oz.	66	17.1
Light syrup	5 oz.	67	17.5

(USDA): United States Department of Agriculture
(HEW/FAO):   Health, Education and Welfare/Food and Agriculture
             Organization
* Prepared as Package Directs

Food and Description	Measure or Quantity	Calories	Carbo-hydrates (grams)
(Del Monte):			
Crushed	½ cup (4 oz.)	94	22.7
Chunks	½ cup	91	22.2
Slices:			
Medium	½ cup	92	22.4
Large	½ cup	103	25.2
Tidbits	½ cup	95	22.9
(Dole):			
Heavy syrup, chunks, crushed, slices or tidbits	½ cup	94	24.7
Juice pack, chunks, crushed or slices	½ cup	70	17.5
Canned, dietetic or low calorie, solids & liq.:			
(USDA)	4 oz.	44	11.6
(Del Monte):			
Chunks	½ cup	70	16.8
Crushed	½ cup	77	18.5
Slices	½ cup	81	19.6
(Diet Delight) juice pack	½ cup (4.4 oz.)	70	18.0
(Featherweight) chunks or slices:			
Juice pack	½ cup	70	18.0
Water pack	½ cup	60	15.0
(S&W) *Nutradiet*, slices	1 slice	30	7.5
PINEAPPLE, CANDIED			
(USDA)	1 oz.	90	22.7
PINEAPPLE-GRAPEFRUIT JUICE, canned (Texsun)	6 fl. oz.	91	22.0
PINEAPPLE & GRAPEFRUIT JUICE DRINK, canned:			
(USDA) 40% fruit juices	½ cup (4.4 oz.)	68	17.0
(Del Monte):			
Regular	6 fl. oz.	98	23.7
Pink	6 fl. oz.	97	23.9
(Dole) pink	6 fl. oz.	101	25.4
PINEAPPLE JUICE:			
Canned, unsweetened:			
(Del Monte):			
Regular	6 fl. oz.	98	23.7

Food and Description	Measure or Quantity	Calories	Carbo-hydrates (grams)
With vitamin C	6 fl. oz.	108	26.2
(Dole)	6 fl. oz.	103	25.4
(Texsun)	6 fl. oz.	97	24.0
*Frozen, unsweetened:			
(USDA)	½ cup (4.4 oz.)	64	15.9
(Minute Maid)	6 fl. oz.	92	22.7
PINEAPPLE & ORANGE JUICE DRINK:			
Canned:			
(USDA) 40% fruit juices	½ cup (4.4 oz.)	67	16.7
(Del Monte)	6 fl. oz.	97	24.0
(Hi-C)	6 fl. oz.	94	23.0
*Frozen (Minute Maid)	6 fl. oz.	94	23.0
PINEAPPLE PRESERVE,			
sweetened (Smucker's)	1 T.	53	13.5
PINE NUT (USDA):			
Pignolias, shelled	4 oz.	626	13.2
Piñon, whole	4 oz. (weighed in shell)	418	13.5
Piñon, shelled	4 oz.	720	23.2
PINOT CHARDONNAY WINE:			
(Louis M. Martini) 12% alcohol	3 fl. oz.	90	.2
(Paul Masson) 12% alcohol	3 fl. oz.	71	2.4
PINOT NOIR WINE:			
(Inglenook) Estate, 12% alcohol	3 fl. oz.	58	.3
(Louis M. Martini) 12½% alcohol	3 fl. oz.	90	.2

(USDA): United States Department of Agriculture
(HEW/FAO): Health, Education and Welfare/Food and Agriculture Organization
* Prepared as Package Directs

Food and Description	Measure or Quantity	Calories	Carbo-hydrates (grams)
PISTACHIO NUT:			
Raw (USDA):			
In shell	4 oz. (weighed in shell)	337	10.8
Shelled	½ cup (2.2 oz.)	368	11.8
Shelled	1 T. (8 grams)	46	1.5
Roasted:			
(Fisher) salted:			
In shell	1 oz.	84	2.7
Shelled	1 oz.	174	5.4
(Flavor House) dry roasted	1 oz.	168	5.4
(Frito-Lay's)	1 oz.	175	5.8
(Planters) dry roasted	1 oz.	170	6.0
PITANGA, fresh (USDA):			
Whole	1 lb. (weighed whole)	187	45.9
Flesh only	4 oz.	58	14.2
PIZZA PIE (See also **PIZZA PIE MIX**):			
Regular (Pizza Hut):			
Beef	½ of 10″ pie (7.6 oz.)	488	55.0
Cheese	½ of 10″ pie	436	53.2
Pepperoni	½ of 10″ pie	459	54.4
Pork	½ of 10″ pie	466	54.6
Supreme	½ of 10″ pie	474	54.4
Frozen:			
Canadian style bacon (Celeste):			
Small	½ of 9-oz. pie	241	25.2
Large	¼ of 9-oz. pie	288	30.0
Cheese:			
(Celeste):			
Small	7-oz. pie	472	57.1
Large	¼ of 19-oz. pie	309	21.6
(Jeno's):			
Regular	½ of 13-oz. pie	420	54.0
Deluxe	⅓ of 20-oz. pie	490	57.0
(La Pizzeria):			
Regular	¼ of 20-oz. pie	330	42.0
Thick crust	⅓ of 18½-oz. pie	410	46.0

Food and Description	Measure or Quantity	Calories	Carbo-hydrates (grams)
(Stouffer's) *French Bread*	½ of 10¼-oz. pkg.	327	42.8
Totino's	½ of pie	440	53.0
(Weight Watchers)	6-oz. pie	364	31.0
Combination:			
(Celeste) Chicago style	¼ of 24-oz. pie	360	36.2
(Jeno's) deluxe	⅓ of 23-oz. pie	560	55.0
(La Pizzeria):			
Small	½ of 13½-oz. pie	420	43.0
Large	¼ of 24½-oz. pie	380	39.0
Totino's:			
Classic	⅓ of pie	520	48.0
Deep crust	⅙ of pie	310	33.0
(Van de Kamp's) thick crust	¼ of 23.4-oz. pie	310	24.0
(Weight Watchers) deluxe	7¼ oz. pie	322	27.9
Deluxe:			
(Celeste):			
Small	9-oz. pie	563	62.7
Large	¼ of 23½-oz. pie	368	37.4
(Stouffer's) *French Bread*	½ of 12⅜-oz. pkg.	404	45.7
Hamburger:			
(Jeno's)	½ of 13½-oz. pie	440	57.0
(Stouffer's) *French Bread*	½ of 12¼-oz. pie	397	37.8
Tostino's	½ of pie	460	41.0
Mexican style (Van de Kamp's)	½ of 11-oz. pkg.	416	27.0
Pepperoni:			
(Celeste):			
Regular:			
Small	7¼-oz. pie	568	54.1
Large	¼ of 20-oz. pie	347	34.8
Chicago style, deluxe	¼ of 24-oz. pie	374	36.7
(Jeno's)	½ of 12-oz. pie	450	57.0
(La Pizzeria)	¼ of 21-oz. pie	330	42.0

(USDA): United States Department of Agriculture
(HEW/FAO): Health, Education and Welfare/Food and Agriculture Organization
* Prepared as Package Directs

Food and Description	Measure or Quantity	Calories	Carbo- hydrates (grams)
(Stouffer's) *French Bread*	½ of 11¼-oz. pkg.	401	43.8
Tostino's:			
Regular	½ of pie	460	52.0
Deep crust	⅙ of pie	300	34.0
(Van de Kamp's) thick crust	¼ of 22-oz. pie	370	38.0
Sausage:			
(Celeste):			
Regular:			
Small	8-oz. pie	525	59.6
Large	¼ of 22-oz. pie	359	34.7
Chicago style deluxe	¼ of 24.-oz. pie	382	36.6
(Jeno's):			
Regular	½ of 13½-oz. pie	450	57.0
Deluxe	⅓ of 21-oz. pie	500	53.0
(La Pizzeria):			
Small	½ of 13-oz. pie	430	41.0
Large	¼ of 23-oz. pie	380	42.0
(Stouffer's) *French Bread*	½ of 12-oz. pkg.	417	43.8
Tostino's:			
Regular	½ of pie	470	54.0
Classic	⅓ of pie	500	50.0
Deep crust	⅙ of pie	300	33.0
(Weight Watchers) veal	6 ¾-oz. pie	350	29.1
Sausage & mushroom:			
(Celeste):			
Small	9-oz. pie	555	56.8
Large	¼ of 24-oz. pie	365	34.1
(Stouffer's) *French Bread*	½ of 12½-oz. pkg.	388	39.8
Sicilian style (Celeste) deluxe	¼ of 26.-oz. pie	408	45.4
Supreme (Celeste):			
Regular:			
Small	10-oz. pie	590	52.2
Large	¼ of 24-oz. pie	354	31.3
Without meat:			
Small	8-oz. pie	434	49.2
Large	¼ of 20-oz. pie	272	30.8
Vegetable (Weight Watchers) supreme	4¼-oz. pie	396	35.0

Food and Description	Measure or Quantity	Calories	Carbo-hydrates (grams)
PIZZA PIE MIX:			
Cheese:			
(Jeno's)	½ of mix	420	62.0
*(Kraft)	4 oz.	265	26.1
Skillet Pizza (General Mills)	¼ of pkg.	210	30.0
Pepperoni:			
(Jeno's)	½ of pkg.	510	67.0
Skillet Pizza (General Mills)	¼ of pkg.	220	31.0
Sausage:			
(Jeno's)	½ of pkg.	530	66.0
*(Kraft)	4 oz.	274	23.9
Skillet Pizza (General Mills)	¼ of pkg.	230	29.0
PIZZA ROLL (Jeno's): frozen, 12 to pkg:			
Cheeseburger	½-oz. roll	45	4.5
Pepperoni & cheese or sausage & cheese	½-oz. roll	43	4.2
Shrimp & cheese	½-oz. roll	37	3.8
PIZZA SAUCE, canned:			
(Contadina)	8 oz.	130	20.0
(Ragu)	5 oz.	120	15.0
PIZZA SEASONING SPICE (French's)	1 tsp. (.1 oz.)	5	1.0
PLANTAIN, raw (USDA):			
Whole	1 lb. (weighed with skin)	389	101.9
Flesh only	4 oz.	135	35.4
PLUM:			
Fresh (USDA):			
Damson:			
Whole	1 lb. (weighed with pits)	272	73.5

(USDA): United States Department of Agriculture
(HEW/FAO): Health, Education and Welfare/Food and Agriculture
Organization
* Prepared as Package Directs

Food and Description	Measure or Quantity	Calories	Carbo-hydrates (grams)
Flesh only	4 oz.	75	20.2
Japanese & hybrid:			
Whole	1 lb. (weighed with pits)	205	52.5
Whole	2.1-oz. plum (2" dia.)	27	6.9
Diced	½ cup (2.9 oz.)	39	10.1
Halves	½ cup (3.1 oz.)	42	10.8
Slices	½ cup (3 oz.)	40	10.3
Prune type:			
Whole	1 lb. (weighed with pits)	320	84.0
Halves	½ cup (2.8 oz.)	60	15.8
Canned, purple, regular pack, solids & liq.:			
(USDA):			
Extra heavy syrup	4 oz.	116	30.3
Heavy syrup, with pits	½ cup (4.5 oz.)	106	27.6
Heavy syrup, without pits	½ cup (4.2 oz.)	100	25.9
Light syrup	4 oz.	71	18.8
(Stokely-Van Camp)	½ cup	120	30.0
Canned, unsweetened or low calorie, solids & liq.:			
(Diet Delight) purple:			
Juice pack	½ cup (4.4 oz.)	70	19.0
Water pack	½ cup (4.4 oz.)	50	13.0
(Featherweight) purple:			
Juice pack	½ cup	80	18.0
Water pack	½ cup	40	9.0
(S&W) *Nutradiet*, purple, juice pack	½ cup	80	20.0
PLUM JELLY:			
Sweetened (Smucker's)	1 T. (.7 oz.)	53	13.5
Dietetic or low calorie (Featherweight)	1 T.	16	4.0
PLUM PRESERVE or JAM, sweetened (Smucker's)	1 T. (.7 oz.)	53	13.5
P.M. FRUIT DRINK, canned (Mott's)	6 fl. oz.	90	22.0

Food and Description	Measure or Quantity	Calories	Carbo-hydrates (grams)
POLISH-STYLE SAUSAGE (See **SAUSAGE**)			
POLYNESIAN-STYLE DINNER, (Swanson)	13-oz. dinner	490	65.0
POMEGRANATE, raw (USDA):			
Whole	1 lb. (weighed whole)	160	41.7
Pulp only	4 oz.	71	18.6
POMPANO, raw (USDA):			
Whole	1 lb. (weighed whole)	423	0.
Meat only	4 oz.	188	0.
POPCORN:0			
Unpopped:			
(USDA)	1 oz.	103	20.4
(3-Minute)	¼ cup (1 oz.)	102	19.8
Popped:			
(USDA):			
Plain	1 oz.	109	21.7
Plain, large kernel	1 cup (6 grams)	23	4.6
Butter or oil & salt added	1 oz.	129	16.8
Butter or oil & salt added	1 cup (9 grams)	41	2.3
Sugar coated	1 cup (1.2 oz.)	134	29.9
(Bachman):			
Plain	1 oz.	160	13.0
Caramel-coated	1 oz.	110	25.0
Cheese flavored	1 oz.	180	14.0
(Jiffy Pop):			
Plain	½ pkg. (2½ oz.)	244	29.8
Buttered	½ pkg. (2½ oz.)	247	29.4
(Jolly Time):			
Plain	1 cup (.5 oz.)	55	10.8

(USDA): United States Department of Agriculture
(HEW/FAO):   Health, Education and Welfare/Food and Agriculture
                        Organization
* Prepared as Package Directs

Food and Description	Measure or Quantity	Calories	Carbohydrates (grams)
Added oil & salt	1 cup (.5 oz.)	64	8.3
(Pillsbury) microwave popcorn	1 cup	60	5.5
(Super Pop Brand) yellow or white, no added oil or salt	1 cup (.2 oz.)	22	4.3
POPOVER:			
Home recipe (USDA)	1 average popover (2 oz.)	128	14.7
*Mix (Flako)	1 popover	170	25.0
POPPY SEED (French's)	1 tsp.	13	.8
POPSICLE, twin	3-fl.-oz. pop	70	17.0
PORGY, raw (USDA):			
Whole	1 lb. (weighed whole)	208	0.
Meat only	4 oz.	127	0.
PORK, medium-fat:			
Fresh (USDA):			
Boston butt:			
Raw	1 lb. (weighed with bone & skin)	1220	0.
Roasted, lean & fat	4 oz.	400	0.
Roasted, lean only	4 oz.	277	0.
Chop:			
Broiled, lean & fat	1 chop (4 oz., weighed with bone)	295	0.
Broiled, lean & fat	1 chop (3 oz., weighed with bone)	332	0.
Broiled, lean only	1 chop (3 oz., weighed without bone)	230	0.
Fat, separable, cooked	1 oz.	219	0.
Ham (See also **HAM**):			
Raw	1 lb. (weighed with bone & skin)	1188	0.

Food and Description	Measure or Quantity	Calories	Carbo-hydrates (grams)
Roasted, lean & fat	4 oz.	424	0.
Roasted, lean only	4 oz.	246	0.
Loin:			
Raw	1 lb. (weighed with bone)	1065	0.
Roasted, lean & fat	4 oz.	411	0.
Roasted, lean only	4 oz.	288	0.
Picnic:			
Raw	1 lb. (weighed with bone & skin)	1083	0.
Simmered, lean & fat	4 oz.	424	0.
Simmered, lean only	4 oz.	240	0.
Spareribs:			
Raw, with bone	1 lb. (weighed with bone)	976	0.
Braised, lean & fat	4 oz.	499	0.
Cured, light commercial cure:			
Bacon (See **BACON**)			
Bacon butt (USDA):			
Raw	1 lb. (weighed with bone & skin)	1227	0.
Roasted, lean & fat	4 oz.	374	0.
Roasted, lean only	4 oz.	276	0.
Ham (See also **HAM**):			
Raw (USDA)	1 lb. (weighed with bone & skin)	1100	0.
Roasted, lean & fat (USDA)	4 oz.	328	0.
Roasted, lean only (USDA)	4 oz.	212	0.
Fully cooked, boneless:			
Parti-Style (Armour Star)	4 oz.	167	.1
(Wilson) rolled	4 oz.	222	0.

(USDA): United States Department of Agriculture
(HEW/FAO):   Health, Education and Welfare/Food and Agriculture
              Organization
* Prepared as Package Directs

Food and Description	Measure or Quantity	Calories	Carbo-hydrates (grams)
Picnic:			
Raw (USDA)	1 lb. (weighed with bone & skin)	1060	0.
Raw (Wilson) smoked	4 oz.	279	0.
Roasted, lean & fat (USDA)	4 oz.	366	0.
Roasted, lean only (USDA)	4 oz.	239	0.
Cured, long-cure, country-style Virginia ham, raw:			
(USDA)	1 lb. (weighed with bone & skin)	1535	1.2
(USDA)	1 lb. (weighed without bone & skin)	1765	1.4
PORK & BEANS (See **BEAN, BAKED**)			
PORK, CANNED, chopped luncheon meat (USDA):			
Regular	1 oz.	83	.4
Chopped	1 cup (4.8 oz.)	400	1.8
Diced	1 cup	415	1.8
PORK DINNER, frozen (Swanson) *TV Brand,* loin of pork	11¼-oz. dinner	470	48.0
PORK RINDS, fried, *Baken-Ets*	1 oz.	150	1.0
PORK SAUSAGE (See **SAUSAGE**)			
PORK STEAK, BREADED, frozen (Hormell)	3-oz. serving	223	11.0
PORK, SWEET & SOUR, frozen (La Choy)	½ of 15-oz. entree	229	45.2

Food and Description	Measure or Quantity	Calories	Carbo-hydrates (grams)
PORT WINE:			
(Great Western) Solera:			
Regular, 18% alcohol	3 fl. oz.	138	11.5
Tawny, 18% alcohol	3 fl. oz.	136	11.4
(Louis M. Martini):			
Regular, 19½% alcohol	3 fl. oz.	165	2.0
Tawny, 19½% alcohol	3 fl. oz.	165	2.0
(Taylor):			
Regular, 18½% alcohol	3 fl. oz.	144	13.2
Tawny, 18½% alcohol	3 fl. oz.	138	12.0
***POSTUM,** cereal beverage			
(General Foods):			
Ground, brewed	6 fl. oz.	8	2.1
Instant, regular or coffee flavored	6 fl. oz.	11	2.5
POTATO (See also **POTATO CHIP, POTATO MIX, POTATO SALAD, POTATO STICK,** etc):			
Raw (USDA):			
Whole	1 lb. (weighed unpared)	279	62.8
Pared, chopped	1 cup (5.2 oz.)	112	25.1
Pared, diced	1 cup (5.5 oz.)	119	26.8
Pared, sliced	1 cup (5.2 oz.)	113	25.5
Cooked (USDA):			
Au gratin or scalloped, with cheese	½ cup (4.3 oz.)	127	17.9
Au gratin or scalloped, without cheese	½ cup (4.3 oz.)	177	16.6
Baked, peeled after baking	2½″ dia. potato (3 raw to 1 lb.)	92	20.9
Boiled, peeled after boiling	1 med. (3 raw to 1 lb.)	103	23.3

(USDA): United States Department of Agriculture
(HEW/FAO): Health, Education and Welfare/Food and Agriculture Organization
* Prepared as Package Directs

Food and Description	Measure or Quantity	Calories	Carbo-hydrates (grams)
Boiled, peeled before boiling:			
Whole	1 med. (3 raw to 1 lb.)	79	17.7
Diced	½ cup (2.8 oz.)	51	11.3
Mashed	½ cup (3.7 oz.)	68	15.1
Riced	½ cup (4 oz.)	74	16.5
Sliced	½ cup (2.8 oz.)	52	11.6
French fried in deep fat	10 pieces (2″ × ½″ × ½″, 2 oz.)	156	20.5
Hash browned, after holding overnight	½ cup (3.4 oz.)	223	28.4
Mashed, milk added	½ cup (3.5 oz.)	64	12.7
Mashed, milk & butter added	½ cup (3.4 oz.)	92	12.1
Pan fried from raw	½ cup (3 oz.)	228	27.7
Scalloped (See Au Gratin)			
Canned:			
(USDA) solids & liq.	1 cup (8.8 oz.)	110	24.5
(Del Monte) white:			
Solids & liq.	1 cup	84	19.8
Drained solids	1 cup	265	28.4
(Stokely-Van Camp) whole, solids & liq.	½ cup (4.4 oz.)	50	11.0
(Sunshine) whole, solids & liq.	1 cup (8.8 oz.)	102	20.9
Dehydrated, mashed (See also POTATO MIX) (USDA):			
Flakes, dry, without milk	½ cup (.8 oz.)	84	19.3
*Flakes, prepared with water, milk & fat	½ cup (3.8 oz.)	100	15.5
Granules, dry, without milk	½ cup	352	80.4
*Granules, prepared with water, milk & butter	½ cup (3.7 oz.)	101	15.1
Frozen:			
(USDA):			
French-fried, heated	10 pieces (2″ × ½″ × ½″, 2 oz.)	125	19.2
Mashed, heated	4 oz.	105	17.8
(Birds Eye):			
Cottage fries	⅓ of 14-oz. pkg.	120	17.0
Crinkle cuts	⅓ of 9 oz. pkg.	115	18.4

Food and Description	Measure or Quantity	Calories	Carbohydrates (grams)
French fries:			
Regular	3-oz. serving	113	16.8
Tasti Fries	2½-oz. serving	140	17.0
Hash browns:			
Regular	4-oz. serving	75	16.6
O'Brien	4-oz. serving	60	14.0
Shredded	3-oz. serving	60	13.0
Shoestring	3.3-oz. serving	140	20.0
Steak fries	3-oz. serving	110	18.0
Tasti Puffs	2½-oz. serving	190	19.0
Tiny Taters	3.2-oz. serving	200	22.0
Whole, peeled	⅒ of 32-oz. pkg.	60	13.0
(Green Giant):			
Au gratin, *Bake'n Serve*	⅓ of 10-oz. pkg.	141	12.1
& sweet peas in bacon cream sauce	⅓ of 10-oz. pkg.	88	12.6
Shoestring, in butter sauce	⅓ of 10-oz. pkg.	123	14.7
Slices in butter sauce	⅓ of 10-oz. pkg.	76	10.9
Stuffed with cheese-flavored topping	5-oz. serving	237	30.0
Stuffed with sour cream & chives	5-oz. serving	232	30.0
Vermicelli, with mushroom & cheese sauce, *Bake'n Serve*	⅓ of 10-oz. pkg.	135	14.3
(McKenzie) white, whole	3½-oz. serving	69	14.9
(Seabrook Farms) white, whole	3½-oz. serving	69	14.9
(Southland) whole	⅕ of 20-oz. pkg.	80	16.0
(Stouffer's):			
Au gratin	⅓ of 11½-oz. pkg.	135	12.9
Scalloped	⅓ of 12-oz. pkg.	130	13.9
POTATO & BACON, canned			
(Hormel) *Short Orders,* au gratin	7½-oz. can	230	20.0

(USDA): United States Department of Agriculture
(HEW/FAO): Health, Education and Welfare/Food and Agriculture Organization
* Prepared as Package Directs

Food and Description	Measure or Quantity	Calories	Carbohydrates (grams)
POTATO & BEEF, canned			
Dinty Moore (Hormel)			
Short Orders, hashed	7½-oz. can	250	25.0
POTATO CHIP:			
(USDA)	1 oz.	161	14.2
(Bachman):			
Regular	1 oz.	160	14.0
BBQ or sour cream & onion flavor	1 oz.	150	14.0
(Featherweight) unsalted	1 oz.	160	14.0
(Frito-Lay's) natural style	1 oz.	157	15.1
Lay's:			
Regular	1 oz.	150	14.0
Bar-B-Q-flavored	1 oz.	160	14.0
Sour cream & onion flavor	1 oz.	160	15.0
(Nalley's):			
Regular	1 oz.	165	14.2
Barbecue flavor	1 oz.	166	14.2
(Planters) stackable	1 oz.	150	17.0
Pringle's:			
Regular	1 oz.	172	11.9
Light	1 oz.	146	16.8
Rippled	1 oz.	159	14.2
Ruffles	1 oz.	150	15.0
POTATO & HAM, canned			
(Hormel) *Short Orders,* scalloped	7½-oz. can	250	18.0
POTATO MIX:			
*Au gratin:			
(Betty Crocker)	½ cup (⅙ of pkg.)	150	21.0
(French's) *Big Tate*	½ cup	160	23.0
*Creamed (Betty Crocker)	½ cup (⅙ of pkg.)	160	20.0
*Hash brown:			
(Betty Crocker) with onion	½ cup (⅙ of pkg.)	150	22.0
(French's) *Big Tate*	½ cup	165	22.0
*Julienne (Betty Crocker)	½ cup (⅙ of pkg.)	140	18.0
*Mashed:			
American Beauty	½ cup	140	16.0

Food and Description	Measure or Quantity	Calories	Carbo-hydrates (grams)
(Betty Crocker) *Buds*	½ cup	130	15.0
(French's):			
Big Tate	½ cup	140	16.0
Idaho	½ cup	120	16.0
(Pillsbury) *Hungry Jack,*			
flakes	½ cup	140	17.0
*Scalloped:			
(Betty Crocker)	½ cup	190	18.0
(French's) *Big Tate*	½ cup	160	25.0
*Sour cream & chive			
(Betty Crocker)	½ cup (⅙ of pkg.)	140	18.0
POTATO PANCAKE MIX			
(French's) *Big Tate*	3″ pancake	43	5.7
POTATO SALAD:			
Home recipe (USDA):			
With cooked salad dressing			
& seasonings	4 oz.	112	18.5
With mayonnaise & French			
dressing, hard-cooked			
eggs, seasonings	4 oz.	164	15.2
Canned (Nalley's):			
Regular	4-oz. serving	139	17.0
German style	4-oz. serving	143	18.2
*POTATO SOUP, canned			
(Campbell) cream of,			
condensed:			
Made with water	10-oz. serving	90	13.0
Made with water & milk	10-oz. serving	140	17.0
POTATO STICK, *O&C*			
(Durkee)	1½-oz. can	231	22.0
POUILLY-FUISSÉ WINE,			
French white Burgundy			
(Barton & Guestier)			
12½% alcohol	3 fl. oz.	64	.3

(USDA): United States Department of Agriculture
(HEW/FAO): Health, Education and Welfare/Food and Agriculture
             Organization
* Prepared as Package Directs

Food and Description	Measure or Quantity	Calories	Carbo-hydrates (grams)
PRALINES 'N CREAM ICE CREAM (Baskin-Robbins)	1 scoop (2½ oz.)	177	23.7
PRESERVE (See also individual listings by flavor) sweetened (Crosse & Blackwell) all flavors	1 T.	60	14.8
PRETZEL:			
(Bachman) regular or butter	1 oz.	110	21.0
(Nabisco) *Mister Salty:*			
Regular	1 piece (.2 oz.)	20	4.0
Dutch	1 piece (.5 oz.)	55	11.0
Little Shapes	1 piece	6	1.2
Veri Thin, sticks	1 piece (.3 grams)	1	.2
(Pepperidge Farm):			
Nuggets	1¼ oz.	148	26.3
Sticks, thin	1¼ oz.	145	26.3
Twist, tiny	1 oz.	116	21.6
(Planters) sticks & twists	1 oz.	110	22.0
(Rokeach):			
Baldies, unsalted, Dutch style	1 oz.	110	20.0
Dutch style	1 oz.	110	24.0
Party cannister	1 oz.	110	23.0
PRICKLY PEAR, fresh (USDA):			
Whole	1 lb. (weighed with rind & seeds)	84	21.8
Flesh only	4 oz.	48	12.4
PRODUCT 19, cereal (Kellogg's)	¾ cup (1 oz.)	110	24.0
PRUNE:			
Canned, regular pack:			
(Del Monte):			
Stewed, with pits, solids & liq.	1 cup (8 oz.)	262	62.5
Moist Pak, with pits	2 oz.	142	33.5
(Sunsweet) stewed, pitted,			

Food and Description	Measure or Quantity	Calories	Carbo-hydrates (grams)
solids & liq.	½ cup	120	32.0
Canned, dietetic (Featherweight) stewed, water pack, solids & liq.	½ cup	130	35.0
Dried:			
(USDA) dried, cooked, with sugar	1 cup (16–18 prunes & ⅔ cup liq.)	504	132.1
(Del Monte):			
Breakfast, with pits	1 oz.	152	35.4
Medium, with pits	2 oz.	152	25.6
Large, with pits	2 oz.	153	36.2
Extra large, with pits	2 oz.	150	35.3
Jumbo, with pits	2 oz.	157	37.0
Pitted	2 oz.	151	35.4
(Sun-Maid):			
With pits	2 oz.	120	32.0
Pitted	2 oz.	140	36.0
(Sunsweet):			
With pits	2 oz.	130	31.3
Pitted	2 oz.	140	36.0
PRUNE JUICE, canned:			
(USDA)	½ cup (4.5 oz.)	99	24.3
(Del Monte)	6 fl. oz.	137	33.2
(Mott's)	6 fl. oz.	140	34.0
(Sunsweet):			
Regular	6 fl. oz.	130	33.0
Home style with pulp	6 fl. oz.	130	32.0
PRUNE NECTAR, canned			
(Mott's)	6 fl. oz.	100	25.0
PRUNE WHIP, home recipe			
(USDA)	1 cup (4.8 oz.)	211	49.8

(USDA): United States Department of Agriculture
(HEW/FAO):   Health, Education and Welfare/Food and Agriculture
                      Organization
* Prepared as Package Directs

Food and Description	Measure or Quantity	Calories	Carbo-hydrates (grams)
PUDDING or PIE FILLING:			
Home recipe (USDA):			
Rice, made with raisins	½ cup (4.7 oz.)	193	35.2
Tapioca:			
Apple	½ cup (4.4 oz.)	146	36.8
Cream	½ cup (2.9 oz.)	110	14.0
Canned, regular pack:			
Banana:			
(Del Monte)	5-oz. container	183	30.1
(Hunt's) *Snack Pack*	5-oz. container	180	24.0
Butterscotch:			
(Del Monte)	5-oz. container	186	30.8
(Hunt's) *Snack Pack*	5-oz. container	170	27.0
(Thank You)	½ cup (4.5 oz.)	169	29.2
Chocolate:			
(Betty Crocker)	½ cup (5 oz.)	180	30.0
(Del Monte):			
Regular	5-oz. container	173	33.0
Fudge	5-oz. container	193	31.0
(Hunt's) *Snack Pack:*			
Regular	5-oz. container	180	28.0
Fudge	5-oz. container	180	26.0
German	5-oz. container	170	25.0
Marshmallow	5-oz. container	170	25.0
Lemon (Hunt's) *Snack Pack*	5-oz. container	150	32.0
Rice:			
(Betty Crocker)	½ cup (4¼ oz.)	150	25.0
(Comstock)	½ of 7½-oz. can	120	23.0
(Hunt's) *Snack Pack*	5-oz. container	190	27.0
(Menner's)	½ of 7½-oz. can	120	23.0
Tapioca:			
(Betty Crocker)	½ cup (4¼ oz.)	150	22.0
(Del Monte)	5-oz. container	174	30.1
(Hunt's) *Snack Pack*	5-oz. container	140	23.0
Vanilla:			
(Del Monte)	5-oz. container	189	32.1
(Hunt's) *Snack Pack*	5-oz. container	180	29.0
Canned, dietetic or low calorie			
(Sego) banana, butterscotch			
or vanilla	8-oz. container	250	39.0
Chilled, *Swiss Miss:*			

Food and Description	Measure or Quantity	Calories	Carbo-hydrates (grams)
Butterscotch	4-oz. container	150	22.0
Chocolate:			
Regular	4-oz. container	160	25.0
Malt	4-oz. container	150	22.0
Sundae	4-oz. container	170	26.0
Double rich	4-oz. container	160	24.0
Rice	4-oz. container	150	24.0
Tapioca	4-oz. container	130	22.0
Vanilla:			
Regular	4-oz. container	150	24.0
Sundae	4-oz. container	170	25.0
Frozen (Rich's):			
Banana	3-oz. container	142	19.3
Butterscotch	4½-oz. container	199	27.4
Chocolate	4½-oz. container	214	27.1
Vanilla	4½-oz. container	199	27.5
*Mix, regular pack:			
Banana:			
(Jell-O) cream:			
Regular	⅙ of 8″ pie, excluding crust	110	18.0
Instant	½ cup	180	30.0
(My-T-Fine) cream, (Royal):	½ cup	175	32.6
Regular	½ cup	160	27.0
Instant	½ cup	180	29.0
Butter pecan (Jell-O) instant	½ cup	180	29.0
Butterscotch:			
(Jell-O) regular or instant	½ cup	180	30.0
(My-T-Fine) regular	½ cup	143	28.0
(Royal):			
Regular	½ cup	160	27.0
Instant	½ cup	180	29.0
Chocolate:			
(Jell-O):			
Regular:			
Plain or milk	½ cup	170	29.0

(USDA): United States Department of Agriculture
(HEW/FAO):   Health, Education and Welfare/Food and Agriculture
             Organization
* Prepared as Package Directs

Food and Description	Measure or Quantity	Calories	Carbo-hydrates (grams)
Fudge	½ cup	170	28.0
Instant:			
Plain	½ cup	190	34.0
Fudge	½ cup	190	33.0
(My-T-Fine) regular:			
Plain	½ cup	133	28.0
Almond	½ cup	169	27.0
Fudge	½ cup	151	27.0
(Royal):			
Regular, plain or *Dark N' Sweet*	½ cup	180	33.0
Instant, plain or *Dark N' Sweet*	½ cup	190	35.0
Coconut:			
(Jell-O) cream:			
Regular	⅙ of 8″ pie (excluding crust)	110	17.0
Instant	½ cup	190	28.0
(Royal) instant	½ cup	170	30.0
Coffee (Royal) instant	½ cup	180	29.0
Custard:			
Jell-O Americana, golden egg	½ cup	170	24.0
(Royal) regular	½ cup	150	22.0
Flan (Royal) regular	½ cup	150	22.0
Lemon:			
(Jell-O):			
Regular	⅙ of 9″ pie (excluding crust)	180	38.0
Instant	½ cup	180	31.0
(My-T-Fine) regular	½ cup	164	30.0
(Royal):			
Regular	½ cup	160	30.0
Instant	½ cup	180	29.0
Lime (Royal) regular, Key Lime	½ cup	160	30.0
Pineapple (Jell-O) cream, instant	½ cup	180	31.0
Pistachio:			
(Jell-O) instant	½ cup	190	30.0
(Royal) instant	½ cup	170	30.0
Rice, *Jell-O Americana*	½ cup	180	30.0

Food and Description	Measure or Quantity	Calories	Carbo-hydrates (grams)
Tapioca:			
Jell-O Americana,			
chocolate or vanilla	½ cup	160	27.0
(My-T-Fine) vanilla	½ cup	130	28.0
(Royal):			
Chocolate	½ cup	180	33.0
Vanilla	½ cup	160	27.0
Vanilla:			
(Jell-O):			
Regular:			
Plain	½ cup	160	27.0
French	½ cup	180	30.0
Instant, plain or French	½ cup	180	30.0
(My-T-Fine) regular	½ cup	133	28.0
(Royal):			
Regular	½ cup	160	27.0
Instant	½ cup	180	29.0
*Mix, dietetic pack:			
Butterscotch:			
(D-Zerta)	½ cup	70	13.0
(Featherweight):			
Regular	4-oz. serving	12	10.0
Artificially sweetened	4-oz. serving	12	3.0
Chocolate:			
(Dia-Mel)	4-oz. serving	60	8.2
(D-Zerta)	4-oz. serving	70	12.0
(Estee)	½ cup	48	11.0
(Featherweight) artificially sweetened	½ cup	60	9.0
Lemon:			
(Dia-Mel)	4-oz. serving	53	8.2
(Estee)	½ cup	53	13.3
Vanilla:			
(Dia-Mel)	4-oz. serving	53	DNA
(D-Zerta)	½ cup	70	13.0
(Estee)	½ cup	39	9.1
(Featherweight) artificially sweetened	½ cup	50	9.0

(USDA): United States Department of Agriculture
(HEW/FAO): Health, Education and Welfare/Food and Agriculture
                    Organization
* Prepared as Package Directs

Food and Description	Measure or Quantity	Calories	Carbo-hydrates (grams)
PUFFED CORN, cereal (USDA)			
with added nutrients	1 oz.	113	22.9
PUFFED OAT, cereal (USDA):			
Plain, added nutrients	1 oz.	113	21.3
Sugar coated, added nutrients	1 oz.	112	24.3
PUFFED RICE, cereal:			
(Malt-O-Meal)	1 cup (½ oz.)	50	12.0
(Quaker)	1 cup (½ oz.)	55	12.7
PUFFED WHEAT, cereal:			
(Malt-O-Meal)	1 cup (½ oz.)	50	11.0
(Quaker)	1 cup (½ oz.)	54	10.8
PUFFS, frozen (Rich's) vanilla	1.8-oz. puff	167	23.4
PUMPKIN:			
Fresh (USDA):			
Whole	1 lb. (weighed with rind & seeds)	83	20.6
Flesh only	4 oz.	29	7.4
Canned:			
(Del Monte)	½ cup (4.3 oz.)	45	9.5
(Festal)	½ cup	45	9.5
(Libby's) solids pack	¼ of 16-oz. can	47	9.9
(Stokely-Van Camp)	½ cup (4.3 oz.)	45	9.5
PUMPKIN SEED, dry (USDA):			
Whole	4 oz. (weighed in hull)	464	12.6
Hulled	4 oz.	627	17.0

Q

Food and Description	Measure or Quantity	Calories	Carbo-hydrates (grams)
QUAIL, raw (USDA):			
Ready-to-cook	1 lb. (weighed with bones)	686	0.
Meat & skin only	4 oz.	195	0.

Food and Description	Measure or Quantity	Calories	Carbo-hydrates (grams)
QUIK (Nestlé):			
Chocolate flavor	1 T. (.4 oz.)	45	9.5
Strawberry flavor	1 T. (.4 oz.)	45	11.0
QUINCE, fresh (USDA):			
Untrimmed	1 lb. (weighed with skin & seeds)	158	42.3
Flesh only	4 oz.	65	17.4
QUINCE JAM, sweetened (Smucker's)	1 T.	53	13.5
QUISP, cereal (Quaker)	1⅙ cups (1 oz.)	121	23.1

R

RABBIT (USDA):			
Domesticated:			
Raw, ready-to-cook	1 lb. (weighed with bones)	581	0.
Stewed, flesh only	4 oz.	245	0.
Wild, ready-to-cook	1 lb. (weighed with bones)	490	0.
RACCOON, roasted, meat only (USDA)	4 oz.	289	0.
RADISH (USDA):			
Common, raw:			
Without tops	½ lb. (weighed untrimmed)	34	7.4
Trimmed, whole	4 small radishes (1.4 oz.)	7	1.4
Trimmed, sliced	½ cup (2 oz.)	10	2.1
Oriental, raw, without tops	½ lb. (weighed unpared)	34	7.4

(USDA): United States Department of Agriculture
(HEW/FAO):   Health, Education and Welfare/Food and Agriculture Organization
* Prepared as Package Directs

Food and Description	Measure or Quantity	Calories	Carbohydrates (grams)
Oriental, raw, trimmed & pared	4 oz.	22	4.8
RAISIN:			
Dried:			
(USDA):			
Whole, pressed down	½ cup (2.9 oz.)	237	63.5
Chopped	½ cup (2.9 oz.)	234	62.7
Ground	½ cup (4.7 oz.)	387	103.7
(Del Monte):			
Golden seedless	3 oz.	287	67.8
Thompson seedless	3 oz.	283	66.5
(Sun-Maid) seedless, natural			
Thompson	½ cup (3 oz.)	290	69.0
Cooked, (USDA) added sugar, solids & liq.	½ cup (4.3 oz.)	260	68.8
RAISINS, RICE & RYE, cereal (Kellogg's)	¾ cup (1 oz.)	140	31.0
RALSTON, cereal, instant and regular	¼ cup (1 oz.)	90	20.0
RASPBERRY:			
Black (USDA):			
Fresh:			
Whole	1 lb. (weighed with caps & stems)	160	34.6
Without caps & stems	½ cup (2.4 oz.)	49	10.5
Canned, water pack, unsweetened, solids & liq.	4 oz.	58	12.1
Red:			
Fresh (USDA):			
Whole	1 lb. (weighed with caps & stems)	126	29.9
Without caps & stems	½ cup (2.5 oz.)	41	9.8
Canned, water pack, unsweetened or low calorie, solids & liq. (USDA)	4 oz.	40	10.0

Food and Description	Measure or Quantity	Calories	Carbo-hydrates (grams)
Frozen (Birds Eye) quick thaw	½ of 10-oz. pkg.	145	34.8
RASPBERRY JELLY, sweetened (Smucker's) black or red	1 T.	53	13.5
RASPBERRY PRESERVE or JAM:			
Sweetened (Smucker's) black or red	1 T.	53	13.5
Dietetic or low calorie:			
(Dia-Mel) black	1 T.	6	0.
(Featherweight)	1 T.	16	4.0
(S&W) *Nutradiet*	1 T.	24	6.0
RASPBERRY SPREAD, low sugar (Smucker's)	1 T.	24	6.0
RAVIOLI:			
Canned, regular pack:			
(Franco-American):			
Beef:			
In meat sauce	7½-oz. serving	230	36.0
In meat sauce, *RavioliOs*	7½-oz. serving	220	32.0
Cheese, in tomato sauce, *RavioliOs*	7½-oz. serving	260	39.0
(Nalley's):			
Beef	8-oz. serving	214	34.1
Chicken	8-oz. serving	225	34.1
Canned, dietetic or low calorie (Dia-Mel) beef, in sauce	8-oz. can	230	35.0

REDFISH (See **DRUM, RED & OCEAN PERCH,** Atlantic)

(USDA): United States Department of Agriculture
(HEW/FAO): Health, Education and Welfare/Food and Agriculture Organization
* Prepared as Package Directs

Food and Description	Measure or Quantity	Calories	Carbo-hydrates (grams)
RED & GRAY SNAPPER, raw (USDA):			
Whole	1 lb. (weighed whole)	219	0.
Meat only	4 oz.	105	0.
RELISH:			
Regular pack:			
Hamburger (Nalley's)	1 T. (.6 oz.)	17	4.1
Hot dog (Nalley's)	1 T. (.7 oz.)	24	4.8
Sour (USDA)	1 T. (.5 oz.)	3	.4
Sweet:			
(USDA) finely chopped	1 T. (.5 oz.)	21	5.1
(Aunt Jane's)	1 rounded tsp. (.4 oz.)	14	3.4
(Lutz & Schramm)	1 T.	14	4.0
(Smucker's)	1 T. (.6 oz.)	23	4.8
Dietetic or low calorie, cucumber			
(Featherweight)	1-oz. serving	11	2.3
RHINESKELLER WINE (Italian Swiss Colony) 12% alcohol	3 fl. oz.	66	3.0
RHINE WINE:			
(Gallo):			
Regular, 12% alcohol	3 fl. oz.	50	.8
Rhine Garten, 12% alcohol	3 fl. oz.	59	3.0
(Great Western):			
Regular, 12% alcohol	3 fl. oz.	73	2.9
Dutchess, 12% alcohol	3 fl. oz.	72	2.9
(Louis M. Martini) 12½% alcohol	3 fl. oz.	90	.2
(Taylor) 12½% alcohol	3 fl. oz.	75	3.0
RHUBARB (USDA):			
Fresh:			
Partly trimmed	1 lb. (weighed with part leaves, ends & trimmings)	54	12.6
Trimmed	4 oz.	18	4.2
Diced	½ cup (2.2 oz.)	10	2.3

Food and Description	Measure or Quantity	Calories	Carbo-hydrates (grams)
Cooked, sweetened, solids & liq.	½ cup (4.2 oz.)	169	43.2
Frozen, sweetened, cooked, added sugar	½ cup (4.4 oz.)	177	44.9
RICE:			
Brown:			
Raw (USDA)	½ cup (3.7 oz.)	374	80.5
Dry, parboiled (Uncle Ben's) long-grain	1 oz.	107	21.2
*(Uncle Ben's) parboiled:			
No added butter or salt	⅔ cup	133	26.4
Added butter & salt	⅔ cup (4.2 oz.)	152	26.4
*(River) natural	½ cup	110	23.0
White:			
Dry:			
(USDA) long grain, instant or precooked	1 oz.	106	23.4
(USDA) regular	½ cup (3.3 oz.)	336	74.7
*Cooked:			
(Carolina) long-grain	½ cup	100	22.0
(Mahatma) long-grain	½ cup	100	22.0
(Minute Rice) no added butter or salt	⅔ cup	120	27.0
(Success Rice) long-grain	½ cup (½ cooking bag)	110	23.0
(Uncle Ben's):			
Long grain, no added butter or salt	⅔ cup (4.2 oz.)	119	27.4
Long grain, with butter & salt	⅔ cup (4.3 oz.)	143	27.4
Converted, no butter or salt	⅔ cup (4.6 oz.)	129	28.9
RICE BRAN (USDA)	1 oz.	78	14.4

(USDA): United States Department of Agriculture
(HEW/FAO):   Health, Education and Welfare/Food and Agriculture Organization
* Prepared as Package Directs

Food and Description	*Measure or Quantity*	*Calories*	*Carbohydrates (grams)*
RICE, FRIED:			
Canned:			
*(La Choy)	⅓ of 11-oz. can	192	39.7
(Chun King) with pork	½ of 10-oz. pkg.	180	24.0
*Seasoning mix (Durkee)	1 cup	213	46.5
RICE, FRIED, & PORK ENTREE, frozen (La Choy)	½ of 12 oz. entree	245	36.8
RICE KRINKLES, cereal (Post)	⅞ cup (1 oz.)	113	26.3
RICE KRISPIES, cereal (Kellogg's)	1 cup (1 oz.)	110	25.0
RICE MIX:			
Beef:			
*(Carolina) *Bake-it-Easy*	¼ of pkg.	110	23.0
Rice-A-Roni	⅙ of 8-oz. pkg.	129	26.0
*Brown & wild (Uncle Ben's):			
Without butter	½ cup	126	24.7
With butter	½ cup	150	24 7
Chicken:			
*(Carolina) *Bake-it-Easy*	¼ of pkg.	110	23.0
Rice-A-Roni	⅕ of 8-oz. pkg.	160	33.2
*Drumstick (Minute Rice)	½ cup	150	25.0
*Fried (Minute Rice)	½ cup	160	25.0
*Oriental (Carolina) *Bake-it-Easy*	¼ of pkg.	120	23.0
*Rib Roast (Minute Rice)	½ cup	150	25.0
Spanish:			
*(Carolina) *Bake-it-Easy*	¼ of pkg.	110	23.0
*(Minute Rice)	½ cup	150	25.0
Rice-A-Roni	⅙ of 7½-oz. pkg.	124	25.9
*White & wild (Carolina)	½ cup	90	20.0
RICE PUDDING (See **PUDDING or PIE FILLING**)			
RICE, SPANISH:			
Home recipe (USDA)	4 oz.	99	18.8

Food and Description	Measure or Quantity	Calories	Carbo- hydrates (grams)
Canned, regular pack:			
(Comstock)	½ of 7½-oz. can	140	27.0
(Libby's)	½ of 15-oz. can	135	27.5
(Menner's)	½ of 7½-oz. can	140	27.0
(Van Camp)	½ cup	95	15.5
RICE & VEGETABLES, frozen:			
(Birds Eye) rice, peas & mushrooms	⅓ of 7-oz. pkg.	106	22.4
(Green Giant):			
& broccoli in cheese sauce	½ of 11-oz. pkg.	149	22.7
Continental, with green beans & almonds	½ of 11-oz. pkg.	138	21.4
Medley, with sweet peas & mushrooms	½ of 11-oz. pkg.	134	23.7
Pilaf, with mushrooms & onions	½ of 11-oz. pkg.	141	28.7
Verdi, with bell peppers & parsley	½ of 11-oz. pkg.	175	32.0
White & wild, medley, with peas, celery, mushroom & almonds	½ of 11½-oz. pkg.	195	27.9
White & wild, oriental, with bean sprouts, pea pods & water chestnuts	⅓ of 12-oz. pkg.	94	16.5
RICE WINE (HEW/FAO):			
Chinese, 20.7% alcohol	3 fl. oz.	114	3.3
Japanese, 10.6% alcohol	3 fl. oz.	215	39.4
ROCK & RYE (Mr. Boston)			
27% alcohol	1 fl. oz.	74	7.2
ROE (USDA):			
Raw:			
Carp, cod, haddock, herring, pike or shad	4 oz.	147	1.7

(USDA): United States Department of Agriculture
(HEW/FAO): Health, Education and Welfare/Food and Agriculture Organization
* Prepared as Package Directs

Food and Description	Measure or Quantity	Calories	Carbo-hydrates (grams)
Salmon, sturgeon or turbot	4 oz.	235	1.6
Baked or broiled, cod & shad	4 oz.	143	2.2
Canned, cod, haddock or herring, solids & liq.	4 oz.	134	.3
ROLAIDS (Warner-Lambert)	1 piece	4	1.4
ROLL or BUN (See also **ROLL DOUGH** and **ROLL MIX**):			
Commercial type:			
Biscuit (Wonder)	1¼-oz. roll	107	17.1
Brown & serve:			
Roman Meal (Wonder):	1-oz. roll	78	12.6
With buttermilk, french style or gen style	1-oz. roll	86	13.6
Half & half or home bake	1-oz. roll	88	13.6
Club (Pepperidge Farm)	1 roll	100	20.0
Crescent, butter (Pepperidge Farm)	1 roll	120	13.0
Deli twist (Arnold)	1.3-oz. roll	110	17.0
Dinner:			
Home Pride	1-oz. roll	93	13.6
(Pepperidge Farm)	1 roll	60	10.0
(Wonder)	1¼-oz. roll	107	17.0
Dinner Party Rounds (Arnold)	.7-oz. roll	55	10.0
Finger (Pepperidge Farm):			
Sesame	1 roll	57	8.7
White poppyseed	1 roll	53	8.0
Frankfurter:			
(Arnold) hot dog	1.3-oz. roll	110	20.0
(Wonder)	2-oz. roll	162	28.9
French:			
(Arnold) *Francisco:*			
Enriched	2-oz. roll	160	31.0
Sourdough	1.1-oz. roll	90	16.0
(Pepperidge Farm):			
Large	1 roll	360	72.0
Small	1 roll	240	46.0
Golden twist (Pepperidge Farm)	1 roll	110	14.0

Food and Description	Measure or Quantity	Calories	Carbo-hydrates (grams)
Hamburger:			
(Arnold)	1.4-oz. roll	110	21.0
(Pepperidge Farm)	1 roll	100	18.0
Roman Meal	1.8-oz. roll	193	36.1
(Wonder)	2-oz. roll	162	29.0
Hearth (Pepperidge Farm)	1 roll	55	10.0
Honey (Hostess)	4¾-oz. serving	579	63.4
Kaiser (Wonder)	6-oz. roll	465	81.8
Old fashioned (Pepperidge Farm)	1 roll	53	7.7
Pan (Wonder)	1¼-oz. roll	107	17.0
Parkerhouse:			
(Arnold) *Dinner Party*	.7-oz. roll	55	10.0
(Pepperidge Farm)	1 roll	57	9.0
Party pan (Pepperidge Farm)	1 roll	32	5.2
Sandwich (Arnold):			
Dutch Egg	1.6-oz. roll	130	22.0
Francisco	2-oz. roll	160	30.0
Soft, plain or poppy seeds	1.3-oz. roll	110	18.0
Soft, sesame seeds	1.3-oz. roll	110	19.0
Sesame crisp (Pepperidge Farm)	1 roll	63	11.0
Frozen:			
Apple crunch (Sara Lee)	1-oz. roll	102	13.5
Caramel pecan (Sara Lee)	1.3-oz. roll	161	17.4
Caramel sticky (Sara Lee)	1-oz. bun	116	15.2
Cinnamon (Sara Lee)	.9-oz. roll	100	13.9
Croissant (Sara Lee)	.9-oz. roll	109	11.2
Crumb (Sara Lee):			
Blueberry	1¾-oz. bun	169	26.8
French	1.7-oz. bun	188	29.9
Danish (Sara Lee):			
Apple	1⅓-oz. roll	120	17.4
Apple country	1.8-oz. roll	156	22.9
Cheese	1⅓-oz. roll	130	13.9
Cheese country	1½-oz. roll	146	13.5
Cherry	1⅓-oz. roll	125	16.4
Cherry country	1.6-oz. roll	135	18.9

(USDA): United States Department of Agriculture
(HEW/FAO): Health, Education and Welfare/Food and Agriculture Organization
* Prepared as Package Directs

Food and Description	Measure or Quantity	Calories	Carbohydrates (grams)
Cinnamon raisin	1⅓-oz. roll	147	17.3
Pecan	1⅓-oz. roll	148	18.3
Honey:			
(Morton):			
Regular	2½-oz. roll	231	30.7
Mini	1.3-oz. roll	133	17.7
(Sara Lee)	1-oz. roll	109	15.2
Parkerhouse (Sara Lee)	1.8-oz. roll	73	10.3
Party (Sara Lee)	.6-oz. roll	55	7.7
Sesame seeds (Sara Lee)	.6-oz. roll	55	7.7
ROLL DOUGH:			
*Frozen (Rich's):			
Cinnamin	1 roll	173	32.8
Danish, round	1 roll	202	24.0
Frankfurter	1 roll	136	24.9
Hamburger:			
Regular	1 roll	134	25.0
Deluxe	1 roll	150	28.2
Onion:			
Regular	1 roll	155	29.1
Deluxe	1 roll	204	38.3
Parkerhouse	1 roll	82	13.4
Refrigerated (Pillsbury):			
Butterflake	1 roll	110	17.0
Cinnamon, with icing:			
Regular	1 roll	115	17.5
Ballard	1 roll	100	17.0
Hungry Jack, Butter Tastin	1 roll	145	19.5
Crescent:			
Regular	1 roll	200	24.0
Ballard	1 roll	190	26.0
Danish:			
Caramel	1 roll	150	19.5
Cinnamon raisin	1 roll	135	20.0
Orange	1 roll	135	19.5
Wheat, bakery style	1 roll	90	16.0
White, bakery style	1 roll	90	18.0
*ROLL MIX (Pillsbury) hot roll	1 roll	95	15.5

Food and Description	Measure or Quantity	Calories	Carbo- hydrates (grams)
ROMAN MEAL CEREAL:			
Regular, 2- or 5-minute	⅓ cups (1 oz.)	103	20.0
With oats, 5-minute	⅓ cup (1 oz.)	105	15.5
ROSEMARY LEAVES			
(French's) dried	1 tsp.	5	.8
ROSÉ WINE:			
(Great Western) 12% alcohol:			
Regular	3 fl. oz.	80	2.4
Isabella	3 fl. oz.	77	4.0
(Louis M. Martini) Gamay, 12½% alcohol	3 fl. oz.	90	.2
(Paul Masson):			
Regular, 11.8% alcohol	3 fl. oz.	76	4.2
Light, 7.1% alcohol	3 fl. oz.	49	3.9
(Taylor) 12½% alcohol	3 fl. oz.	72	3.0
ROSÉ WINE, SPARKLING			
(Chanson)	3 fl. oz.	72	3.6
ROTINI, canned (Franco-American):			
In tomato sauce	½ of 15-oz. can	200	36.0
& meatballs in tomato sauce	½ of 14 ¾-oz. can	240	29.0
ROYAL FUDGE ICE CREAM			
(Good Humor)	4 fl. oz.	120	14.0
RUM (See DISTILLED LIQUOR)			
RUTABAGA:			
Raw (USDA):			
Without tops	1 lb. (weighed with skin)	177	42.4
Diced	½ cup (2.5 oz.)	32	7.7
Boiled (USDA) drained, diced	½ cup (3 oz.)	30	7.1
Canned (Sunshine) solids & liq.	½ cup (4.2 oz.)	32	6.9
Frozen (Southland)	⅓ of 20-oz. pkg.	50	13.0

(USDA): United States Department of Agriculture
(HEW/FAO): Health, Education and Welfare/Food and Agriculture Organization
* Prepared as Package Directs

Food and Description	Measure or Quantity	Calories	Carbo- hydrates (grams)
RYE, whole grain (USDA)	1 oz.	95	20.8
RYE FLOUR (See FLOUR)			
RYE WHISKEY (See **DISTILLED LIQUOR**)			

S

Food and Description	Measure or Quantity	Calories	Carbo- hydrates (grams)
SABLEFISH, raw (USDA):			
Whole	1 lb. (weighed whole)	362	0.
Meat only	4 oz.	215	0.
SAFFLOWER SEED KERNELS, dry (USDA)	1 oz.	174	3.5
SAGE (French's)	1 tsp. (.9 grams)	4	.6
SAINT-EMILION WINE, French Bordeaux (Barton & Guestier) 12% alcohol	3 fl. oz.	63	.7
SAKE WINE (HEW/FAO) 19.8% alcohol	3 fl. oz.	116	4.3
SALAD DRESSING (See also **SALAD DRESSING MIX**):			
Regular:			
Bacon (Seven Seas) creamy	1 T.	60	1.0
Bell pepper (Seven Seas) *Viva*	1 T.	45	1.0
Blue or bleu cheese:			
(Bernstein's) Danish	1 T. (.5 oz.)	60	.6
(Seven Seas) chunky	1 T.	70	1.0
(Wish-Bone) chunky	1 T. (.5 oz.)	70	1.0
Boiled, home recipe (USDA)	1 T. (.6 oz.)	26	2.4
Caesar:			
(Pfeiffer)	1 T. (.5 oz.)	70	.5
(Seven Seas) regular or *Viva*	1 T.	60	1.0

Food and Description	Measure or Quantity	Calories	Carbo-hydrates (grams)
(Wish-Bone)	1 T. (.5 oz.)	80	1.0
Capri (Seven Seas)	1 T.	70	3.0
Cucumber (Wish-Bone) creamy	1 T. (.5 oz.)	80	2.0
French:			
Home recipe (USDA) made with corn or cottonseed oil	1 T. (.6 oz.)	101	.6
(Bernstein's):			
Creamy	1 T. (.5 oz.)	56	2.1
Chutney	1 T. (.5 oz.)	62	3.6
(Nalley's):			
Regular	1 T. (.6 oz.)	56	2.1
Chutney	1 T. (.5 oz.)	62	3.6
Original	1 T. (.5 oz.)	60	3.1
(Pfeiffer) homo	1 T. (.5 oz.)	55	3.5
(Seven Seas):			
Creamy	1 T. (.5 oz.)	60	2.0
Family style	1 T. (.5 oz.)	60	3.0
(Wish-Bone):			
Deluxe	1 T. (.5 oz.)	60	3.0
Garlic	1 T. (.5 oz.)	60	2.0
Sweet'n Spicy	1 T. (.5 oz.)	60	3.0
Garlic (Wish-Bone) creamy	1 T. (.5 oz.)	80	2.0
Green Goddess:			
(Nalley's)	1 T. (.5 oz.)	68	1.2
(Seven Seas)	1 T.	60	0.
(Wish-Bone)	1 T. (.5 oz.)	70	1.0
Herb & spice (Seven Seas)	1 T.	60	1.0
Italian:			
(Bernstein's):			
Regular	1 T. (.5 oz.)	50	.8
With cheese	1 T. (.5 oz.)	56	.8
(Pfeiffer) chef	1 T. (.5 oz.)	60	.5
(Seven Seas):			
Regular, creamy or *Viva*	1 T.	70	1.0
Family style	1 T.	70	
(Wish-Bone)	1 T. (.5 oz.)	80	1.0

(USDA): United States Department of Agriculture
(HEW/FAO):   Health, Education and Welfare/Food and Agriculture
                        Organization
* Prepared as Package Directs

Food and Description	Measure or Quantity	Calories	Carbohydrates (grams)
Louis dressing (Nalley's)	1 T.	69	1.8
Mayonnaise-type (USDA)	1 T. (.5 oz.)	65	2.2
Onion & chive (Seven Seas) creamy	1 T.	60	1.0
Potato salad (Marzetti)	1 T. (.5 oz.)	62	2.9
Red wine vinegar & oil (Seven Seas)	1 T. (.6 oz.)	60	1.0
Roquefort (Bernstein's)	1 T. (.5 oz.)	65	.8
Russian:			
(Pfeiffer)	1 T. (.5 oz.)	65	2.0
(Seven Seas) creamy	1 T.	80	1.0
(Wish-Bone)	1 T. (.5 oz.)	50	7.0
(Saffola)	1 T. (.5 oz.)	51	2.2
Spin Blend (Hellmann's)	1 T. (.6 oz.)	57	2.6
Sweet'n Sour (Dutch Pantry):			
Regular	1 T.	80	3.9
Creamy	1 T.	77	4.0
Thousand Island:			
(Bernstein's)	1 T. (.5 oz.)	63	1.7
(Nalley's)	1 T. (.5 oz.)	59	2.3
(Pfeiffer)	1 T. (.5 oz.)	65	2.0
(Seven Seas)	1 T.	50	2.0
(Wish-Bone)	1 T. (.5 oz.)	70	3.0
Vinaigrette (Bernstein's) French	1 T. (.5 oz.)	49	.2
Dietetic or low calorie:			
Bleu or blue cheese:			
(Dia-Mel)	1 T. (.5 oz.)	15	0.
(Featherweight) imitation	1 T.	4	1.0
(Tillie Lewis) *Tasti Diet*	1 T. (.5 oz.)	12	<1.0
(Walden Farms) chunky	1 T.	27	1.5
(Wish-Bone) chunky	1 T. (.5 oz.)	40	3.0
Caesar:			
(Dia-Mel)	1 T. (.5 oz.)	50	.5
(Estee) garlic	1 T. (.5 oz.)	4	1.0
(Pfeiffer)	1 T. (.5 oz.)	10	1.0
Cucumber & onion (Featherweight) creamy	1 T.	4	1.0
French:			
(Dia-Mel)	1 T. (.5 oz.)	30	1.0

Food and Description	Measure or Quantity	Calories	Carbo-hydrates (grams)
(Featherweight) imitation	1 T.	6	1.0
(Pfeiffer)	1 T. (.5 oz.)	17	2.5
(Tillie Lewis) *Tasti Diet*	1 T. (.5 oz.)	6	<1.0
(Walden Farms) creamy	1 T.	33	3.0
(Wish-Bone)	1 T. (.5 oz.)	30	2.0
Herb & spice (Featherweight)	1 T.	6	1.0
Italian:			
(Dia-Mel)	1 T.	2	.5
(Estee) spicy	1 T. (.5 oz.)	4	1.0
(Featherweight)	1 T.	4	1.0
(Pfeiffer)	1 T. (.5 oz.)	10	1.5
(Tillie Lewis) *Tasti Diet*	1 T. (.5 oz.)	2	0.
(Weight Watchers)	1 T. (.5 oz.)	50	2.0
(Wish-Bone)	1 T. (.5 oz.)	30	1.0
Red wine (Pfeiffer)	1 T. (.5 oz.)	10	1.0
Red wine/vinegar (Featherweight)	1 T.	6	1.0
Russian:			
(Dia-Mel)	1 T. (.5 oz.)	9	.5
(Featherweight) creamy	1 T.	6	1.0
(Pfeiffer)	1 T. (.5 oz.)	15	2.0
(Tillie Lewis) *Tasti Diet*	1 T. (.5 oz.)	6	<1.0
(Weight Watchers)	1 T. (.5 oz.)	50	2.0
(Wish-Bone)	1 T.	25	5.0
Thousand Island:			
(Dia-Mel)	1 T. (.5 oz.)	530	1.0
(Pfeiffer)	1 T. (.5 oz.)	15	2.0
(Walden Farms) tangy	1 T.	24	3.0
(Weight Watchers)	1 T. (.5 oz.)	50	2.0
(Wish-Bone)	1 T.	25	3.0
2-calorie low sodium (Featherweight)	1 T.	2	0.
Whipped:			
(Dia-Mel)	1 T.	22	2.1
(Tillie Lewis) *Tasti Diet*	1 T. (.5 oz.)	18	1.0

(USDA): United States Department of Agriculture
(HEW/FAO): Health, Education and Welfare/Food and Agriculture Organization
* Prepared as Package Directs

Food and Description	Measure or Quantity	Calories	Carbohydrates (grams)
SALAD DRESSING MIX:			
*Regular (Good Seasons):			
Bleu or blue cheese:			
Regular	1 T.	90	.5
Thick'n Creamy	1 T.	80	.5
Buttermilk, farm style	1 T.	60	1.0
French:			
Regular	1 T.	80	3.0
Old-fashioned	1 T.	80	1.0
Riviera	1 T.	90	3.0
Thick'n Creamy	1 T.	75	2.0
Garlic:			
Regular	1 T.	80	1.0
With cheese	1 T.	90	1.0
Italian:			
Regular	1 T.	80	1.0
Cheese or mild	1 T.	90	1.0
Thick'n Creamy	1 T.	85	1.0
Onion	1 T.	80	1.0
Thousand Island, *Thick'n Creamy*	1 T. (.6 oz.)	75	2.0
Dietetic or low calorie:			
*Blue cheese (Weight Watchers)	1 T.	10	1.0
French:			
(Dia-Mel)	½-oz. packet	18	0.
(Louis Sherry)	½-oz. packet	18	0.
*(Weight Watchers)	1 T.	4	1.0
Garlic (Dia-Mel) creamy	½-oz. packet	21	1.0
Italian:			
(Dia-Mel)	½-oz. packet	2	1.0
*(Good Seasons)	1 T.	8	2.0
(Louis Sherry)	½-oz. packet	2	0.
*(Weight Watchers):			
Regular	1 T.	2	0.
Creamy	1 T.	4	1.0
Russian:			
(Louis Sherry)	½-oz. packet	20	0.
*(Weight Watchers)	1 T.	4	1.0
Thousand Island:			
(Dia-Mel)	½-oz. packet	20	0.
*(Weight Watchers)	1 T.	12	1.0

Food and Description	Measure or Quantity	Calories	Carbo-hydrates (grams)
SALAD LIFT, spice (French's)	1 tsp. (4 grams)	6	1.0
SALAMI:			
Dry (USDA)	1 oz.	128	.3
Cooked (USDA)	1 oz.	88	.4
Packaged:			
(Best's Kosher):			
Chub	1-oz. serving	91	.9
Sliced, low fat	1-oz. serving	70	.9
(Hormel):			
Cotto	1 oz.	65	0.
Genoa:			
DiLusso	1 oz.	100	Tr.
Sliced	1 oz.	126	.6
Hard:			
Regular	1 oz.	117	.2
Sliced	1 oz.	118	.4
Party sliced	1 oz.	94	.1
(Oscar Mayer):			
For beer:			
Regular	.8-oz. slice	54	.4
Beer	.8-oz. slice	76	.2
Cotto:			
Regular	.8-oz. slice	52	.4
Regular	1-oz. slice	63	.5
Beef	.5-oz. slice	34	.4
Beef	.8-oz. slice	52	.6
Hard, all meat	.3-oz. slice	3	.2
(Oscherwitz):			
Chub	1-oz. serving	91	.9
Sliced, low fat	1-oz. serving	70	.9
(Swift):			
Genoa	1 oz.	114	.3
Hard	1 oz.	115	.9
(Vienna) beef	1 oz.	79	.8
SALISBURY STEAK:			
Canned (Morton House)	⅓ of 12½-oz. can	160	7.0

(USDA): United States Department of Agriculture
(HEW/FAO):   Health, Education and Welfare/Food and Agriculture
                     Organization
* Prepared as Package Directs

Food and Description	Measure or Quantity	Calories	Carbo-hydrates (grams)
Frozen:			
(Banquet):			
Regular	11-oz. dinner	390	24.0
Buffet Supper, and gravy	2-lb. pkg.	1454	48.2
Cookin' Bag, and gravy	5-oz. pkg.	246	7.8
Man-Pleaser	19-oz. dinner	873	71.7
(Green Giant):			
Boil-in-bag, with tomato sauce	9-oz. entree	390	22.0
Oven bake, with gravy	7-oz. entree	290	14.0
(Morton):			
Regular	11-oz. dinner	287	25.1
Country Table:			
Dinner	15-oz. dinner	515	37.9
Entree	10¼-oz. entree	494	60.0
King Size	19-oz. dinner	772	64.8
(Stouffer's) with onion gravy	12-oz. pkg.	470	9.8
(Swanson):			
Regular, with gravy	10-oz. entree	430	16.0
Hungry Man	17-oz. dinner	890	63.0
3-course	16-oz. dinner	490	47.0
TV Brand:			
Dinner	11½-oz. dinner	500	40.0
Entree, with crinkle cut potatoes	5½-oz. entree	350	27.0
SALMON:			
Atlantic (USDA):			
Raw:			
Whole	1 lb. (weighed whole)	640	0.
Meat only	4 oz.	246	0.
Canned, solids & liq., including bones	4 oz.	230	0.
Chinook or King (USDA):			
Raw:			
Steak	1 lb. (weighed whole)	886	0.
Meat only	4 oz.	252	0.
Canned, solids & liq., including bones	4 oz.	238	0.

Food and Description	Measure or Quantity	Calories	Carbo-hydrates (grams)
Chum, canned (USDA), solids & liq., including bones	4 oz.	158	0.
Coho, canned (USDA) solids & liq., including bones	4 oz.	174	0.
Keta, canned (Bumble Bee) solids & liq., including bones	½ cup (3.9 oz.)	153	0.
Pink or Humpback (USDA):			
Raw:			
Steak	1 lb. (weighed whole)	475	0.
Meat only	4 oz.	135	0.
Canned, solids & liq.:			
(USDA) including bones	4 oz.	160	0.
(Bumble Bee) including bones	½ cup (4 oz.)	155	0.
(Del Monte)	7¾-oz. can	277	0.
Sockeye or Red or Blueback, canned, solids & liq.:			
(USDA)	4 oz.	194	0.
(Bumble Bee) including bones	½ cup (4 oz.)	188	0.
(Del Monte)	½ of 7¾-oz. can	165	0.
Unspecified kind of salmon (USDA) baked or broiled	4.2-oz. steak (approx. 4″ × 3″ × ½″)	218	0.
SALMON, SMOKED (USDA)	4 oz.	200	0.
SALT:			
Regular:			
Butter-flavored (French's) imitation	1 tsp. (3.6 grams)	8	0.
Garlic (Lawry's)	1 tsp. (4 grams)	5	1.0
Hickory smoke (French's)	1 tsp. (4 grams)	2	Tr.
Onion (Lawry's)	1 tsp.	4	.9
Seasoned (Lawry's)	1 tsp.	1	.1
Table:			
(USDA)	1 tsp. (6 grams)	0	0.

(USDA): United States Department of Agriculture
(HEW/FAO): Health, Education and Welfare/Food and Agriculture Organization
* Prepared as Package Directs

Food and Description	Measure or Quantity	Calories	Carbo-hydrates (grams)
(Morton) iodized	1 tsp. (7 grams)	0	0.
Lite Salt (Morton) iodized	1 tsp. (6 grams)	0	0.
Substitute:			
(Adolph's):			
Regular	1 tsp. (6 grams)	1	Tr.
Packet	8-gram packet	<1	Tr.
Seasoned	1 tsp.	6	1.1
(Dia-Mel) *Salt-It*	⅛ tsp.	0	0.
(Morton):			
Regular	1 tsp. (6 grams)	Tr.	Tr.
Seasoned	1 tsp. (6 grams)	3	.5
SALT PORK, raw (USDA):			
With skin	1 lb. (weighed with skin)	3410	0.
Without skin	1 oz.	222	0.
SANDWICH SPREAD:			
Regular:			
(USDA)	1 T. (.5 oz.)	57	2.4
(Bennett's)	1 T. (.5 oz.)	44	3.7
(Best Foods/Hellmann's)	1 T. (.5 oz.)	65	2.2
(Nalley's)	1 T. (.5 oz.)	38	3.0
(Oscar Mayer)	1-oz. serving	68	3.2
Dietetic or low calorie			
(USDA)	1 T. (.5 oz.)	17	1.2
SANGRIA (Taylor) 11.6% alcohol	3 fl. oz.	99	10.8
SARDINE:			
Raw (HEW/FAO):			
Whole	1 lb. (weighed whole)	321	0.
Meat only	4 oz.	146	0.
Canned:			
Atlantic:			
(USDA) in oil:			
Solids & liq.	3¾-oz. can	330	.6
Drained solids, with skin & bones	3¾-oz. can	187	DNA
(Del Monte) in tomato sauce, solids & liq.	7½-oz. can	330	4.0

Food and Description	Measure or Quantity	Calories	Carbo- hydrates (grams)
Imported (Underwood):			
In mustard sauce	3¾-oz. can	230	Tr.
In tomato sauce	3¾-oz. can	230	1.0
Norwegian:			
King Oscar Brand:			
In mustard sauce, solids & liq.	3¾-oz. can	240	2.0
In oil, drained	3-oz. can	260	1.0
In tomato sauce, solids & liq.	3¾-oz. can	240	2.0
(Underwood)	3¾-oz. can	380	Tr.
Pacific (USDA) in brine or mustard, solids & liq.	4 oz.	222	1.9
SAUCE (See also **SAUCE MIX**):			
A-1	1 T. (.6 oz.)	12	3.1
Barbecue:			
Chris & Pitt's	1 T.	15	4.0
(French's) regular or smoky	1 T.	25	5.0
(Gold's)	1 T.	16	3.9
Open Pit:			
Regular	1 T. (.6 oz.)	15	3.6
Hickory smoked flavor	1 T.	16	4.0
With minced onions	1 T.	18	4.0
Chili (See **CHILI SAUCE**)			
Cocktail (See also Seafood):			
(Gold's)	1 oz.	31	7.5
(Nalley's)	2 oz.	66	14.2
(Pfeiffer)	2 oz.	100	12.0
Escoffier Sauce:			
Diable	1 T. (.6 oz.)	17	4.3
Robert	1 T.	20	5.1
Famous (Durkee)	1 T.	69	2.2
Hot, *Frank's*	1 tsp.	1	0.
Italian:			
(Carnation)	2 fl. oz.	43	7.0
(Ragu) red cooking	3½ fl. oz.	45	6.0
Marinara (Ragu)	5 oz.	120	15.0

(USDA): United States Department of Agriculture
(HEW/FAO):   Health, Education and Welfare/Food and Agriculture
            Organization
* Prepared as Package Directs

Food and Description	Measure or Quantity	Calories	Carbo-hydrates (grams)
Mushroom (Nalley's)	1 oz.	17	2.0
Pizza (See **PIZZA SAUCE**)			
Salsa Picante, hot table sauce (Del Monte)	¼ cup (2 oz.)	12	3.0
Salsa Roja, mild table sauce (Del Monte)	¼ cup (2 oz.)	18	4.0
Seafood (See also Cocktail) (Del Monte) cocktail	1 T. (.6 oz.)	22	4.9
Soy:			
(Gold's)	1 T.	10	1.0
(Kikkoman)	1 T. (.6 oz.)	11	1.1
(La Choy)	1 T. (.5 oz.)	8	.9
Spare rib (Gold's)	1 T.	51	11.7
Steak (Dawn Fresh) with mushrooms	2 oz.	18	3.5
Steak Supreme	1 T.	20	5.1
Sweet & sour:			
(Carnation)	2 fl. oz.	20	4.5
(La Choy)	1 oz.	51	12.6
Swiss steak (Carnation)	2 fl. oz.	20	4.5
Taco:			
(Del Monte):			
Hot	¼ cup (2 oz.)	16	4.0
Mild	¼ cup (2 oz.)	14	4.0
Old El Paso	1 oz.	11	2.3
(Ortega)	1 T (.6 oz.)	22	5.1
Tartar:			
Hellmann's (Best Foods)	1 T. (.5 oz.)	73	.2
(Nalley's)	1 T. (.5 oz.)	89	.3
Teriyaki (Kikkoman)	1 T. (.6 oz.)	15	2.8
Tomato (See **TOMATO SAUCE**)			
"V-8"	1 oz.	25	6.0
White (USDA) medium	1 cup (9 oz.)	413	22.4
Worcestershire:			
(French's) regular or smoke	1 T.	10	2.0
(Gold's)	1 T.	42	3.3
(Lea & Perrins)	1 T. (.6 oz.)	12	3.0
SAUCE MIX:			
Regular:			
A la King (Durkee)	1.1-oz. pkg.	133	14.0

Food and Description	Measure or Quantity	Calories	Carbo-hydrates (grams)
*Cheese:			
(Durkee)	½ cup	168	9.5
(French's)	½ cup	160	14.0
Hollandaise:			
(Durkee)	1-oz. pkg.	173	11.0
*(French's)	1 T.	15	.7
*Sour cream:			
(Durkee)	⅔ cup	214	15.0
(French's)	2½ T.	60	5.0
*Stroganoff (French's)	⅓ cup	110	11.0
*Sweet & sour:			
(Durkee)	½ cup	115	22.5
(French's)	½ cup	55	14.0
*Teriyaki (French's)	1 T.	17	3.5
*White (Durkee)	1 cup	218	41.0
*Dietetic, lemon butter (Weight Watchers)	1 T.	8	1.0
SAUERKRAUT, canned:			
(USDA):			
Solids & liq.	1 cup (8.3 oz.)	42	9.4
Drained solids	1 cup (5 oz.)	31	6.2
(Blue Boy) solids & liq.	1 cup (8.7 oz.)	60	16.0
(Claussen) drained	½ cup (2.7 oz.)	16	2.8
(Del Monte) solids & liq.	1 cup (8 oz.)	55	10.7
(Libby's) solids & liq.	⅛ of 32-oz. jar	21	4.0
(Silver Floss):			
Regular:			
Can	½ cup (4 oz.)	30	5.0
Jar	½ cup	25	5.0
Polybag	½ cup (4 oz.)	20	4.0
Bavarian Kraut	½ cup	35	8.0
Krispy Kraut	½ cup (4 oz.)	25	5.0
(Stokely-Van Camp) solids & liq.:			
Bavarian style	½ cup (4.2 oz.)	35	7.0
Chopped or shredded	½ cup (4.2 oz.)	25	4.5

(USDA): United States Department of Agriculture
(HEW/FAO):   Health, Education and Welfare/Food and Agriculture
                      Organization
* Prepared as Package Directs

Food and Description	Measure or Quantity	Calories	Carbo-hydrates (grams)
SAUERKRAUT JUICE, canned (USDA)	½ cup (4.3 oz.)	12	2.8
SAUSAGE:			
Brown & serve:			
(USDA):			
Before browning	1-oz. serving	111	.8
After browning	1-oz. serving	120	.8
*(Swift):			
Bacon & sausage	.7-oz. link	72	.4
Beef	.7-oz. link	86	.5
Kountry Kured	.7-oz. link	86	.3
Original flavor	.7-oz. link	77	.5
Italian-style (Best's Kosher; Oscherwitz)	3-oz. link	271	.7
Polish-style:			
(Best's Kosher; Oscherwitz)	3-oz. piece	271	1.8
(Frito-Lay's) smoked beef	1-oz. serving	73	.6
(Vienna) beef	3-oz. piece	240	1.3
Pork:			
(USDA) link or bulk:			
Uncooked	1-oz. serving	141	Tr.
Cooked	1-oz. serving	135	Tr.
(Hormel):			
*Little Sizzlers	1 sausage	65	Tr.
Smoked	1-oz. serving	98	.2
(Jimmy Dean) uncooked	2-oz. serving	227	Tr.
*(Oscar Mayer) Little Friers	.6-oz. link	64	.4
Canned (USDA):			
Solids & liq.	1 oz.	118	.7
Drained	1 oz.	108	.5
Smoked:			
(Best's Kosher; Oscherwitz)	3-oz. piece	274	2.4
(Eckrich):			
Beef or maple flavor, Smok-Y-Links	.8-oz. link	75	1.0
Meat	1-oz. serving	105	.5
Skinless:			
Regular	1.2-oz. link	115	1.0
Regular	2-oz. link	190	2.0
Smok-Y-Links	.8-oz. link	85	1.0
(Hormel):			
Pork	3-oz. serving	295	.7

Food and Description	Measure or Quantity	Calories	Carbo-hydrates (grams)
Smokies	1 sausage	80	1.0
(Oscar Mayer):			
Regular	1½-oz. link	137	.6
Regular	4-oz. link	359	1.5
Beef	1½-oz. link	132	.9
Cheese	1½-oz. link	142	.4
(Vienna)	2½-oz. serving	196	.9
Summer (See **THURINGER**)			
Turkey (Louis Rich) links or			
tube, cooked	1-oz. serving	45	<1.0
Vienna (see **VIENNA** **SAUSAGE**)			
SAUTERNES:			
(Gallo) 12% alcohol:			
Regular	3 fl. oz.	50	.9
Haut	3 fl. oz.	67	2.1
(Great Western) Aurora, 12% alcohol	3 fl. oz.	79	4.5
(Louis M. Martini) dry, 12½% alcohol	3 fl. oz.	90	.2
(Taylor) 12½% alcohol	3 fl. oz.	81	4.8
SAVORY (French's)	1 tsp. (1.4 grams)	5	1.0
SCALLION (See **ONION,** **GREEN**)			
SCALLOP:			
Raw (USDA) muscle only	4 oz.	92	3.7
Steamed (USDA)	4 oz.	127	DNA
Frozen:			
(USDA) breaded, fried, reheated	4 oz.	220	11.9
(Mrs. Paul's):			
Batter fried	½ of 7-oz. pkg.	203	20.8
Breaded & fried	½ of 7-oz. pkg.	201	24.1
With butter & cheese	7-oz. serving	267	11.2

(USDA): United States Department of Agriculture
(HEW/FAO): Health, Education and Welfare/Food and Agriculture Organization
* Prepared as Package Directs

Food and Description	Measure or Quantity	Calories	Carbo-hydrates (grams)
(Van de Kamp's) country seasoned	½ of 7-oz. pkg.	270	19.0
SCHAV SOUP, canned (Gold's)	8-oz. serving	11	2.1
SCHNAPPS, CINNAMON (Mr. Boston) 27% alcohol	1 fl. oz.	76	8.0
SCHNAPPS, PEPPERMINT (Mr. Boston) 50% alcohol	1 fl. oz.	115	8.0
SCHNAPPS, SPEARMINT (Mr. Boston) 27% alcohol	1 fl. oz.	76	8.0
*SCOTCH BROTH, canned (Campbell) condensed	10-oz. serving	100	11.0
SCRAPPLE (USDA)	4 oz.	244	16.6
SCREWDRIVER COCKTAIL: Canned (Mr. Boston) 12% alcohol	3 fl. oz.	111	12.0
Mix (Bar-Tender's)	⅝-oz. serving	70	17.4
SCUP (See **PORGY**)			
SEA BASS, WHITE, raw USDA) meat only	4 oz.	109	0.
SEAFOOD PLATTER, frozen (Mrs. Paul's) combination, breaded & fried	9 oz. pkg.	507	57.1
SEAFOOD SEASONING (French's)	1 tsp. (.2 oz.)	2	Tr.
SEGO DIET FOOD, canned: Milk chocolate, very chocolate, very chocolate fudge, very chocolate malt, very chocolate marshmallow, very coconut or very Dutch chocolate	10-fl.-oz. can	225	39.0

Food and Description	Measure or Quantity	Calories	Carbo-hydrates (grams)
Very banana, very butterscotch, very cherry vanilla, very French vanilla, very strawberry, very vanilla	10-fl.-oz. can	225	34.0
SESAME NUT MIX, canned (Planters) oil roasted	1 oz.	160	8.0
SESAME SEEDS, dry (USDA):			
Whole	1 oz.	160	6.1
Hulled	1 oz.	165	5.0
SHAD (USDA):			
Raw:			
Whole	1 lb. (weighed whole)	370	0.
Meat only	4 oz.	193	0.
Cooked, home recipe:			
Baked with butter or margarine & bacon slices	4 oz.	228	0.
Creole	4 oz.	172	1.8
Canned, solids & liq.	4 oz.	172	0.
SHAD, GIZZARD, raw (USDA):			
Whole	1 lb. (weighed whole)	229	0.
Meat only	4 oz.	227	0.
SHAKE 'n BAKE:			
Regular:			
Chicken:			
Regular	2.4-oz. pkg.	291	43.0
Barbecue style	3¾-oz. pkg.	377	82.2
Crispy country mild	2.4-oz. pkg.	321	50.1
Italian flavor	2.4-oz. pkg.	294	41.4
Fish	2-oz. pkg.	234	33.9
Hamburger	2-oz. pkg.	169	33.2

(USDA): United States Department of Agriculture
(HEW/FAO):   Health, Education and Welfare/Food and Agriculture
Organization
* Prepared as Package Directs

Food and Description	Measure or Quantity	Calories	Carbohydrates (grams)
Pork	2.4-oz. pkg.	255	47.1
Pork & ribs, barbecue style	2.9-oz. pkg.	305	61.2
& home style gravy mix:			
Beef	3.1-oz. pkg.	304	51.4
Pork	3.7-oz. pkg.	327	67.4
SHALLOT, raw (USDA):			
With skin	1 oz.	18	4.2
With skin removed	1 oz.	20	4.8
SHERBET:			
(Baskin-Robbins):			
Daiquiri ice	1 scoop	99	20.9
Orange	1 scoop	84	20.9
(Dean) 1.7% fat	¼ pt.	137	30.6
SHERRY:			
Regular (Great Western) Solera, 18% alcohol	3 fl. oz.	120	8.5
Cream:			
(Great Western) Solera, 18% alcohol	3 fl. oz.	141	12.2
(Louis M. Martini) 19½% alcohol	3 fl. oz.	138	1.2
(Taylor) 17½% alcohol	3 fl. oz.	138	13.2
Dry:			
(Great Western) Solera, 18% alcohol	3 fl. oz.	109	4.6
(Louis M. Martini) 19½% alcohol	3 fl. oz.	138	1.2
(Taylor) 19½% alcohol	3 fl. oz.	104	2.8
Dry Sack (Williams & Humbert) 20½% alcohol	3 fl. oz.	120	4.5
Medium:			
(Great Western) cooking, 18% alcohol	3 fl. oz.	111	6.4
(Taylor) 17½% alcohol	3 fl. oz.	123	9.0
SHERRY FLAVORING			
(French's)	1 tsp.	17	

Food and Description	Measure or Quantity	Calories	Carbo-hydrates (grams)
SHREDDED WHEAT:			
(Nabisco):			
Regular	.8-oz. biscuit	90	19.0
Spoon Size	⅔ cup (1 oz.)	110	23.0
(Quaker)	.7-oz. biscuit	52	11.0
SHRIMP:			
Raw (USDA):			
Whole	1 lb. (weighed in shell)	285	4.7
Meat only	4 oz.	103	1.7
Canned:			
(USDA):			
Wet pack, solids & liq.	4 oz.	91	.9
Dry pack or drained	4 oz.	132	.8
(Bumble Bee) baby, solids & liq.	4½-oz. can	90	.9
Cooked, french fried (USDA)	4 oz.	255	11.3
Frozen (Mrs. Paul's) breaded & fried	½ of 6 oz. pkg.	198	16.8
SHRIMP DINNER, frozen (Van de Kamp's)	10 oz. dinner	370	40.0
SHRIMP PASTE, canned (USDA)	1 oz.	51	.4
SHRIMP PUFF, frozen (Durkee)	1 piece	44	3.0
SHRIMP SOUP, canned:			
*(Campbell) condensed, cream of:			
Made with milk	10-oz. serving	210	17.0
Made with water	10-oz. serving	110	10.0
(Crosse & Blackwell)	½ of 13-oz. can	90	7.0
SIRLOIN BURGER SOUP, canned (Campbell)			
Chunky	9½-oz. serving	200	20.0

(USDA): United States Department of Agriculture
(HEW/FAO):   Health, Education and Welfare/Food and Agriculture
                      Organization
* Prepared as Package Directs

Food and Description	Measure or Quantity	Calories	Carbo-hydrates (grams)
SKATE, raw (USDA) meat only	4 oz.	111	0
SLENDER (Carnation):			
Bar:			
Chocolate	1 bar	138	11.5
Cinnamon & vanilla	1 bar	138	12.0
Liquid, all flavors	10-fl.-oz. can	225	34.0
Mix:			
Chocolate, chocolate malt or dutch chocolate	1-oz. pkg.	110	20.0
Coffee, french vanilla or wild strawberry	1-oz. pkg.	110	21.0
SLOE GIN (See **GIN, SLOE**)			
SLOPPY HOT DOG SEASONING MIX (French's)	1½-oz. pkg.	160	28.0
SLOPPY JOE:			
Canned:			
(Hormel) *Short Orders*	7½-oz. can	340	15.0
(Libby's):			
Beef	⅔ cup (2½ oz.)	119	6.0
Pork	⅔ cup (2½ oz.)	103	5.7
(Morton House) barbecue sauce with beef	⅓ of 15-oz. can	240	19.0
(Nalley's)	8-oz. serving	348	24.0
Frozen:			
(Banquet) *Cookin' Bag*	5-oz. pkg.	199	11.2
(Green Giant) with tomato sauce & beef, *Toast Topper*	5 oz. serving	154	14.3
SLOPPY JOE SEASONING MIX:			
*(Durkee):			
Regular	1¼ cups	726	30.0
Pizza flavor	1¼ cups	746	26.0
(French's)	1½-oz. pkg.	128	32.0

Food and Description	Measure or Quantity	Calories	Carbo-hydrates (grams)
SMELT, Atlantic, jack & bar (USDA):			
Raw:			
Whole	1 lb. (weighed whole)	244	0.
Meat only	4 oz.	111	0.
Canned, solids & liq.	4 oz.	227	0.
SMOKED SAUSAGE (See **SAUSAGE**)			
SNACK (See **CRACKER, POPCORN, POTATO CHIP,** etc.)			
SNAIL, raw (USDA):			
Unspecified kind	4 oz.	102	2.3
Giant African	4 oz.	83	5.0
SNAPPER (See **RED SNAPPER**)			
SNO BALLS (HOSTESS)	1½-oz. piece	140	25.1
SOAVE WINE (Antinori) 12% alcohol	3 fl. oz.	84	6.3
SOFT DRINK:			
Sweetened:			
Apple (Welch's)	6 fl. oz.	90	23.5
Aspen	6 fl. oz.	76	18.6
Birch beer:			
(Pennsylvania Dutch)	6 fl. oz.	84	19.7
(Yukon Club)	6 fl. oz.	89	22.3
Bitter lemon:			
(Canada Dry)	6 fl. oz.	77	19.2
(Schweppes)	6 fl. oz.	84	20.3
Bubble Up	6 fl. oz.	73	18.4

(USDA): United States Department of Agriculture
(HEW/FAO): Health, Education and Welfare/Food and Agriculture Organization
* Prepared as Package Directs

Food and Description	Measure or Quantity	Calories	Carbo-hydrates (grams)
Cherry:			
(Canada Dry) wild	6 fl. oz.	96	24.0
(Shasta) black	6 fl. oz.	86	21.7
Chocolate (Yoo-Hoo) high protein	6 fl. oz.	108	24.1
Club (all brands)	6 fl. oz.	0	0.
Coconut (Yoo-Hoo)	6 fl. oz.	89	18.0
Coffee (Hoffman)	6 fl. oz.	70	17.5
Cola:			
(Canada Dry) *Jamaica*	6 fl. oz.	79	19.8
Coca-Cola	6 fl. oz.	72	18.0
Pepsi-Cola	6 fl. oz.	79	19.8
(Royal Crown)	6 fl. oz.	78	19.4
(Shasta):			
Regular	6 fl. oz.	72	19.5
Cherry	6 fl. oz.	68	18.5
Cream:			
(Canada Dry) vanilla	6 fl. oz.	96	24.0
(Schweppes) red	6 fl. oz.	86	21.3
(Shasta)	6 fl. oz.	75	20.5
Dr. Nehi (Royal Crown)	6 fl. oz.	73	18.3
Dr. Pepper	6 fl. oz.	75	19.4
Fruit punch:			
(Nehi)	6 fl. oz.	91	22.8
(Shasta)	6 fl. oz.	84	23.0
Ginger Ale:			
(Canada Dry)	6 fl. oz.	65	15.6
(Fanta)	6 fl. oz.	63	15.8
(Nehi)	6 fl. oz.	69	16.6
(Royal Crown)	6 fl. oz.	66	16.4
(Schweppes)	6 fl. oz.	66	16.3
(Shasta)	6 fl. oz.	59	16.0
Ginger beer (Schweppes)	6 fl. oz.	72	16.8
Grape:			
(Canada Dry) concord	6 fl. oz.	96	24.0
(Fanta)	6 fl. oz.	86	21.8
(Hi-C)	6 fl. oz.	89	22.0
(Nehi)	6 fl. oz.	87	21.3
(Patio)	6 fl. oz.	96	24.0
(Schweppes)	6 fl. oz.	96	24.0
(Shasta)	6 fl. oz.	97	15.7
(Welch's) sparkling	6 fl. oz.	90	23.0
Hi Spot (Canada Dry)	6 fl. oz.	74	18.6

Food and Description	Measure or Quantity	Calories	Carbo-hydrates (grams)
Kick (Royal Crown)	6 fl. oz.	89	22.1
Lemonade:			
(Hi-C)	6 fl. oz.	80	20.0
(Shasta)	6 fl. oz.	71	19.0
Lemon-lime (Shasta)	6 fl. oz.	69	19.0
Mello Yellow	6 fl. oz.	87	22.5
Mt. Dew	6 fl. oz.	89	22.2
Mr. PiBB	6 fl. oz.	70	18.8
Orange:			
(Canada Dry) *Sunripe*	6 fl. oz.	90	14.1
(Fanta)	6 fl. oz.	88	22.5
(Hi-C)	6 fl. oz.	92	23.0
(Nehi)	6 fl. oz.	95	23.8
(Patio)	6 fl. oz.	96	24.0
(Schweppes) sparkling	6 fl. oz.	89	22.0
(Shasta)	6 fl. oz.	86	23.5
(Sunkist)	6 fl. oz.	96	7.6
(Welch's)	6 fl. oz.	90	23.5
Peach (Nehi)	6 fl. oz.	92	23.0
Quinine or tonic water:			
(Canada Dry)	6 fl. oz.	70	16.1
(Schweppes)	6 fl. oz.	66	16.5
(Shasta)	6 fl. oz.	59	16.0
Ronda (Schweppes)	6 fl. oz.	77	19.6
Root beer:			
Barrelhead (Canada Dry)	6 fl. oz.	79	19.8
(Dad's)	6 fl. oz.	79	19.6
(Fanta)	6 fl. oz.	77	20.3
(Nehi)	6 fl. oz.	87	21.8
On Tap	6 fl. oz.	81	20.4
(Patio)	6 fl. oz.	83	21.0
Rooti (Canada Dry)	6 fl. oz.	79	19.8
(Schweppes)	6 fl. oz.	79	19.3
(Shasta) draft	6 fl. oz.	75	20.5
Seven-Up	6 fl. oz.	72	18.1
Sprite	6 fl. oz.	71	18.0
Strawberry:			
(Canada Dry) California	6 fl. oz.	89	22.3

(USDA): United States Department of Agriculture
(HEW/FAO):   Health, Education and Welfare/Food and Agriculture
                        Organization
* Prepared as Package Directs

Food and Description	Measure or Quantity	Calories	Carbo-hydrates (grams)
(Nehi)	6 fl. oz.	87	21.8
(Shasta)	6 fl. oz.	72	19.5
(Welch's)	6 fl. oz.	90	23.5
(Yoo-Hoo)	6 fl. oz.	95	20.9
Tahitian Treat (Canada Dry)	6 fl. oz.	96	24.1
Teem	6 fl. oz.	74	18.6
Tom Collins or collins mix			
(Canada Dry)	6 fl. oz.	60	15.0
Upper Ten (Royal Crown)	6 fl. oz.	76	19.0
Vanilla:			
(Canada Dry) cream	6 fl. oz.	88	22.0
(Yoo-Hoo) shake	6 fl. oz.	93	20.4
Wink (Canada Dry)	6 fl. oz.	91	22.7
Dietetic or low calorie:			
Bubble Up	6 fl. oz.	1	.2
Cherry:			
(Shasta) black	6 fl. oz.	< 1	Tr.
Tab, black	6 fl. oz.	2	Tr.
Chocolate mint (No-Cal)	6 fl. oz.	2	<.1
Citrus, *Flair*	6 fl. oz.	1	.2
Cola:			
(Canada Dry)	6 fl. oz.	<1	.6
Diet Rite	6 fl. oz.	<1	Tr.
(No-Cal)	6 fl. oz.	0	<.1
Pepsi, diet or Light	6 fl. oz.	<1	<.1
(Shasta) regular or cherry	6 fl. oz.	<1	Tr.
Tab	6 fl. oz.	<1	<.1
Cream:			
(No-Cal)	6 fl. oz.	0	<.1
(Shasta)	6 fl. oz.	<1	Tr.
Dr. Pepper	6 fl. oz.	<2	.4
Fresca	6 fl. oz.	1	0.
Ginger Ale:			
(Canada Dry)	6 fl. oz.	<1	0.
(No-Cal)	6 fl. oz.	0	Tr.
(Shasta)	6 fl. oz.	<1	Tr.
Tab	6 fl. oz.	2	Tr.
Grape:			
(Shasta)	6 fl. oz.	<1	Tr.
Tab	6 fl. oz.	2	0.
Grapefruit (Shasta)	6 fl. oz.	<1	.2
Lemon-lime:			
(Shasta)	6 fl. oz.	<1	Tr.

Food and Description	Measure or Quantity	Calories	Carbo-hydrates (grams)
Tab	6 fl. oz.	2	0.
Mr. PiBB	6 fl. oz.	<1	0.
Orange:			
(No-Cal)	6 fl. oz.	0	0.
(Shasta)	6 fl. oz.	<1	Tr.
Tab	6 fl. oz.	<1	0.
RC 100 (Royal Crown)	6 fl. oz.	< 1	Tr.
Red Pop (No-Cal)	6 fl. oz.	0	0.
Rondo (Schweppes)	6 fl. oz.	<1	Tr.
Root beer:			
Barrelhead (Canada Dry)	6 fl. oz.	<1	.8
(Dad's)	6 fl. oz.	<1	.2
(No-Cal)	6 fl. oz.	0	Tr.
(Shasta) draft	6 fl. oz.	<1	.2
Tab	6 fl. oz.	1	.2
Seven-Up	6 fl. oz.	2	0.
Shape-Up (No-Cal)	6 fl. oz.	0	0.
Sprite	6 fl. oz.	2	0.
Strawberry:			
(Shasta)	6 fl. oz.	<1	Tr.
Tab	6 fl. oz.	<2	0.
Tab	6 fl. oz.	<1	.1
Tea (No-Cal)	6 fl. oz.	0	0.
TNT (No-Cal)	6 fl. oz.	0	0.
SOLE:			
Raw (USDA):			
Whole	1 lb. (weighed whole)	118	0.
Meat only	4 oz.	90	0.
Frozen:			
(Mrs. Paul's) fillets, with lemon butter	½ of 8½-oz. pkg.	155	9.7
(Van de Kamp's) batter dipped, french fried	2-oz. piece	140	12.0
(Weight Watchers) in lemon sauce, 2 compartment meal	9¼-oz. pkg.	201	17.0

(USDA): United States Department of Agriculture
(HEW/FAO):   Health, Education and Welfare/Food and Agriculture Organization
* Prepared as Package Directs

Food and Description	Measure or Quantity	Calories	Carbo-hydrates (grams)
SORGHUM (USDA):			
Grain	1 oz.	94	20.7
Syrup	1 T. (.7 oz.)	54	12.2
SORREL (See **DOCK**)			
SOUFFLÉ, frozen (Stouffer's):			
Cheese	⅓ of 12-oz. pkg.	241	9.3
Corn	⅓ of 12-oz. pkg.	154	18.9
SOUP (See individual listings by kind)			
SOUP GREENS, canned (Durkee)	2½-oz. jar	216	43.0
SOURSOP, raw (USDA):			
Whole	1 lb. (weighed with skin & seeds)	200	50.3
Flesh only	4 oz.	74	18.5
SOUSE (USDA)	1 oz.	51	.3
SOUTHERN COMFORT:			
80 proof	1 fl. oz.	79	3.4
90 proof	1 fl. oz.	84	3.5
100 proof	1 fl. oz.	97	3.5
SOYBEAN:			
(USDA):			
Young seeds:			
Raw	1 lb. (weighed in pod)	322	31.7
Boiled, drained	4 oz.	134	11.5
Canned:			
Solids & liq.	4 oz.	85	7.1
Drained solids	4 oz.	117	8.4
Mature seeds:			
Raw	1 lb.	1828	152.0
Raw	1 cup (7.4 oz.)	846	70.4
Cooked	4 oz.	147	12.2

Food and Description	Measure or Quantity	Calories	Carbo-hydrates (grams)
Oil roasted:			
(Soy Ahoy) regular, barbecue or garlic	1 oz.	152	4.8
(Soytown)	1 oz.	152	4.8
SOYBEAN CURD or TOFU (USDA):			
Regular	4 oz.	82	2.7
Cake	4.2-oz. cake	86	2.9
SOYBEAN FLOUR (See FLOUR)			
SOYBEAN GRITS, high fat (USDA)	1 cup (4.9 oz.)	524	46.0
SOYBEAN MILK (USDA):			
Fluid	4 oz.	37	1.5
Powder	1 oz.	122	7.9
SOYBEAN PROTEIN (USDA)	1 oz.	91	4.3
SOYBEAN PROTEINATE (USDA)	1 oz.	88	2.2
SOYBEAN SPROUT (See BEAN SPROUT)			
SOY SAUCE (See SAUCE, Soy)			

SPAGHETTI (Plain spaghetti products are essentially the same in caloric value and carbohydrate content on the same weight basis. The longer the cooking, the more water is absorbed and this affects the nutritive value):

(USDA): United States Department of Agriculture
(HEW/FAO): Health, Education and Welfare/Food and Agriculture Organization
* Prepared as Package Directs

Food and Description	Measure or Quantity	Calories	Carbo-hydrates (grams)
Dry (USDA):			
Whole	1 oz.	105	21.3
Broken	1 cup (2.5 oz.)	262	53.4
Cooked:			
8-10 minutes, "al dente"	1 cup (5.1 oz.)	216	53.9
8-10 minutes, "al dente"	4 oz.	168	34.1
14-20 minutes, tender	1 cup (4.9 oz.)	155	35.2
14-20 minutes, tender	4 oz.	126	26.1
Canned, regular pack:			
(Franco-American):			
Regular:			
With meatballs in tomato sauce	7⅜-oz. can	210	26.0
In meat sauce	7½-oz. serving	230	26.0
In tomato sauce with cheese	7⅜-oz. serving	170	33.0
SpaghettiOs:			
With little meatballs in tomato sauce	7⅜-oz. serving	210	24.0
With sliced franks in tomato sauce	7⅜-oz. serving	210	26.0
In tomato & cheese sauce	7⅜-oz. serving	160	33.0
(Hormel) Short Orders, & meatballs in tomato sauce	7½-oz. can	210	24.0
(Libby's) & meatballs in to-mato sauce	7½-oz. serving	189	27.5
(Nalley's) & meatballs	8-oz. serving	245	31.8
Canned, dietetic pack (Dia-Mel) & meatballs in tomato sauce	8-oz. can	200	24.0
Frozen:			
(Banquet):			
Regular:			
& meatballs	11½-oz. dinner	450	62.9
With meat sauce	8-oz. entree	311	31.3
Buffet Supper, & meatballs	2 lb. pkg.	1127	129.1
(Green Giant) & meatballs in tomato sauce	9-oz. entree	269	29.1
(Morton) & meatballs	11-oz. dinner	344	59.4
(Stouffer's) & meat sauce	14-oz. pkg.	442	61.6
(Swanson) TV Brand:			
Dinner	12½-oz. dinner	410	57.0
Entree, in tomato sauce with breaded veal	8¼-oz. entree	290	24.0

Food and Description	Measure or Quantity	Calories	Carbohydrates (grams)
SPAGHETTI SAUCE (See also **SPAGHETTI SAUCE MIX** and **SAUCE,** Italian):			
Regular:			
Clam (Ragu) chopped	5-oz. serving	110	14.0
Marinara:			
(Prince)	4-oz. serving	80	12.4
(Ragu)	5-oz. serving	120	15.0
Meat-flavored:			
(Ann Page)	¼ of 15½-oz. jar	81	12.3
(Ragu)	5-oz. serving	115	14.0
Meat:			
(Prince)	½ cup (4.9 oz.)	101	11.1
(Ragu) extra thick & zesty	5-oz. serving	130	14.0
(Ronzoni)	4-oz. serving	87	11.0
Meatless or plain:			
(Hain) Italian style	4-oz. serving	72	14.2
(Prince)	½ cup (4.6 oz.)	90	11.4
(Ragu):			
Regular	5-oz. serving	105	14.0
Extra thick & zesty	5-oz. serving	120	13.0
(Ronzoni)	4-oz. serving	78	13.0
Mushroom:			
(Hain) Italian style	4-oz. serving	80	14.3
(Prince)	4-oz. serving	77	11.3
(Ragu):			
Regular	5-oz. serving	105	13.0
Extra thick & zesty	5-oz. serving	110	14.0
Pepperoni (Ragu)	5-oz. serving	120	14.0
Dietetic (Featherweight) low sodium	⅔ cup	30	10.0
*SPAGHETTI SAUCE MIX:			
(Durkee):			
Regular	½ cup	45	10.4
Mushroom	1⅓ cups	104	24.0
(French's):			
Italian style	⅝ cup	100	15.0

(USDA): United States Department of Agriculture
(HEW/FAO): Health, Education and Welfare/Food and Agriculture Organization
* Prepared as Package Directs

Food and Description	Measure or Quantity	Calories	Carbohydrates (grams)
Mushroom	⅝ cup	100	13.0
(Spatini)	2-oz. serving	40	8.0
SPAM (Hormel):			
Regular	1-oz. serving	88	1.1
& cheese chunks	1-oz. serving	87	.7
Deviled	1-oz. serving	79	0.
Smoked flavored	1-oz. serving	88	.3
SPANISH MACKEREL, raw (USDA):			
Whole	1 lb. (weighed whole)	490	0.
Meat only	4 oz.	201	0.
SPECIAL K, cereal (Kellogg's)	1 cup (1 oz.)	110	21.0
SPINACH:			
Raw (USDA):			
Untrimmed	1 lb. (weighed with large stems & roots)	85	14.0
Trimmed or packaged	1 lb.	118	19.5
Trimmed, whole leaves	1 cup (1.2 oz.)	9	1.4
Trimmed, chopped	1 cup (1.8 oz.)	14	2.2
Boiled (USDA) whole leaves, drained	1 cup (5.5 oz.)	36	5.6
Canned, regular pack:			
(USDA):			
Solids & liq.	½ cup (4.1 oz.)	21	3.5
Drained solids	½ cup	27	4.0
(Del Monte) solids & liq.	½ cup (4.1 oz.)	28	3.4
(Libby's) solids & liq.	½ cup (4.2 oz.)	27	3.6
(Sunshine) whole leaf, solids & liq.	½ cup (4.1 oz.)	24	2.9
Canned, dietetic or low calorie:			
(USDA) low sodium:			
Solids & liq.	4 oz.	24	3.9
Drained solids	4 oz.	29	4.5
(Blue Boy) solids & liq.	4-oz. serving	22	2.4
(Featherweight) low sodium	½ cup	35	4.0

Food and Description	Measure or Quantity	Calories	Carbo- hydrates (grams)
Frozen:			
(USDA) chopped, boiled, drained	4 oz.	26	4.2
(Birds Eye):			
Chopped or leaf	⅓ of 10-oz. pkg.	23	2.7
Creamed	⅓ of 9-oz. pkg.	57	4.0
(Green Giant):			
In butter sauce	⅓ of 10.-oz. pkg.	43	2.3
Creamed	⅓ of 10-oz. pkg.	69	7.8
Souffle, *Bake'n Serve*	⅓ of 10-oz. pkg.	109	8.2
(McKenzie)	⅓ of 10-oz. pkg.	27	3.3
(Seabrook Farms) chopped or whole	⅓ of 10-oz. pkg.	27	3.3
(Stouffer's) souffle	⅓ of 12-oz. pkg.	130	11.9

SPINY LOBSTER (See CRAYFISH)

SPLEEN, raw (USDA):

Beef & calf	4 oz.	118	0.
Hog	4 oz.	121	0.
Lamb	4 oz.	130	0.

SQUAB, pigeon, raw (USDA):

Dressed	1 lb. (weighed with feet, inedible viscera & bones)	569	0.
Meat & skin	4 oz.	333	0.
Meat only	4 oz.	161	0.
Light meat only, without skin	4 oz.	142	0.
Giblets	1 oz.	44	.3

SQUASH SEEDS, dry (USDA):

In hull	4 oz.	464	12.6
Hulled	1 oz.	157	4.3

(USDA): United States Department of Agriculture
(HEW/FAO): Health, Education and Welfare/Food and Agriculture Organization
* Prepared as Package Directs

Food and Description	Measure or Quantity	Calories	Carbo- hydrates (grams)
SQUASH, SUMMER:			
Fresh (USDA):			
Crookneck & straightneck, yellow:			
Whole	1 lb. (weighed untrimmed)	89	19.1
Boiled, drained:			
Diced	½ cup (3.6 oz.)	15	3.2
Slices	½ cup (3.1 oz.)	13	2.7
Scallop, white & pale green:			
Whole	1 lb. (weighed untrimmed)	93	22.7
Boiled, drained, mashed	½ cup (4.2 oz.)	19	4.5
Zucchini & cocazelle, green:			
Whole	1 lb. (weighed untrimmed)	73	15.5
Boiled, drained slices	½ cup (2.7 oz.)	9	1.9
Canned (Del Monte) zucchini, in tomato sauce	½ cup (4.1 oz.)	37	7.9
Frozen:			
(USDA):			
Unthawed	4 oz.	24	5.3
Boiled, drained	4 oz.	24	5.3
(Birds Eye):			
Sliced	⅓ of 10-oz. pkg.	18	4.0
Zucchini	⅓ of 10-oz. pkg.	16	3.0
(Green Giant) in cheese sauce, Southern recipe	⅓ of 10-oz. pkg.	41	5.1
(McKenzie):			
Crookneck, yellow	3.3-oz. serving	22	3.8
Zucchini	3½-oz. serving	20	3.6
(Mrs. Paul's):			
Zucchini parmesan	⅓ of 11-oz. pkg.	84	7.0
Zucchini sticks, batter fried	⅓ of 9-oz. pkg.	65	23.1
(Seabrook Farms):			
Crookneck, yellow	⅓ of 10-oz. pkg.	22	3.8
Zucchini	3½-oz. serving	20	3.6
(Southland):			
Crookneck	⅕ of 16-oz. pkg.	20	4.0
Crookneck, with onion	⅕ of 16-oz. pkg.	20	5.0
Zucchini, with onion	⅕ of 16-oz. pkg.	15	3.0
Zucchini, sliced	⅕ of 16-oz. pkg.	15	3.3

Food and Description	Measure or Quantity	Calories	Carbo-hydrates (grams)
SQUASH, WINTER:			
Fresh (USDA):			
Acorn:			
Whole	1 lb. (weighed with skin & seeds)	152	38.6
Baked, flesh only, mashed	½ cup (3.6 oz.)	56	14.3
Boiled, mashed	½ cup (4.1 oz.)	39	9.7
Butternut:			
Whole	1 lb. (weighed with skin & seeds)	171	44.4
Baked, flesh only	4 oz.	77	19.8
Boiled, flesh only	4 oz.	46	11.8
Hubbard:			
Whole	1 lb. (weighed with skin & seeds)	117	28.1
Baked, flesh only	4 oz.	57	13.3
Boiled, flesh only, diced	½ cup (4.2 oz.)	35	8.1
Boiled, flesh only, mashed	½ cup (4.3 oz.)	37	8.4
Frozen:			
(USDA) heated	½ cup (4.2 oz.)	46	11.0
(Birds Eye)	⅓ of pkg.	50	11.0
(Southland) butternut	⅓ of 20-oz. pkg.	60	16.0
SQUID, raw (USDA) meat only	4 oz.	95	1.7
STARCH (See **CORNSTARCH**)			
START, instant breakfast drink	½ cup	51	12.7
STEAK & GREEN PEPPERS, frozen (Swanson) in oriental-style sauce	8½-oz. entree	200	11.0
STEAK & POTATO SOUP, canned (Campbell) *Chunky*	9½-oz. serving	170	21.0

(USDA): United States Department of Agriculture
(HEW/FAO):   Health, Education and Welfare/Food and Agriculture
                    Organization
* Prepared as Package Directs

Food and Description	Measure or Quantity	Calories	Carbohydrates (grams)
STOCK BASE (French's):			
Beef	1 tsp. (4 grams)	8	2.0
Chicken	1 tsp. (3.2 grams)	8	1.0
*STOCKPOT SOUP (Campbell) condensed, vegetable & beef	10-oz. serving	120	12.0
STOMACH, PORK, scalded (USDA)	4 oz.	172	0.
STRAINED FOOD (See **BABY FOOD**)			
STRAWBERRY:			
Fresh (USDA):			
Whole	1 lb. (weighed with caps & stems)	161	36.6
Whole, capped	1 cup (5.1 oz.)	53	2.1
Canned (USDA) unsweetened or low calorie, water pack, solids & liq.	4 oz.	25	6.4
Frozen (Birds Eye):			
Halves	⅓ of 16-oz. pkg.	196	48.2
Whole	¼ of 16-oz. pkg.	97	23.2
Whole, quick thaw	½ of 10-oz. pkg.	123	29.7
STRAWBERRY DRINK (Hi-C):			
Canned	6 fl. oz.	89	22.0
*Mix	6 fl. oz.	68	17.0
STRAWBERRY ICE CREAM:			
(Baskin-Robbins)	1 scoop (2½ oz.)	141	15.6
(Breyer's)	¼ pt.	130	17.0
(Good Humor)	4-fl. oz.	120	15.0
(Swift's) sweet cream	½ cup	124	15.3
STRAWBERRY JELLY:			
Sweetened (Smucker's)	1 T.	53	13.5
Dietetic (Featherweight)	1 T.	16	4.0

Food and Description	Measure or Quantity	Calories	Carbo-hydrates (grams)
STRAWBERRY PRESERVES or JAM:			
Sweetened:			
(Smucker's)	1 T.	53	13.5
(Welch's)	1 T.	52	13.5
Dietetic or low calorie:			
(Dia-Mel)	1 tsp. (6 grams)	2	0.
(Diet Delight)	1 T.	13	3.0
(Estee)	1 T. (.6 oz.)	18	4.8
(Featherweight):			
Regular	1 T.	16	4.0
Artificially sweetened	1 T.	6	1.0
(S&W) *Nutradiet*	1 T.	12	3.0
(Tillie Lewis) *Tasti Diet*	1 T.	12	3.0
STRAWBERRY SPREAD, low sugar:			
(Smucker's)	1 T.	24	6.0
(Welch's) Lite	1 T.	30	6.2
STUFFING MIX:			
*Chicken, *Stove Top*	½ cup	170	21.0
Cornbread:			
(Pepperidge Farm)	8-oz. pkg.	880	168.0
Stove Top	½ cup	170	20.0
Herb seasoned (Pepperidge Farm)	8-oz. pkg.	880	168.0
*Pork, *Stove Top*	½ cup	170	20.0
*With rice, *Stove Top*	½ cup	180	23.0
White bread, *Mrs. Cubbison's*	1 oz.	101	20.5
STURGEON (USDA):			
Raw:			
Section	1 lb. (weighed with skin & bones)	362	0.
Meat only	4 oz.	107	0.

(USDA): United States Department of Agriculture
(HEW/FAO): Health, Education and Welfare/Food and Agriculture Organization
* Prepared as Package Directs

Food and Description	Measure or Quantity	Calories	Carbohydrates (grams)
Smoked	4 oz.	169	0.
Steamed	4 oz.	181	0.
SUCCOTASH:			
Canned:			
(Libby's):			
Cream style	½ cup (4.6 oz.)	111	22.8
Whole kernel	¼ of 16-oz. can	82	16.0
(Stokely-Van Camp) solids & liq.	½ cup (4.5 oz.)	85	17.5
Frozen:			
(USDA) boiled, drained	½ cup (3.4 oz.)	89	19.7
(Birds Eye)	⅓ of 10-oz. pkg.	80	17.0
SUCKER, CARP (USDA) raw:			
Whole	1 lb. (weighed whole)	196	0.
Meat only	4 oz.	126	0.
SUCKER, including **WHITE MULLET** (USDA) raw:			
Whole	1 lb. (weighed whole)	203	0.
Meat only	4 oz.	118	0.
SUET, raw (USDA)	1 oz.	242	0.
SUGAR, beet or cane (there are no differences in calories and carbohydrates among brands) (USDA):			
Brown:			
Regular	1 lb.	1692	437.3
Brownulated	1 cup (5.4 oz.)	567	146.5
Firm-packed	1 cup (7.5 oz.)	791	204.4
Firm-packed	1 T. (.5 oz.)	48	12.5
Confectioners':			
Unsifted	1 cup (4.3 oz.)	474	122.4
Unsifted	1 T. (8 grams)	30	7.7
Sifted	1 cup (3.4 oz.)	366	94.5
Sifted	1 T. (6 grams)	23	5.9
Stirred	1 cup (4.2 oz.)	462	119.4

Food and Description	Measure or Quantity	Calories	Carbo-hydrates (grams)
Stirred	1 T. (8 grams)	29	7.5
Granulated	1 lb.	1746	451.3
Granulated	1 cup (6.9 oz.)	751	194.0
Granulated	1 T. (.4 oz.)	46	11.9
Granulated	1 lump (1⅛" × ¾" × ⅜", 6 grams)	23	6.0
Maple	1 lb.	1579	408.0
Maple	1¾" × 1¼" × ½" piece (1.2 oz.)	104	27.0
SUGAR APPLE, raw (USDA):			
Whole	1 lb. (weighed with skin & seeds)	192	48.4
Flesh only	4 oz.	107	26.9
SUGAR CORN POPS, cereal (Kellogg's)	½ cup (1 oz.)	110	26.0
SUGAR PUFFS, cereal (Malt-O-Meal)	⅞ cup (1 oz.)	110	26.0
SUGAR SMACKS, cereal (Kellogg's)	¾ cup (1 oz.)	110	25.0
SUGAR SUBSTITUTE:			
(Featherweight) any type	Any quantity	0	0.
Sprinkle Sweet (Pillsbury)	1 tsp.	2	.5
Sugar-Like (Dia-Mel)	1-gram packet	3	1.0
Suprose (Whitlock)	1-gram packet	4	.9
(S&W) *Nutradiet*	1 tsp.	0	0.
Sweet'ner (Weight Watchers)	1-gram packet	3	1.0
Sweet'n-it (Dia-Mel) liquid	5 drops	0	0.
*Sweet*10* (Pillsbury)	⅛ tsp.	0	0.
***SUKIYAKI DINNER** (Chun King) stir fry	⅕ of pkg.	100	3.0

(USDA): United States Department of Agriculture
(HEW/FAO): Health, Education and Welfare/Food and Agriculture Organization
* Prepared as Package Directs

Food and Description	Measure or Quantity	Calories	Carbohydrates (grams)
SUNFLOWER SEED:			
(USDA):			
In hulls	4 oz. (weighed in hull)	343	12.2
Hulled	1 oz.	159	5.6
(Fisher):			
In hull, roasted, salted	1 oz.	86	3.0
Hulled, roasted:			
Dry, salted	1 oz.	164	5.6
Oil, salted	1 oz.	167	5.6
(Flavor House) dry roasted	1 oz.	179	4.0
(Frito-Lay's)	1 oz.	181	4.7
(Planter's):			
Dry roasted	1 oz.	160	5.0
Unsalted	1 oz.	170	5.0
SUNFLOWER SEED FLOUR (See **FLOUR**)			
SUZY Q (Hostess):			
Banana	2¼-oz. cake	244	38.4
Chocolate	2½-oz. cake	237	36.4
SWAMP CABBAGE (USDA):			
Raw, whole	1 lb. (weighed untrimmed)	107	19.8
Boiled, trimmed, drained	4 oz.	24	4.4
SWEETBREADS (USDA):			
Beef:			
Raw	1 lb.	939	0.
Braised	4 oz.	363	0.
Calf:			
Raw	1 lb.	426	0.
Braised	4 oz.	191	0.
Hog (See **PANCREAS**)			
Lamb:			
Raw	1 lb.	426	0.
Braised	4 oz.	198	0.
SWEET POTATO:			
Raw (USDA):			
All kinds, unpared	1 lb. (weighed whole)	419	96.6

Food and Description	Measure or Quantity	Calories	Carbo-hydrates (grams)
All kinds, pared	4 oz.	129	29.8
Firm-fleshed, Jersey types, pared	4 oz.	116	25.5
Soft-fleshed, Puerto Rico variety, pared	4 oz.	133	31.0
Baked (USDA) peeled after baking	3.9-oz. sweet potato (5″ × 2″)	155	35.8
Baked (USDA) peeled after boiling	5-oz. sweet potato (5″ × 2″)	168	38.7
Candied (USDA) home recipe	6.2-oz. sweet potato (3½″ × 2¼″)	294	59.8
Canned, regular pack (USDA):			
In syrup, solids & liq.	4 oz.	129	31.2
Vacuum or solid pack	4 oz.	118	27.1
Canned, dietetic or low calorie, without added sugar & salt (USDA)	4 oz.	52	12.2
Dehydrated flakes (USDA):			
Dry	½ cup (2 oz.)	220	52.2
*Prepared with water	½ cup (4.4 oz.)	120	28.5
Frozen:			
(Green Giant) glazed, Southern recipe	⅓ of 10-oz. pkg.	120	22.7
(Mrs. Paul's):			
Regular	⅓ of 12-oz. pkg.	153	36.1
With apple	⅓ of 12-oz. pkg.	180	44.1

SWEETSOP (See **SUGAR APPLE**)

*SWEET & SOUR DINNER

| (Chun King) stir fry | ⅕ of pkg. | 140 | 10.0 |

SWEET & SOUR ORIENTAL,
canned (La Choy):

| With chicken | ½ of 15-oz. can | 240 | 50.0 |

(USDA): United States Department of Agriculture
(HEW/FAO):   Health, Education and Welfare/Food and Agriculture Organization
* Prepared as Package Directs

Food and Description	Measure or Quantity	Calories	Carbo-hydrates (grams)
With pork	½ of 15-oz. can	260	48.0
SWISS STEAK, frozen (Swanson) *TV Brand*	10 oz. dinner	350	40.0
SWORDFISH (USDA):			
Raw, meat only	1 lb.	535	0.
Broiled, with butter or margarine	3″ × 3″ × ½″ steak (4.4 oz.)	218	0.
Canned, solids & liq.	4 oz.	116	0.
SYLVANDER WINE (Louis M. Martini) 12½% alcohol	3 fl. oz.	90	.2
SYRUP:			
Sweetened:			
Apricot (Smucker's)	1 T.	50	13.0
Blackberry (Smucker's)	1 T.	50	13.0
Blueberry (Smucker's)	1 T.	50	13.0
Boysenberry (Smucker's)	1 T.	50	13.0
Chocolate:			
Bosco	1 T. (.7 oz.)	55	13.3
(Hershey's)	1 T. (.7 oz.)	52	11.7
Corn, *Karo:*			
Dark	1 T. (.7 oz.)	58	14.6
Light	1 T. (.7 oz.)	48	14.5
Cane (USDA)	1 T. (.7 oz.)	55	14.0
Maple, imitation, *Karo*	1 T. (.7 oz.)	57	14.2
Pancake & waffle:			
Aunt Jemima	1 T. (.7 oz.)	53	13.1
Golden Griddle	1 T. (.7 oz.)	54	13.3
Karo	1 T. (.7 oz.)	54	13.3
Log Cabin:			
Regular	1 T. (.7 oz.)	52	13.1
Buttered	1 T. (.7 oz.)	55	13.0
Maple-honey	1 T. (.7 oz.)	56	13.9
Mrs. Butterworth's	1 T. (.7 oz.)	55	13.0
Raspberry (Smucker's) red	1 T. (.6 oz.)	43	11.1
Strawberry (Smucker's)	1 T. (.6 oz.)	50	13.0
Dietetic or low calorie:			
Blueberry (Featherweight)	1 T.	14	3.0

Food and Description	Measure or Quantity	Calories	Carbo-hydrates (grams)
Chocolate:			
(Diet Delight)	1 T. (.6 oz.)	8	2.0
(Featherweight)	1 T.	30	7.0
Coffee (No-Cal)	1 T.	6	1.2
Cola (No-Cal)	1 T.	Tr.	Tr.
Maple (S&W) *Nutradiet,* imitation	1 T.	12	3.0
Pancake or waffle:			
Aunt Jemima	1 T. (.6 oz.)	29	7.3
(Diet Delight)	1 T. (.6 oz.)	6	4.0
(Featherweight)	1 T.	12	3.0
(Tillie Lewis) *Tasti Diet*	1 T. (.5 oz.)	4	1.0

T

*TACO (Ortega)	1 taco	150	15.0
TACO SEASONING MIX:			
*(Durkee)	1 cup	641	7.5
(French's)	1¼-oz. pkg.	120	24.0
TACO SHELL (Ortega)	1 shell (.4 oz.)	50	7.7
TAMALE:			
Canned:			
(Derby) beef, with sauce	1 tamale (2.2 oz.)	120	6.5
(Hormel) beef:			
Regular	¼ of 15-oz. can	144	8.6
Short Orders	½ of 7½-oz. can	135	8.5
(Nalley's):			
Beef	4-oz. serving	134	12.5
Chicken	4-oz. serving	104	12.5
Olive, ripe	4-oz. serving	124	13.6
Old El Paso, with chili gravy	1 tamale	116	11.5

(USDA): United States Department of Agriculture
(HEW/FAO): Health, Education and Welfare/Food and Agriculture Organization
* Prepared as Package Directs

Food and Description	Measure or Quantity	Calories	Carbo-hydrates (grams)
Frozen (Hormel) beef	1 tamale (3.1 oz.)	130	11.3
TAMALE PIE, canned (Nalley's)	4-oz. serving	113	12.5
TAMARIND, fresh (USDA):			
Whole	1 lb. (weighed with pods & seeds)	520	136.1
Flesh only	4 oz.	271	70.9
TANG, instant breakfast drink:			
Grape	½ cup (4 oz.)	64	16.0
Grapefruit	½ cup (4 oz.)	61	15.0
Orange	½ cup (4 oz.)	62	15.3
TANGELO, fresh (USDA):			
Whole	1 lb. (weighed with peel, membrane & seeds)	104	24.6
Juice	½ cup (4.4 oz.)	51	12.0
TANGERINE or MANDARIN ORANGE:			
Fresh (USDA):			
Whole	1 lb. (weighed with peel, membrane & seeds)	154	38.9
Whole	4.1-oz. tangerine (2 ⅜″ dia.)	39	10.0
Sections (without membranes)	1 cup (6.8 oz.)	89	22.4
Canned, regular pack (Del Monte) solids & liq.	¼ of 22-oz. can	106	25.3
Canned, dietetic or low calorie, solids & liq.:			
(Diet Delight) juice pack	½ cup (4.3 oz.)	50	13.0
(Featherweight) water pack	½ cup	35	8.0
(S&W) *Nutradiet*	½ cup	28	7.0
TANGERINE DRINK, canned (Hi-C)	6 fl. oz.	90	23.0

Food and Description	Measure or Quantity	Calories	Carbo-hydrates (grams)
TANGERINE JUICE:			
Fresh (USDA)	½ cup (4.4 oz.)	53	12.5
Canned (USDA):			
Unsweetened	½ cup (4.4 oz.)	53	12.6
Sweetened	½ cup (4.4 oz.)	62	14.9
*Frozen:			
(USDA)	½ cup (4.4 oz.)	57	13.4
(Minute Maid) sweetened	6 fl. oz.	85	20.8
TAPIOCA, dry, quick cooking, granulated:			
(USDA)	1 cup (5.4 oz.)	535	131.3
(USDA)	1 T. (10 grams)	35	8.6
TARO, raw (USDA):			
Tubers, whole	1 lb. (weighed with skin)	373	90.3
Tubers, skin removed	4 oz.	111	26.9
Leaves & stems	1 lb.	181	33.6
TARRAGON (French's)	1 tsp.	5	.7
TASTEEOS, cereal (Ralston-Purina)	1¼ cups (1 oz.)	110	22.0
TAUTUG or BLACKFISH, raw (USDA):			
Whole	1 lb. (weighed whole)	149	0.
Meat only	4 oz.	101	0.
TEA (See also **TEA, ICED**):			
Bag:			
(Lipton)	1 bag	2	0.
(Tender Leaf)	1 bag	1	0.
Mix, instant:			
(USDA) dry powder, slightly sweetened	1 tsp.	1	.4
*(USDA) beverage, slightly sweetened	1 cup (8.4 oz.)	5	.9

(USDA): United States Department of Agriculture
(HEW/FAO):   Health, Education and Welfare/Food and Agriculture
                        Organization
* Prepared as Package Directs

Food and Description	Measure or Quantity	Calories	Carbo-hydrates (grams)
*(Lipton):	1 cup (8 fl. oz.)	4	1.0
Lemon flavored	1 cup (8 fl. oz.)	4	1.0
100% tea	8 fl. oz.	0	0.
*Nestea	1 tsp.	2	Tr.
(Tender Leaf)	1 tsp.	1	Tr.
TEA, FLAVORED BAG (Lipton)			
Black Rum, Cinnamon, Lemon & Spice, Mint and Orange & Spice	1 bag	2	<1.0
***TEA, HERBAL**			
(Lipton):			
Almond Pleasure, Dessert Mint, Gentle Orange and Cinnamon Apple	1 cup	2	0.
Quietly Chamomile or Toasty Spice	1 cup	4	<1.0
(Sahadi):			
Spicy Almond, Distinctly Mint, Wild Hibiscus, Orchard Orange, Rosehips and Peppermint	6 oz.	2	0.
Chamomile	6 oz.	0	0.
Spearmint	6 oz.	4	<1.0
TEA, ICED:			
Canned, sweetened:			
(Lipton) lemon flavored	6 fl. oz.	67	16.5
(Shasta) lemon flavored	6 fl. oz.	61	16.5
Canned, unsweetened (Lipton)	6 fl. oz.	1.0	0.
*Mix:			
Presweetened, lemon flavored:			
Country Time	8 fl. oz.	121	30.2
(Lipton)	8 fl. oz.	60	16.0
(Nestea)	8 fl. oz.	93	22.6
Unsweetened, dietetic or low calorie:			
(Lipton) lemon flavored	1 cup (8 fl. oz.)	2	0.
Nestea:			
Plain	6 fl. oz.	0	0.
Lemon flavored	8 fl. oz.	2	.2
Light, lemon & sugar flavored	6 fl. oz.	40	11.0

Food and Description	Measure or Quantity	Calories	Carbohydrates (grams)
TEAM, cereal (Nabisco)	1 cup (1 oz.)	110	24.0
TENDERGREEN (See **MUSTARD SPINACH**)			
TERIYAKI, frozen (Stouffer's) beef, with rice & vegetables	½ of 10-oz. pkg.	183	20.4
TEQUILA (See **DISTILLED LIQUOR**)			
TEQUILA SUNRISE COCKTAIL, canned (Mr. Boston) 12½% alcohol	3 fl. oz.	120	14.4
***TEXTURED VEGETABLE PROTEIN** (Morningstar Farms):			
Breakfast links	¾-oz. link	62	.3
Breakfast patties	1.3-oz. pattie	109	3.2
Breakfast strips	.2-oz. strip	34	.2
Grillers, hamburger-like patties	2.1-oz. pattie	189	4.5
THURINGER, sausage:			
(USDA)	1-oz. serving	87	.5
(Best's Kosher)	1-oz. serving	104	1.1
(Hormel):			
Buffet	1-oz. serving	95	.3
Old Smokehouse	1-oz. serving	100	.1
Summer sausage	1-oz. slice	76	.2
(Louis Rich) turkey	1-oz. slice	50	<1.0
(Oscar Mayer) summer sausage:			
Regular	.8-oz. slice	75	.2
Beef	.8-oz. slice	72	.7
(Oscherwitz)	1-oz. slice	104	1.1
THYME, dried (French's)	1 tsp.	5	1.0
***TIA MARIA,** liqueur (Hiram Walker) 63 proof	1 fl. oz.	92	10.0

(USDA): United States Department of Agriculture
(HEW/FAO): Health, Education and Welfare/Food and Agriculture
                        Organization
* Prepared as Package Directs

Food and Description	Measure or Quantity	Calories	Carbo-hydrates (grams)
TIGER TAILS (Hostess)	2.2-oz. piece	222	38.1
TILEFISH (USDA):			
Raw, whole	1 lb. (weighed whole)	183	0.
Baked, meat only	4 oz.	156	0.
TOASTER CAKE or PASTRY:			
Flavor Kist (Schulze and Burch):			
Regular:			
All flavors except brown sugar cinnamon	1 piece	190	35.0
Brown sugar cinnamon	1 piece	200	25.0
Frosted:			
Apple, blueberry, cherry or strawberry	1 piece	190	36.0
Brown sugar cinnamon	1 piece	200	36.0
Fudge	1 piece	195	34.0
(Nabisco) all varieties	1.7-oz. piece	190	35.0
Pop Tarts (Kellogg's):			
Regular:			
Blueberry or cherry	1 piece (1.83 oz.)	210	36.0
Brown sugar cinnamon	1 piece (1 ¾ oz.)	210	33.0
Chocolate chip	1 piece (1¾ oz.)	200	34.0
Strawberry	1 piece (1.83 oz.)	200	37.0
Frosted:			
Blueberry or strawberry	1 piece (1.83 oz.)	200	38.0
Brown sugar cinnamon	1 piece (1¾ oz.)	210	34.0
Cherry	1 piece (1.83 oz.)	210	37.0
Chocolate fudge	1 piece (1.83 oz.)	200	36.0
Chocolate-vanilla creme	1 piece (1.83 oz.)	220	37.0
Concord grape, dutch apple, raspberry	1 piece (1.83 oz.)	210	36.0
Toast-r-Cake (Thomas'):			
Blueberry	1.3-oz. piece	116	17.7
Bran	1.3-oz. piece	119	19.9
Corn	1.3-oz. piece	124	18.7
TOASTY O's, cereal (Malt-O-Meal)	1¼ cups (1 oz.)	110	20.0

Food and Description	Measure or Quantity	Calories	Carbohydrates (grams)
TODDLER BABY FOOD (See **BABY FOOD**)			
TOFFEE FUDGE			
Swirl ice cream (Good Humor)	4-fl. oz.	130	18.0
TOFU (See **SOYBEAN CURD**)			
TOMATO:			
Fresh (USDA):			
Green:			
Whole, untrimmed	1 lb. (weighed with core & stem end)	99	21.1
Trimmed, unpeeled	4 oz.	27	5.8
Ripe:			
Whole:			
Eaten with skin	1 lb.	100	21.3
Peeled	1 lb. (weighed with skin, stem ends & hard core)	88	18.8
Peeled	1 med. (2″ × 2½″, 5.3 oz.)	33	7.0
Peeled	1 small (1 ¾″ × 2½″, 3.9 oz.)	24	5.2
Sliced, peeled	½ cup (3.2 oz.)	20	4.2
Boiled (USDA)	½ cup (4.3 oz.)	31	6.7
Canned, regular pack:			
(USDA) whole, solids & liq.	½ cup (4.2 oz.)	25	5.1
(Contadina):			
Sliced, baby	4 oz.	35	8.0
Stewed	4 oz.	35	8.0
Whole, round & pear	1 cup	53	10.6
(Del Monte) solids & liq.:			
Stewed	½ cup (4.2 oz.)	39	8.2
Wedges	½ cup (4.1 oz.)	35	7.2
Whole, peeled	½ cup (4.2 oz.)	27	5.3

(USDA): United States Department of Agriculture
(HEW/FAO):   Health, Education and Welfare/Food and Agriculture
                        Organization
* Prepared as Package Directs

Food and Description	Measure or Quantity	Calories	Carbo-hydrates (grams)
(Hunt's):			
Stewed	4 oz.	30	8.0
Whole, peeled	4 oz.	25	5.0
(Libby's)			
Stewed	½ of 16-oz. can	61	12.7
Whole, peeled, solids & liq.	½ of 16-oz. can	50	9.8
(Stokely-Van Camp) solids & liq.:			
Stewed	½ cup (4.2 oz.)	35	7.5
Whole	½ cup (4.3 oz.)	25	5.0
Canned, dietetic or low calorie:			
(USDA) low sodium	4 oz.	23	4.8
(Diet Delight) whole, peeled, solids & liq.	½ cup (4.3 oz.)	25	5.0
(Featherweight)	½ cup	20	4.0
(S&W) Nutradiet	½ cup	25	5.0
TOMATO JUICE:			
Canned, regular pack:			
(USDA)	½ cup (4.3 oz.)	23	5.2
(Campbell)	6 fl. oz.	40	8.0
(Del Monte)	6 fl. oz.	36	7.4
(Libby's)	6 fl. oz.	38	7.5
Mussleman's	6 fl. oz.	30	7.0
(Ocean Spray)	6 fl. oz.	35	7.0
(Stokely-Van Camp)	½ cup (4.2 oz.)	23	4.5
Canned, dietetic or low calorie:			
(USDA)	4 oz. (by wt.)	22	4.9
(Diet Delight)	6 fl. oz. (6.4 oz.)	35	7.0
(Featherweight)	6 fl. oz.	35	8.0
(S&W) Nutradiet	6 fl. oz.	35	8.0
Concentrate (USDA):			
Canned	4 oz. (by wt.)	86	19.4
*Canned, diluted with 3 parts water by volume	4 oz. (by wt.)	23	5.1
*Dehydrated (USDA)	½ cup (4.3 oz.)	24	5.4
TOMATO JUICE COCKTAIL:			
(USDA)	4 oz. (by wt.)	14	5.7
(USDA)	6-fl.-oz. can	139	31.6
(Ocean Spray) Firehouse Jubilee	6 fl. oz.	44	9.1
Snap-E-Tom	6 fl. oz.	40	7.0

Food and Description	Measure or Quantity	Calories	Carbo-hydrates (grams)
TOMATO PASTE, canned:			
Regular pack:			
(USDA)	6-oz. can	139	31.6
(USDA)	½ cup (4.6 oz.)	106	24.0
(USDA)	1 T. (.6 oz.)	13	3.0
(Contadina)	6 oz.	150	35.0
(Del Monte)	6 oz.	164	33.8
(Hunt's)	6 oz.	140	30.0
Dietetic (Featherweight) low sodium	6 oz.	150	35.0
TOMATO & PEPPERS, hot chili (Ortega) Jalapeno	1-oz. serving	7	1.1
TOMATO, PICKLED, canned (Claussen) Kosher, green, halves	1-oz. piece	6	1.1
TOMATO PUREE:			
Canned, regular pack:			
(USDA)	1 cup (8.8 oz.)	98	22.2
(Contadina) heavy	1 cup (8.8 oz.)	110	26.4
Canned, dietetic or low calorie:			
(USDA)	8 oz. (by wt.)	88	20.0
(Featherweight)	1 cup	90	20.0
TOMATO SAUCE, canned:			
Regular pack:			
(Contadina)	½ cup	43	9.8
(Del Monte):			
Regular	½ cup	42	13.5
Hot	½ cup	40	8.5
With mushroom	½ cup	51	10.7
With onions	½ cup	54	11.5
With tomato tidbits	½ cup	65	2.9
(Hunt's):			
With bits	4 oz.	35	8.0
With cheese	4 oz.	70	10.0
With herbs	4 oz.	80	12.0

(USDA): United States Department of Agriculture
(HEW/FAO): Health, Education and Welfare/Food and Agriculture
                Organization
* Prepared as Package Directs

Food and Description	Measure or Quantity	Calories	Carbo- hydrates (grams)
With mushroom	4 oz.	40	9.0
With onion	4 oz.	45	10.0
Plain	4 oz.	35	8.0
Prima Salsa:			
Regular	4 oz.	110	20.0
With meat	4 oz.	120	20.0
With mushroom	4 oz.	110	20.0
Special	4 oz.	40	10.0
(Libby's)	½ of 8-oz. can	35	6.5
(Stokely-Van Camp)	½ cup (4.5 oz.)	35	6.5
TOMATO SOUP:			
Canned, regular pack:			
*(USDA) condensed:			
Prepared with equal volume water	1 cup (8.6 oz.)	88	15.7
Prepared with equal volume milk	1 cup (8.8 oz.)	172	22.5
*(Campbell):			
Condensed:			
Regular:			
Prepared with milk	10-oz. serving	210	27.0
Prepared with water	10-oz. serving	110	20.0
& rice, old fashioned	10-oz. serving	150	29.0
Semi-condensed, *Soup For One, Royale*	11-oz. serving	180	34.0
*(Rokeach) condensed:			
Regular:			
Made with milk	10-oz. serving	190	27.0
Made with water	10-oz. serving	90	20.0
& rice	10-oz. serving	160	25.0
Canned, dietetic or low calorie:			
(Campbell) low sodium	7¼-oz. can	130	22.0
(Dia-Mel)	8-oz. serving	50	11.0
*Mix (Lipton) *Cup-A-Soup*	6 fl. oz.	80	17.0
TOMATO-VEGETABLE JUICE COCKTAIL, canned (Ocean Spray)	6 fl. oz.	44	9.1

Food and Description	Measure or Quantity	Calories	Carbohydrates (grams)
TOMCOD, ATLANTIC, raw (USDA):			
Whole	1 lb. (weighed whole)	136	0.
Meat only	4 oz.	87	0.
TOM COLLINS, canned (Mr. Boston) 12½% alcohol	3 fl. oz.	105	10.8
TONGUE (USDA):			
Beef, medium fat:			
Raw, untrimmed	1 lb.	714	1.4
Braised	4 oz.	277	.5
Calf:			
Raw, untrimmed	1 lb.	454	3.1
Braised	4 oz.	181	1.1
Hog:			
Raw, untrimmed	1 lb.	741	1.7
Braised	4 oz.	287	.6
Lamb:			
Raw, untrimmed	1 lb.	659	1.7
Braised	4 oz.	288	.6
Sheep:			
Raw, untrimmed	1 lb.	877	7.9
Braised	4 oz.	366	2.7
TONGUE, CANNED (USDA):			
Pickled	1 oz.	76	<.1
Potted or deviled	1 oz.	82	.2
TOPPING:			
Sweetened:			
Butterscotch (Smucker's)	1 T.	70	16.5
Caramel (Smucker's)	1 T.	70	16.5
Cherry (Smucker's)	1 T.	65	16.0
Chocolate:			
(Hershey's) fudge	1 T.	49	7.3
(Smucker's):			
Regular or fudge	1 T.	65	13.5
Fudge nut or milk	1 T.	70	15.5

(USDA): United States Department of Agriculture
(HEW/FAO): Health, Education and Welfare/Food and Agriculture Organization
* Prepared as Package Directs

Food and Description	Measure or Quantity	Calories	Carbo-hydrates (grams)
Marshmallow (See **MARSHMALLOW FLUFF**)			
Peanut butter caramel (Smucker's)	1 T.	75	14.5
Pecan (Smucker's) in syrup	1 T.	65	14.0
Pineapple (Smucker's)	1 T.	65	16.0
Strawberry (Smucker's)	1 T.	60	15.0
Walnuts, in syrup (Smucker's)	1 T.	65	13.5
Dietetic or low calorie, chocolate:			
(Diet Delight)	1 T. (.6 oz.)	16	3.6
(Tillie Lewis) *Tasti Diet*	1 T. (.5 oz.)	8	2.0
TOPPING, WHIPPED:			
Canned or aerosol:			
Regular pack:			
(USDA):			
Pressurized	1 cup (2.5 oz.)	190	9.0
Pressurized	1 T. (4 grams)	10	Tr.
Cool Whip (Birds Eye) frozen, nondairy	1 T. (.2 oz.)	19	1.3
Lucky Whip, aerosol	1 T. (.2 oz.)	12	.5
Spoon'N Serve (Rich's), frozen, non-dairy	1 T. (.14 oz.)	14	1.1
Whip Topping (Rich's) aerosol	¼-oz. serving	20	1.2
Dietetic (Featherweight)	1 T.	3	.5
*Mix:			
Regular (Dream Whip)	1 T. (.2 oz.)	10	1.0
Dietetic (D-Zerta)	1 T.	8	0.
TOP RAMEN, beef (Nissin Foods)	3-oz. serving	390	50.5
TORTILLA:			
(USDA)	.7-oz. tortilla	42	9.7
(Amigos)	1-oz. tortilla	111	19.7
TOSTADA SHELL, canned (Ortega)	.4-oz. shell	50	6.0
TOTAL, cereal (General Mills)	1 cup (1 oz.)	110	23.0

Food and Description	Measure or Quantity	Calories	Carbohydrates (grams)
TOWEL GOURD, raw (USDA):			
Unpared	1 lb. (weighed with skin)	69	15.8
Pared	4 oz.	20	4.6
TRIPE:			
Beef (USDA):			
Commercial	4 oz.	113	0.
Pickled	4 oz.	70	0.
Canned (Libby's)	¼ of 24-oz. can	290	1.1
TRIPLE SEC LIQUEUR (Mr. Boston)	1 fl. oz.	79	8.5
TRIX, cereal (General Mills)	1 cup (1 oz.)	110	25.0
TROUT (USDA):			
Brook, fresh:			
Whole	1 lb. (weighed whole)	224	0.
Meat only	4 oz.	115	0.
Lake (See **LAKE TROUT**)			
Rainbow:			
Fresh, meat with skin	4 oz.	221	0.
Canned	4 oz.	237	0.
TUNA:			
Raw (USDA):			
Bluefin, meat only	4 oz.	165	0.
Yellowfin, meat only	4 oz.	151	0.
Canned, in oil:			
(USDA):			
Solids & liq.	6½-oz. can	530	0.
Drained solids	6½-oz. can	309	0.
(Breast O' Chicken) solids & liq.	6½-oz. can	427	0.
(Bumble Bee) drained solids:			
Chunk light	6½-oz. can	309	0.
Solid, white	7-oz. can	333	0.

(USDA): United States Department of Agriculture
(HEW/FAO): Health, Education and Welfare/Food and Agriculture Organization
* Prepared as Package Directs

Food and Description	Measure or Quantity	Calories	Carbo-hydrates (grams)
(Carnation) solids & liq.	6½-oz. can	427	0.
(Chicken of the Sea) chunk, light:			
Solids & liq.	6½-oz. can	405	<1.8
Drained solids	6½-oz. can	294	0.
(Star Kist) solids & liq.:			
Chunk:			
Light	6½-oz. can	427	0.
White	6½-oz. can	467	0.
Flakes or grated	6¼-oz. can	426	0.
Solids, light:			
Regular	7-oz. can	459	0.
In Tonno olive oil	7-oz. can	443	0.
Solid, white	7-oz. can	503	0.
Canned in water, solids & liq.:			
(USDA)	6½-oz. can	234	0.
(Breast O' Chicken)	6½-oz. can	211	0.
(Bumble Bee):			
Chunk, light	6½-oz. can	234	0.
Solid, white	7-oz. can	251	0.
(Carnation)	6½-oz. can	211	0.
(Star-Kist):			
Chunk:			
Light	6½-oz. can	194	0.
White	6½-oz. can	240	0.
Solid:			
Light	7-oz. can	235	0.
White, imported Albacore	7-oz. can	235	0.
White, local Albacore	7-oz. can	334	0.
*TUNA HELPER (General Mills):			
Country dumplings	⅕ of pkg.	230	31.0
Creamy noodles	⅕ of pkg.	280	31.0
Noodles & cheese sauce	⅕ of pkg.	230	28.0
TUNA & PEAS, frozen (Green Giant) creamed, *Toast Toppers*	5-oz. serving	136	9.8
TUNA PIE, frozen:			
(Banquet)	8-oz. pie	434	42.7
(Morton)	8-oz. pie	373	36.4

Food and Description	Measure or Quantity	Calories	Carbo-hydrates (grams)
TUNA SALAD:			
Home recipe (USDA) made with tuna, celery, mayonnaise, pickle, onion & egg	4-oz. serving	193	4.0
Canned (Swanson) *Spreadable*	1½-oz. serving	81	3.2
TURBOT, GREENLAND (USDA) raw:			
Whole	1 lb. (weighed whole)	344	0.
Meat only	4 oz.	166	0.
TURKEY:			
Raw (USDA):			
Ready-to-cook	1 lb. (weighed with bones)	722	0.
Dark meat	4 oz.	145	0.
Light meat	4 oz.	132	0.
Skin only	4 oz.	459	0.
Barbecued (Louis Rich) breast, half	1-oz. slice	40	0.
Roasted (USDA):			
Flesh, skin & giblets	From 13½-lb. raw, ready-to-cook turkey	9678	0.
Flesh & skin	From 13½-lb. raw, ready-to-cook turkey	7872	0.
Flesh & skin	4 oz.	253	0.
Meat only:			
Chopped	1 cup (5 oz.)	268	0.
Diced	4 oz.	200	0.
Light	4 oz.	200	0.
Light	1 slice (4″ × 2″ × ¼″, 3 oz.)	75	0.
Dark	4 oz.	230	0.
Dark	1 slice (2½″ × 1⅝″ × ¼″, .7 oz.)	43	0.

(USDA): United States Department of Agriculture
(HEW/FAO): Health, Education and Welfare/Food and Agriculture
 Organization
* Prepared as Package Directs

Food and Description	Measure or Quantity	Calories	Carbo-hydrates (grams)
Skin only	1 oz.	128	0.
Giblets, simmered (USDA)	1 slice	132	.9
Canned, boned:			
(USDA)	4 oz.	229	0.
(Hormel) chunk	6 ¾-oz. can	223	.6
(Swanson) chunk	4 oz.	229	0.
Packaged:			
(Eckrich) sliced	1-oz. slice	47	1.3
(Hormel) breast	.8-oz. slice	29	.1
(Louis Rich):			
Turkey bologna	1-oz. slice	60	1.0
Turkey breast:			
Oven roasted	1-oz. slice	30	0.
Smoked	.7-oz. slice	25	0.
Turkey ham:			
Chopped	1-oz. slice	45	<1.0
Cured	1-oz. slice	35	<1.0
Turkey luncheon loaf	1-oz. slice	45	<1.0
Turkey pastrami, chunk or sliced	1-oz. serving	35	<1.0
Turkey salami, regular or cotto	1-oz. slice	50	<1.0
Turkey, smoked	1-oz. slice	35	<1.0
(Oscar Mayer) breast	.75-oz. slice	21	0.
Smoked (Louis Rich):			
Breast	1-oz. serving	35	0.
Drumstick, without bone	1-oz. serving	40	<1.0
Wing drumette, without bone	1-oz. serving	45	<1.0
TURKEY DINNER or ENTREE, frozen:			
(USDA) sliced turkey, mashed potatoes & peas	12-oz. dinner	381	43.2
(Banquet):			
Regular	11-oz. dinner	293	27.8
Man Pleaser	19-oz. dinner	620	72.8
(Morton):			
Regular	11-oz. dinner	338	34.4
Country Table, sliced:			
Dinner	15-oz. dinner	580	81.1
Entree	12¼-oz. entree	390	34.9
King Size	19-oz. dinner	583	64.8

Food and Description	Measure or Quantity	Calories	Carbo- hydrates (grams)
(Swanson):			
Regular, with gravy & dressing	9¼-oz. entree	310	21.0
Hungry Man	18¾-oz. dinner	740	79.0
3-course	16-oz. dinner	520	62.0
TV Brand:			
Dinner	11½-oz. dinner	360	45.0
Entree, with gravy & dressing & whipped potatoes	8¾-oz. entree	260	26.0
(Weight Watchers) sliced, with gravy & stuffing, 3-compartment	15¼-oz. meal	390	37.3
TURKEY GIZZARD (USDA):			
Raw	4 oz.	178	1.2
Simmered	4 oz.	222	1.2
TURKEY PIE:			
Home recipe (USDA) baked	⅓ of 9" pie	550	42.2
Frozen:			
(Banquet)	8-oz. pie	415	40.6
(Morton)	8-oz. pie	334	31.8
(Stouffer's)	10-oz. pie	451	34.7
(Swanson):			
Regular	8-oz. pie	460	47.0
Hungry Man	16-oz. pie	800	64.0
TURKEY, POTTED (USDA)	1 oz.	70	0
TURKEY SALAD, canned (Carnation) Spreadable	1½-oz. serving	86	3.0
TURKEY SOUP, canned:			
Regular pack:			
*(USDA) condensed, prepared with equal volume water	1 cup (8.8 oz.)	82	8.8

(USDA): United States Department of Agriculture
(HEW/FAO):   Health, Education and Welfare/Food and Agriculture
                      Organization
* Prepared as Package Directs

Food and Description	Measure or Quantity	Calories	Carbohydrates (grams)
(Campbell):			
Chunky	9¼-oz. serving	140	15.0
*Condensed:			
& noodle	10-oz. serving	80	10.0
& vegetable	10-oz. serving	90	10.0
*Semi-condensed, *Soup*			
For One, Royale	11-oz. serving	180	34.0
Dietetic (Campbell) low sodium	7¼-oz. can	130	22.0
TURKEY TETRAZZINI, frozen:			
(Stouffer's)	½ of 12-oz. pkg.	248	16.9
(Weight Watchers)	13-oz. pkg.	403	36.9
TURMERIC (French's)	1 tsp.	7	1.3
TURNIP (USDA):			
Fresh:			
Without tops	1 lb. (weighed with skins)	117	25.7
Pared, diced	½ cup (2.4 oz.)	20	4.4
Pared, slices	½ cup (2.3 oz.)	19	4.2
Boiled, drained:			
Diced	½ cup (2.8 oz.)	18	3.8
Mashed	½ cup (4 oz.)	26	5.6
TURNIP GREENS, leaves & stems:			
Fresh (USDA):	1 lb. (weighed untrimmed)	107	19.0
Boiled (USDA):			
In small amount water, short time, drained	½ cup (2.5 oz.)	14	2.6
In large amount water, long time, drained	½ cup (2.5 oz.)	14	2.4
Canned:			
(USDA) solids & liq.	½ cup (4.1 oz.)	21	3.7
(Stokely-Van Camp) chopped	½ cup (4.1 oz.)	23	3.5
(Sunshine) solids & liq:			
Chopped	½ cup (4.1 oz.)	19	2.5
& diced turnips	½ cup (4.1 oz.)	21	3.2
Frozen:			
(Birds Eye):			
Chopped	⅓ of 10.-oz. pkg.	20	3.0

Food and Description	Measure or Quantity	Calories	Carbohydrates (grams)
Chopped, with sliced turnips	⅓ of 10-oz. pkg.	20	3.0
(McKenzie or Seabrook Farms):			
Chopped	⅓ of 10-oz. pkg.	25	3.4
Diced	1-oz. serving	4	.8
(Southland):			
Chopped	⅕ of 16-oz. pkg.	20	4.0
With diced turnips	⅕ of 16-oz. pkg.	20	5.0
TURNOVER:			
Frozen (Pepperidge Farm):			
Apple	1 turnover	310	30.0
Blueberry	1 turnover	320	32.0
Cherry	1 turnover	340	30.0
Peach	1 turnover	320	33.0
Raspberry	1 turnover	340	37.0
Refrigerated (Pillsbury):			
Apple	1 turnover	170	23.0
Blueberry	1 turnover	170	22.0
Cherry	1 turnover	180	24.0
TURTLE GREEN (USDA):			
Raw:			
In shell	1 lb. (weighed in shell)	97	0.
Meat only	4 oz.	101	0.
Canned	4 oz.	120	0.
TWINKIE (Hostess):			
Regular	1½-oz. cake	147	26.0
Devil's food	1½-oz. cake	150	24.7

Food and Description	Measure or Quantity	Calories	Carbo-hydrates (grams)

V

Food and Description	Measure or Quantity	Calories	Carbo-hydrates (grams)
VALPOLICELLA WINE, Italian red (Antinori)	3 fl. oz.	84	6.3
VANDERMINT, Dutch liqueur (Park Avenue Imports) 60 proof	1 fl. oz.	90	10.2
VANILLA EXTRACT (Virginia Dare) 35% alcohol	1 tsp.	10	Tr.
VANILLA ICE CREAM:			
(Baskin-Robbins):			
Regular	1 scoop (2½ oz.)	147	15.6
French	1 scoop (2½ oz.)	181	15.9
(Good Humor)	4-fl. oz.	140	14.0
(Meadow Gold)	¼ pt.	140	16.0
(Swift's) sweet cream	½ cup (2.3 oz.)	127	15.7
VEAL, medium fat (USDA):			
Chuck:			
Raw	1 lb. (weighed with bone)	628	0.
Braised, lean & fat	4 oz.	266	0.
Flank:			
Raw	1 lb. (weighed with bone)	1410	0.
Stewed, lean & fat	4 oz.	442	0.
Foreshank:			
Raw	1 lb. (weighed with bone)	368	0.
Stewed, lean & fat	4 oz.	245	0.
Loin:			
Raw	1 lb. (weighed with bone)	681	0.
Broiled, medium done, chop, lean & fat	4 oz.	265	0.
Plate:			
Raw	1 lb. (weighed with bone)	828	0.

Food and Description	Measure or Quantity	Calories	Carbo-hydrates (grams)
Stewed, lean & fat	4 oz.	344	0.
Rib:			
Raw, lean & fat	1 lb. (weighed with bone)	723	0.
Roasted, medium done, lean & fat	4 oz.	305	0.
Round & rump:			
Raw	1 lb. (weighed with bone)	573	0.
Broiled, steak or cutlet, lean & fat	4 oz. (weighed without bone)	245	0.
VEAL DINNER or ENTREE, frozen:			
(Banquet) parmigiana:			
Buffet Supper	2-lb. pkg.	1563	119.1
Cookin' Bag	5-oz. pkg.	287	19.5
Dinner:			
Regular	11-oz. dinner	421	42.1
Man-Pleaser	20-oz. dinner	982	110.2
(Green Giant) parmigiana, breaded	14-oz. pkg.	621	36.6
(Morton) parmigiana	11-oz. dinner	272	28.1
(Swanson) parmigiana:			
Regular	12¼-oz. dinner	460	41.1
Hungry Man	20½-oz. dinner	990	75.0
TV Brand	12¼-oz. dinner	243	12.0
(Weight Watchers) parmigiana, patty, two-compartment	9-oz. meal	243	12.0
VEAL STEAK, frozen (Hormel):			
Regular	4-oz. serving	131	2.1
Breaded	4-oz. serving	242	13.1
VEGETABLE BOUILLON:			
(Herb-Ox):			
Cube	1 cube	6	.5

(USDA): United States Department of Agriculture
(HEW/FAO):   Health, Education and Welfare/Food and Agriculture
                        Organization
* Prepared as Package Directs

Food and Description	Measure or Quantity	Calories	Carbo-hydrates (grams)
Packet	1 packet	12	2.2
MBT	6-gram packet	12	2.0
VEGETABLE FAT (See **FAT**)			
VEGETABLE FLAKES, dehydrated (French's)	1 T.	12	3.0
VEGETABLE JUICE COCKTAIL:			
Canned, regular pack:			
(USDA)	4 oz. (by wt.)	19	4.1
V-8 (Campbell):			
Regular	6 fl. oz.	35	8.0
Spicy hot	6 fl. oz.	40	8.0
Canned, low sodium:			
(S&W) *Nutradiet*	6 fl. oz.	35	8.0
V-8 (Campbell)	6 fl. oz.	35	8.0
VEGETABLES, MIXED:			
Canned, regular pack:			
(Chun King) chow mein, solids & liq.	¼ of 16-oz. can	20	2.0
(Del Monte):			
Solids & liq.	½ cup (4 oz.)	38	6.9
Drained solids	½ cup (3.2 oz.)	41	7.4
(La Choy):			
Chinese style	1 cup (5.5 oz.)	24	1.6
Chop suey	1 cup (5.5 oz.)	36	6.9
(Libby's) solids & liq.	½ cup (4.2 oz.)	40	8.5
(Stokely-Van Camp) solids & liq.	½ cup (4.3 oz.)	40	8.5
Canned, dietetic or low calorie (Featherweight)	½ cup	35	8.0
Frozen:			
(USDA) boiled, drained	½ cup (3.2 oz.)	58	12.2
(Birds Eye):			
Americana Recipe:			
New England style	⅓ of 10-oz. pkg.	69	11.7
New Orleans style	⅓ of 10-oz. pkg.	69	13.8
Pennsylvania Dutch style	½ of 10-oz. pkg.	44	7.3
San Francisco style	⅓ of 10-oz. pkg.	42	6.4

Food and Description	Measure or Quantity	Calories	Carbo-hydrates (grams)
Wisconsin style	⅓ of 10-oz. pkg.	44	6.4
Bavarian style beans & spaetzle with seasoned sauce	⅓ of 10-oz. pkg.	63	10.6
Cantonese style, stir fry	⅓ of 10-oz. pkg.	50	10.2
Chinese style, with seasoned sauce	⅓ of 10-oz. pkg.	28	5.2
Chinese style, stir fry	⅓ of 10-oz. pkg.	37	7.0
(Kounty Kist):			
Regular	⅕ of 20-oz. pkg.	55	10.4
California blend	⅕ of 18-oz. pkg.	29	4.6
(La Choy):			
Chinese style	½ of 10-oz. pkg.	36	5.3
Japanese style	½ of 10-oz. pkg.	36	5.8
(La Sueur):			
Pea, pea pod & water chestnuts in sauce	⅓ of 10-oz. pkg.	72	8.9
Pea, onion & carrots in butter sauce	⅓ of 10-oz. pkg.	67	7.6
(Southland):			
California blend	⅕ of 16-oz. pkg.	35	7.0
Gumbo	⅕ of 16-oz. pkg.	45	10.0
Oriental	⅕ of 16-oz. pkg.	30	6.0
Stew	⅕ of 20-oz. pkg.	60	14.0
VEGETABLE SOUP:			
Canned, regular pack:			
*(USDA) beef, prepared with equal volume water	1 cup (8.6 oz.)	78	9.6
*(USDA) with beef broth, prepared with equal volume water	1 cup (8.8 oz.)	80	13.8
*(USDA) vegetarian, prepared with equal volume water	1 cup (8.6 oz.)	78	13.2
(Campbell):			
Chunky:			
Regular	9½-oz. serving	130	21.0

(USDA): United States Department of Agriculture
(HEW/FAO): Health, Education and Welfare/Food and Agriculture Organization
* Prepared as Package Directs

Food and Description	Measure or Quantity	Calories	Carbo-hydrates (grams)
Regular	10¾-oz. can	140	24.0
Beef, old fashioned	9½-oz. serving	160	18.0
Beef, old fashioned	10¾-oz. can	180	21.0
*Condensed:			
Regular	10-oz. serving	100	16.0
Beef	10-oz. serving	90	10.0
Old fashioned	10-oz. serving	80	12.0
Vegetarian	10-oz. serving	90	14.0
*Semicondensed, *Soup for One:*			
Burly, with beef	11-oz. serving	150	20.0
Old World	11-oz. serving	120	18.0
*(Rokeach) condensed, vegetarian	10-oz. serving	90	15.0
Canned, dietetic or low calorie:			
(Campbell) low sodium:			
Regular	7¼-oz. can	90	15.0
Beef	7½-oz. can	90	9.0
*(Dia-Mel):			
Regular	8-oz. serving	60	12.0
Beef	8-oz. serving	80	11.0
*Frozen:			
(USDA) with beef, prepared with equal volume water	8 oz. (by wt.)	79	7.7
(Mother's Own)	8 oz. serving	40	<1.0
*Mix (Lipton):			
Beef	8 fl. oz.	50	7.0
Beef, *Cup-A-Soup*	6 fl. oz.	50	8.0
Country	8 fl. oz.	80	14.0
Spring, *Cup-A-Soup*	6 fl. oz.	40	7.0
VEGETABLE STEW, canned, *Dinty Moore* (Hormel)	7½-oz. serving	163	18.3
"VEGETARIAN FOODS":			
Canned or dry:			
Chicken, fried (Loma Linda) with gravy	1½-oz. piece	109	1.9
Chili (Worthington)	½ cup (4.9 oz.)	190	20.0
Choplet (Worthington)	1.6-oz. slice	50	3.0

Food and Description	Measure or Quantity	Calories	Carbo-hydrates (grams)
Cutlet (Worthington)	2.2-oz. slice	63	2.6
Dinner cuts (Loma Linda):			
Regular	1½-oz. piece	54	1.6
No salt added	1½-oz. piece	44	2.6
Franks (Loma Linda):			
Big	1.9-oz. piece	100	4.1
Sizzle	2.2-oz. piece	167	4.6
FriChik (Worthington)	1.6-oz. piece	95	1.0
Granburger (Worthington)	6 T. (1.2 oz.)	130	12.0
Linketts (Loma Linda)	1.3-oz. link	74	2.2
Little links (Loma Linda)	.8-oz. link	45	1.3
Nonmeat balls (Worthington)	.6-oz. piece	40	2.3
Numete (Worthington)	½" slice (2.4 oz.)	160	9.0
Nuteena (Loma Linda)	½" slice (2.4 oz.)	165	7.6
Peanuts & soya (USDA)	4 oz.	269	15.2
Proteena (Loma Linda)	½" slice (2.5 oz.)	144	6.5
Protose (Worthington)	½" slice (2.7 oz.)	190	7.0
Redi-burger (Loma Linda)	½" slice (2.4 oz.)	132	8.8
Sandwich spread:			
(Loma Linda)	1 T. (.6 oz.)	24	1.7
(Worthington)	1.2-oz. link	65	1.5
Savorex (Loma Linda)	1 T. (.5 oz.)	32	2.0
Skallops (Worthington) drained	½ cup (3 oz.)	70	3.0
Soyalac (Loma Linda):			
Concentrate, liquid	1 cup (9 oz.)	177	17.0
Powder	1 oz.	136	12.4
Ready-to-use	1 cup (8.5 oz.)	166	15.9
Soyameat (Worthington):			
Beef-like slices	1-oz. slice	55	1.5
Chicken-like:			
Diced	¼ cup (2 oz.)	120	2.0
Sliced	1.1-oz. slice	65	1.0
Salisbury steak-like slices	2.3-oz. slice	160	2.0
Soyamel (Worthington):			
Regular	1 oz.	140	15.2
Low fat	1 oz.	110	14.0

(USDA): United States Department of Agriculture
(HEW/FAO): Health, Education and Welfare/Food and Agriculture Organization
* Prepared as Package Directs

Food and Description	Measure or Quantity	Calories	Carbo-hydrates (grams)
Stew pac (Loma Linda)	.2-oz. piece	7	.6
Super links (Worthington)	1.9-oz. link	120	4.0
Swiss steak & gravy (Loma Linda)	2 ¾ oz. steak	138	8.9
Tender bits (Loma Linda)	6-oz. piece	23	1.1
Tender rounds (Loma Linda)	1-oz. piece	39	2.4
VegeBurger (Loma Linda):			
Regular	½ cup (3.8 oz.)	116	4.3
No salt added	½ cup (3.8 oz.)	119	6.9
Vegelona (Loma Linda)	½" slice (2.4 oz.)	102	7.0
Vegetable steak (Worthington)	1.3-oz. piece	40	2.8
Vegetarian burger (Worthington)	⅓ cup (3.3 oz.)	130	6.0
Veja-Bits (Worthington)	4.3-oz. serving	70	4.0
Veja-Links (Worthington)	1.1-oz. link	70	1.5
Vita-Burger (Loma Linda)	1 T. (¼ oz.)	23	2.1
Wheat protein, nuts or peanuts (USDA)	4 oz.	240	20.1
Wheat protein, vegetable oil (USDA)	4 oz.	214	5.9
Wheat soy protein, soy or other vegetable oil (USDA)	4 oz.	170	10.8
Wheat or soy protein (USDA)	4 oz.	118	8.6
Wheat protein (USDA)	4 oz.	124	10.0
Worthington 209, turkey-like flavor	1.1-oz. slice	75	1.5
Frozen:			
Beef-like roll (Worthington)	2½-oz. slice	140	4.0
Beef-like slices (Worthington)	1-oz. slice	60	2.0
Beef pie (Worthington)	8-oz. pie	470	51.0
Bologna (Loma Linda)	1-oz. slice	77	2.8
Bolono (Worthington)	.7-oz. slice	35	1.5
Chicken (Loma Linda)	1-oz. slice	57	1.5
Chicken, fried (Loma Linda)	2-oz. piece	188	3.6
Chicken-like pie (Worthington)	8-oz. pie	450	42.0
Chicken-like roll (Worthington)	2½-oz. piece	170	2.0
Chicken-like slices (Worthington)	1-oz. slice	70	1.0
Chic-Ketts (Worthington)	½ cup (3 oz.)	180	6.0

Food and Description	Measure or Quantity	Calories	Carbo-hydrates (grams)
Corned beef-like roll (Worthington)	2½-oz. piece	190	6.0
Corned beef-like, sliced (Worthington)	.5-oz. slice	40	2.3
Croquettes (Worthington)	1-oz. piece	75	5.0
Fillets (Worthington)	1.7-oz. piece	108	5.0
FriPats (Worthington)	2.5-oz. piece	180	3.0
Meatballs (Loma Linda)	¾-oz. piece	46	2.2
Meatless salami (Worthington)	.7-oz. slice	50	1.5
Prosage (Worthington):			
Links	.8-oz. link	60	1.7
Patties	1.3-oz. piece	100	3.5
Roll	⅜" slice (1.2 oz.)	90	3.0
Roast beef (Loma Linda)	1-oz. slice	65	1.3
Salami (Loma Linda)	1-oz. slice	65	1.7
Sausage, breakfast (Loma Linda)	⅓" slice (1 oz.)	72	1.4
Sizzle burger (Loma Linda)	2½-oz. piece	210	13.3
Smoked beef-like roll (Worthington)	2½-oz. piece	170	7.0
Smoked beef-like luncheon slice (Worthington)	.3-oz. slice	22	1.0
Smoked turkey-like roll (Worthington)	2½-oz. piece	180	3.0
Smoked turkey-like slices (Worthington)	3-oz. piece	50	.8
Stakelets (Worthington)	3-oz. piece	180	8.0
Stripples (Worthington)	.3-oz. strip	25	.8
Tuno (Worthington)	2-oz. serving	90	3.0
Tuno pot pie (Worthington)	8-oz. pie	460	43.0
Turkey (Loma Linda)	1-oz. slice	61	1.6
Wham (Worthington):			
Roll	2½-oz. piece	140	4.0
Sliced	.8-oz. slice	47	1.3
VENISON (USDA) raw, lean meat only	4 oz.	143	0.

(USDA): United States Department of Agriculture
(HEW/FAO): Health, Education and Welfare/Food and Agriculture Organization
* Prepared as Package Directs

Food and Description	Measure or Quantity	Calories	Carbo-hydrates (grams)
VERMOUTH:			
Dry:			
(Gallo) 18% alcohol	3 fl. oz.	75	1.7
(Great Western) 16% alcohol	3 fl. oz.	87	1.6
(Taylor) 17% alcohol	3 fl. oz.	99	3.0
Sweet:			
(Great Western) 16% alcohol	3 fl. oz.	132	12.4
(Taylor) 17% alcohol	3 fl. oz.	132	12.3
VICHYSSOISE SOUP, canned			
(Crosse & Blackwell) cream of	½ of 13-oz. can	70	5.0
VIENNA SAUSAGE, CANNED:			
(USDA)	1 oz.	68	<.1
(Hormel):			
Regular	1 piece	53	Tr.
Chicken	1-oz. serving	60	.2
(Libby's):			
In barbecue sauce	.7-oz. sausage	50	.5
In beef broth	.7-oz. sausage	45	.2
VINEGAR:			
Cider:			
(USDA)	1 T. (.5 oz.)	2	.9
(USDA)	½ cup (4.2 oz.)	17	7.1
Distilled:			
(USDA)	1 T. (.5 oz.)	2	.8
(USDA)	½ cup (4.2 oz.)	14	6.0
Red, red with garlic or white wine (Regina)	1 T. (.5 oz.)	<1	Tr.
VINESPINACH or BASELLA			
(USDA) raw	4 oz.	22	3.9
VODKA, unflavored (See **DISTILLED LIQUOR**)			

Food and Description	Measure or Quantity	Calories	Carbohydrates (grams)

W

WAFER (See **COOKIE** or **CRACKER**)

Food and Description	Measure or Quantity	Calories	Carbohydrates (grams)
WAFFELOS, cereal (Ralston Purina)	1 cup (1 oz.)	110	25.0
WAFFLE:			
Home recipe (USDA)	7" waffle (2.6 oz.)	209	28.1
Frozen:			
(USDA)	1.6-oz. waffle (8 in 13-oz. pkg.)	116	19.3
USDA)	.8-oz. waffle (6 in 5-oz. pkg.)	61	10.1
(Aunt Jemima) jumbo, any flavor	1¼-oz. waffle	86	14.5
(Eggo):			
Regular	1.4-oz. waffle	120	17.0
Blueberry or strawberry	1.4-oz. waffle	130	18.0
Roman Meal:			
Regular	1½-oz. waffle	140	16.5
Golden Delights	1.4 oz. piece	131	15.1
WAFFLE MIX (See also **PANCAKE & WAFFLE MIX**) (USDA):			
Complete mix:			
Dry	1 oz.	130	18.5
*Prepared with water	2.6-oz. waffle	229	30.2
Incomplete mix:			
Dry	1 oz.	101	21.5
*Prepared with egg & milk	2.6-oz. waffle	206	27.2

(USDA): United States Department of Agriculture
(HEW/FAO):   Health, Education and Welfare/Food and Agriculture
                      Organization
* Prepared as Package Directs

Food and Description	Measure or Quantity	Calories	Carbohydrates (grams)
*Prepared with egg & milk	7.1-oz. waffle (9" × 9" × ⅝", 1⅛ cups batter)	550	72.4
WAFFLE SYRUP (See **SYRUP**)			
WALLBANGER COCKTAIL, canned (Mr. Boston) 12½% alcohol	3 fl. oz.	102	9.6
WALNUT: (USDA):			
Black, in shell, whole	1 lb. (weighed in shell)	627	14.8
Black, shelled, whole	4 oz. (weighed whole)	712	16.8
Black, chopped	½ cup (2.1 oz.)	377	8.9
English or Persian, in shell, whole	1 lb. (weighed in shell)	1327	32.2
English or Persian, shelled, whole	4 oz.	738	17.9
English or Persian, chopped	½ cup (2.1 oz.)	391	9.5
English or Persian, halves	½ cup (1.8 oz.)	326	7.9
(California) halves & pieces	½ cup (1.8 oz.)	356	6.5
(Fisher):			
Black	½ cup (2.1 oz.)	374	8.8
English	½ cup (2.1 oz.)	389	9.5
WATER CHESTNUT, CHINESE: Raw (USDA):			
Whole	1 lb. (weighed unpeeled)	272	66.5
Peeled	4 oz.	90	21.5
Canned:			
(Chun King) solids & liq.	½ of 8½-oz. can	70	11.0
(La Choy) sliced, drained	¼ of 8-oz. can	16	3.9
WATERCRESS, raw (USDA):			
Untrimmed	½ lb. (weighed untrimmed)	40	6.2
Trimmed	½ cup (.6 oz.)	3	.5

Food and Description	Measure or Quantity	Calories	Carbo-hydrates (grams)
WATERMELON, fresh (USDA):			
Whole	1 lb. (weighed with rind)	54	13.4
Wedge	2 lb. wedge (4″ × 8″ measured with rind)	111	27.3
Diced	1 cup (5.6 oz.)	42	10.2
WAX GOURD, raw (USDA):			
Whole	1 lb. (weighed with skin & cavity contents)	41	9.4
Flesh only	4 oz.	15	3.4
WEAKFISH (USDA):			
Raw, whole	1 lb. (weighed whole)	263	0.
Broiled, meat only	4 oz.	236	0.
WEINER WRAP, refrigerated (Pillsbury) plain or cheese	1 wrap	60	10.0
WELSH RAREBIT:			
Home recipe (USDA)	1 cup (8.2 oz.)	415	14.6
Frozen:			
(Green Giant) with cheddar & swiss cheese, *Toast Topper*	5-oz. serving	219	11.4
(Stouffer's)	½ of 10-oz. pkg.	359	16.9
WESTERN DINNER, frozen:			
(Banquet)	11-oz. dinner	417	32.4
(Morton) *Round-up*	11¾-oz. dinner	426	33.5
(Swanson):			
Hungry Man	17¾-oz. dinner	820	67.0
TV Brand	11¾-oz. dinner	440	42.0

(USDA): United States Department of Agriculture
(HEW/FAO):   Health, Education and Welfare/Food and Agriculture
                    Organization
* Prepared as Package Directs

Food and Description	Measure or Quantity	Calories	Carbo-hydrates (grams)
WHALE MEAT, raw (USDA)	4 oz.	177	0.
WHEAT CEREAL (Elam's) cooked	1 oz.	100	20.2
WHEATENA, dry	¼ cup (1.1 oz.)	112	22.5
WHEAT FLAKES, cereal:			
(USDA) crushed	1 cup (2½ oz.)	248	56.4
(Van Brode)	¾ cup (1 oz.)	106	22.7
WHEAT GERM:			
(USDA) crude, commercial, milled	1 oz.	103	13.2
(Elam's) raw	1 oz	112	12.8
WHEAT GERM CEREAL:			
(USDA)	¼ cup (1 oz.)	110	14.0
(Kretschmer):			
Regular	¼ cup (1 oz.)	99	8.8
Brown sugar & honey	¼ cup (1 oz.)	114	17.0
WHEATIES, cereal (General Mills)	1 cup (1 oz.)	110	23.0
WHEAT & OATMEAL CEREAL, hot (Elam's)	1-oz. serving	105	18.8
WHEAT, ROLLED (USDA):			
Uncooked	1 cup (3.1 oz.)	296	66.3
Cooked	1 cup (7.7 oz.)	163	36.7
WHEAT, SHREDDED, cereal (See **SHREDDED WHEAT**)			
WHEAT, WHOLE-GRAIN (USDA) hard red spring	1 oz.	94	19.6
WHEAT, WHOLE-MEAL, cereal (USDA):			
Dry	1 oz.	96	20.5
Cooked	4 oz.	51	10.7

Food and Description	Measure or Quantity	Calories	Carbo-hydrates (grams)
WHEY (USDA):			
Dry	1 oz.	99	20.8
Fluid	1 cup (8.6 oz.)	63	12.4
WHISKEY or WHISKY (See **DISTILLED LIQUOR**)			
WHISKEY SOUR COCKTAIL:			
Canned (Mr. Boston) 12½% alcohol	3 fl. oz.	120	14.4
Mix:			
(Bar-Tender's)	⅝-oz. serving	70	17.2
(Holland House) dry	.6-oz. pkg.	69	17.0
WHITEFISH, LAKE (USDA):			
Raw:			
Whole	1 lb. (weighed whole)	330	0.
Meat only	4 oz.	176	0.
Baked, stuffed, made with bacon, butter, onion, celery & bread crumbs, home recipe	4 oz.	244	6.6
Smoked	4 oz.	176	0.
WHITEFISH & PIKE, (See **GEFILTE FISH**)			
WIENER (See **FRANKFURTER**)			
WILD BERRY, fruit drink (Hi-C)	6 fl. oz.	88	22.0
WILD RICE, raw (USDA)	½ cup (2.9 oz.)	289	61.7
WINE (most wines are listed by kind, brand, vineyard, region or grape name):			
Cooking (Regina):			
Burgundy or sauterne	¼ cup (1 fl. oz.)	2	Tr.

(USDA): United States Department of Agriculture
(HEW/FAO):   Health, Education and Welfare/Food and Agriculture
                      Organization
* Prepared as Package Directs

Food and Description	Measure or Quantity	Calories	Carbo-hydrates (grams)
Sherry	¼ cup (1 fl. oz.)	20	5.0
Dessert (USDA) 18.8% alcohol	3 fl. oz.	122	6.9
Table (USDA) 12.2% alcohol	3 fl. oz.	75	3.7
*WON TON SOUP:			
Canned (Campbell) condensed	10-oz. serving	50	6.0
Frozen (La Choy)	1 cup	92	12.3
WORCESTERSHIRE SAUCE (See **SAUCE**)			
WRECKFISH, raw (USDA) meat only	4 oz.	129	0.

Y

Food and Description	Measure or Quantity	Calories	Carbo-hydrates (grams)
YAM (USDA):			
Raw:			
Whole	1 lb. (weighed with skin)	394	90.5
Flesh only	4 oz.	115	26.3
Canned & frozen (See **SWEET POTATO**)			
YAM BEAN, raw (USDA):			
Unpared tuber	1 lb. (weighed unpared)	225	52.2
Pared tuber	4 oz.	62	14.5
YEAST:			
Baker's:			
Compressed:			
(USDA)	1 oz.	24	3.1
(Fleischmann's)	⅗ oz. cake	19	1.9
Dry:			
(USDA)	1 oz.	80	11.0
(USDA)	7-gram pkg.	20	2.7
(Fleischmann's)	¼ oz. (pkg. or jar)	24	2.9

Food and Description	Measure or Quantity	Calories	Carbo-hydrates (grams)
Brewer's dry, debittered:			
(USDA)	1 oz.	80	10.9
(USDA)	1 T. (8 grams)	23	3.1
YELLOWTAIL, raw, meat only			
(USDA)	4 oz.	156	0.
YOGURT:			
Regular:			
Plain:			
(Bison)	8-oz. container	160	16.8
(Colombo) Natural Lite	8-oz. container	110	17.0
(Dannon)	8-oz. container	150	17.0
(Friendship)	8-oz. container	170	15.0
(Sweet'n Low)	8-oz. container	90	15.0
Yoplait	6-oz. container	130	14.0
Apple:			
(Bison)	8-oz. container	262	45.9
(Colombo) Spiced	8-oz. container	240	39.0
(Dannon) Dutch	8-oz. container	260	49.0
Mélangé (Dannon)	6-oz. container	180	31.0
(New Country)	8-oz. container	240	42.0
Apricot:			
(Bison) dutch	8-oz. container	262	45.9
(Dannon)	8-oz. container	260	49.0
Banana:			
(Dannon)	8-oz. container	262	49.0
LeShake (Kellogg)	8-oz. container	170	28.0
Banana-strawberry			
(Colombo)	8-oz. container	235	38.0
Blueberry:			
(Bison):			
Regular	8-oz. container	262	45.9
Light	6-oz. container	162	28.1
(Colombo)	8-oz. container	250	38.0
(Dannon)	8-oz. container	260	49.0
(Friendship)	8-oz. container	230	57.0
LeShake (Kellogg)	8-oz. container	170	28.0

(USDA): United States Department of Agriculture
(HEW/FAO): Health, Education and Welfare/Food and Agriculture Organization
* Prepared as Package Directs

Food and Description	Measure or Quantity	Calories	Carbo-hydrates (grams)
Mélangé (Dannon)	6-oz. container	180	31.0
(Sweet'n Low)	8-oz. container	150	33.0
Yoplait (General Mills)	6 oz. container	190	32.0
Boysenberry:			
(Bison)	8-oz. container	262	45.9
(Dannon)	8-oz. container	260	49.0
(Sweet'n Low)	8-oz. container	150	33.0
Cherry:			
(Bison) Light	6-oz. container	162	28.1
(Colombo) black	8-oz. container	230	34.0
(Dannon)	8-oz. container	260	49.0
(Friendship)	8-oz. container	230	57.0
Mélangé (Dannon)	6-oz. container	180	31.0
(New Country) Supreme	8-oz. container	240	44.0
(Sweet'n Low)	8-oz. container	150	33.0
Yoplait	6-oz. container	190	32.0
Cherry-vanilla (Colombo)	8-oz. container	250	40.0
Coffee:			
(Colombo)	8-oz. container	200	29.0
(Dannon)	8-oz. container	200	32.0
Date-walnut-raisin (Bison)	8-oz. container	262	45.9
Fruit Crunch (New Country)	8-oz. container	240	42.0
Granola strawberry (Colombo)	8-oz. container	240	40.0
Guava:			
(Colombo)	8-oz. container	240	40.0
(Dannon)	8-oz. container	260	49.0
Hawaiian salad (New Country)	8-oz. container	250	42.0
Honey'n Berries (New Country)	8-oz. container	240	43.0
Honey vanilla (Colombo)	8-oz. container	220	30.0
Lemon:			
(Dannon)	8-oz. container	200	32.0
(New Country)	8-oz. container	240	43.0
(Sweet'N Low)	8-oz. container	150	33.0
Yoplait	6-oz. container	190	32.0
Orange, *Yoplait*	6-oz. container	190	32.0
Orange supreme (New Country)	8-oz. container	240	43.0
Peach:			
(Bison)	8-oz. container	262	45.9

Food and Description	Measure or Quantity	Calories	Carbohydrates (grams)
(Dannon)	8-oz. container	260	49.0
(Friendship)	8-oz. container	230	57.0
(New Country) 'n cream	8-oz. container	240	43.0
(Sweet'N Low)	8-oz. container	150	33.0
Peach Melba (Colombo)	8-oz. container	230	37.0
Piña Colada:			
(Colombo)	8-oz. container	240	40.0
(Dannon)	8-oz. container	260	49.0
(Friendship)	8-oz. container	230	57.0
Pineapple:			
(Bison) light	6-oz. container	162	28.1
Mélangé (Dannon)	6-oz. container	180	31.0
Raspberry:			
(Colombo)	8-oz. container	250	45.9
(Dannon) red	8-oz. container	260	49.0
(Friendship)	8-oz. container	230	57.0
LeShake (Kellogg)	8-oz. container	180	29.0
Mélangé (Dannon)	6-oz. container	180	31.0
(Sweet'N Low)	8-oz. container	150	33.0
Yoplait	6-oz. container	190	32.0
Raspberry ripple (New Country)	8-oz. container	240	43.0
Strawberry:			
(Bison) Light	6-oz. container	162	28.1
(Colombo)	8-oz. container	230	36.0
(Dannon)	8-oz. container	260	49.0
(Friendship)	8-oz. container	230	57.0
Mélangé (Dannon)	6-oz. container	180	31.0
(Sweet'N Low)	8-oz. container	150	33.0
Yoplait	6-oz. container	190	32.0
Strawberry banana (Sweet'N Low)	8-oz. container	150	33.0
Strawberry Colada (Colombo)	8-oz. container	230	36.0
Strawberry supreme (New Country)	8-oz. container	240	43.0
Tropical Fruit (Sweet'N Low)	8-oz. container	150	33.0

(USDA): United States Department of Agriculture
(HEW/FAO): Health, Education and Welfare/Food and Agriculture Organization
* Prepared as Package Directs

Food and Description	Measure or Quantity	Calories	Carbo-hydrates (grams)
Vanilla:			
(Dannon)	8-oz. container	200	32.0
LeShake (Kellogg)	8-oz. container	190	32.0
(New Country) French, ripple	8-oz. container	240	43.0
Frozen, hard:			
Banana:			
Danny-Yo	3½-oz. serving	110	21.0
Danny-in-a-Cup	8-oz. cup	210	42.0
Boysenberry:			
Danny-On-A-Stick, carob coated	2½-fl.-oz. bar	135	13.0
Danny-Yo	3½-oz. serving	110	21.0
Boysenberry swirl (Bison)	¼ of 16-oz. container	116	24.0
Cherry vanilla (Bison)	¼ of 16-oz. container	116	24.0
Chocolate:			
(Bison)	¼ of 16-oz. container	116	24.0
(Colombo) bar, chocolate coated	1 bar	145	17.0
(Dannon):			
Danny-in-a-Cup	8-fl.-oz. cup	210	42.0
Danny-On-A-Stick, chocolate coated	2½-fl.-oz. bar	135	13.0
Chocolate chip (Bison)	¼ of 16-oz. container	116	24.0
Chocolate chocolate chip (Colombo)	4-oz. serving	150	28.0
Mocha (Colombo) bar	1 bar	80	14.0
Pinã Colada:			
(Colombo)	4-oz. serving	110	20.0
(Dannon):			
Danny-in-a-Cup	8-oz. cup	210	42.0
Danny-On-A-Stick	2½-fl.-oz. bar	65	13.0
Raspberry, red (Dannon)			
Danny-On-A-Stick, chocolate coated	2½-fl.-oz. bar	135	13.0
Danny-in-a-Cup	8-oz. container	210	42.0
Danny-Yo	3½ fl. oz	110	21.0
Raspberry swirl (Bison)	¼ of 16-oz. container	116	24.0

Food and Description	Measure or Quantity	Calories	Carbo-hydrates (grams)
Strawberry:			
(Bison)	¼ of 16-oz. container	116	24.0
(Colombo):			
Regular	4-oz. serving	110	20.0
Bar	1 bar	80	14.0
(Dannon):			
Danny-in-a-Cup	8 fl. oz.	210	42.0
Danny-Yo	3½ fl. oz.	110	21.0
Vanilla:			
(Bison)	¼ of 16-oz. container	116	24.0
(Colombo):			
Regular	4-oz. serving	110	20.0
Bar, chocolate covered	1 bar	145	17.0
(Dannon):			
Danny-in-a-Cup	8 fl. oz.	180	20.0
Danny-On-A-Stick	2½-fl.-oz. bar	65	13.0
Danny-Yo	3½-oz. serving	110	21.0
Frozen, soft (Colombo)	6-fl.-oz. serving	130	24.0

Z

ZINFANDEL WINE (Inglenook)			
Vintage	3 fl. oz.	59	.3
ZITI, frozen (Weight Watchers)	12½-oz. pkg.	342	41.2
ZWIEBACK (Gerber; Nabisco)	1 piece	30	5.0

nited States Department of Agriculture
    Health, Education and Welfare/Food and Agriculture
    Organization
    kage Directs

Bibliography

Dawson, Elsie H., Gilpin, Gladys L., and Fulton, Lois H. *Average weight of a measured cup of various foods*. U.S.D.A. ARS 61–6, February 1969. 19 pp.

Leung, W. T. W., Busson, F., and Jardin, C. *Food composition table for use in Africa*. U.S. Department of Health, Education and Welfare and Food and Agriculture Organization of the United Nations. 1968. 306 pp.

Leung, W. T. W., Butrum, R. V., and Chang, F. H. *Food composition table for use in East Asia*. U.S. Department of Health, Education and Welfare and Food and Agriculture Organization of the United Nations. December 1972. 334 pp.

Merrill, A. L. and Watt, B. K., *Energy value of foods— basis and derivation*. U.S.D.A. Handb. 74, 105 pp. 1955.

Pecot, Rebecca K., Jaeger, Carol M., and Watt, Bernice K., *Proximate composition of beef from carcass to cooked meat: Method of derivation and tables of values*. U.S.D.A. Home Economics Research Report 31, 32 pp. 1965.

Pecot, Rebecca K. and Watt, Bernice K., *Food yields: Summarized by different stages of preparation*. U.S.D.A. Handb. 102, 93 pp. 1956.

U.S.D.A. Nutritive value of foods. Home and Garden Bul. 72, 36 pp. 1964 and revised edition, 1970. 41 pp.

U.S.D.A. Unpubl. Data 1969.

Watt, Bernice K., Merrill, Annabel L., et al., *Composition of foods: Raw, processed, prepared*. U.S.D.A. Agriculture Handb. 8, 190 pp. 1963.